Metaphor, Cancer and the End of Life

This book presents the methodology, findings and implications of a large-scale corpus-based study of the metaphors used to talk about cancer and the end of life (including care at the end of life) in the UK. It focuses on metaphor as a central linguistic and cognitive tool that is frequently used to talk and think about sensitive and subjective experiences, such as illness, emotions, death and dying, and that can both help and hinder communication and well-being, depending on how it is used. The book centres on a combination of qualitative analyses and innovative corpus linguistic methods. This methodological assemblage was applied to the systematic study of the metaphors used in a 1.5-million-word corpus. The corpus consists of interviews with, and online forum posts written by, members of three stakeholder groups, namely: patients diagnosed with advanced cancer; unpaid carers looking after a relative with a diagnosis of advanced cancer; and healthcare professionals. The book presents a range of qualitative and quantitative findings that have implications for: metaphor theory and analysis; corpus linguistic and computational approaches to metaphor; and training and practice in cancer care and hospice, palliative and end-of-life care.

Elena Semino is Professor of Linguistics and Verbal Art in the Department of Linguistics and English Language at Lancaster University, and Visiting Professor at the University of Fuzhou (China).

Zsófia Demjén is Senior Lecturer in Applied Linguistics at the UCL Centre for Applied Linguistics.

Andrew Hardie is a Reader in Linguistics at Lancaster University.

Sheila Payne is Emeritus Chair in Palliative Care at the International Observatory on End of Life Care at Lancaster University, and Visiting Professor at Ulster University and Zurich University of Applied Sciences.

Paul Rayson is Director of the UCREL Research Centre and Reader in Natural Language Processing at Lancaster University.

Routledge Advances in Corpus Linguistics
Edited by Tony McEnery
Lancaster University, UK
Michael Hoey
Liverpool University, UK

For a full list of titles in this series, please visit www.routledge.com

11 Corpus-Based Contrastive Studies of English and Chinese
Richard Xiao and Tony McEnery

12 The Discourse of Teaching Practice Feedback
A Corpus-Based Investigation of Spoken and Written Modes
Fiona Farr

13 Corpus Approaches to Evaluation
Susan Hunston

14 Corpus Stylistics and Dickens's Fiction
Michaela Mahlberg

15 Spoken Corpus Linguistics
From Monomodal to Multimodal
Svenja Adolphs and Ronald Carter

16 Digital Literary Studies
Corpus Approaches to Poetry, Prose, and Drama
David L. Hoover, Jonathan Culpeper, and Kieran O'Halloran

17 Triangulating Methodological Approaches in Corpus Linguistics Research
Edited by Paul Baker and Jesse Egbert

18 The Language of Hate
A Corpus Linguistic Analysis of White Supremacist Language
Andrew Brindle

19 Metaphor, Cancer and the End of Life
A Corpus-Based Study
Elena Semino, Zsófia Demjén, Andrew Hardie, Sheila Payne and Paul Rayson

Metaphor, Cancer and the End of Life

A Corpus-Based Study

Elena Semino, Zsófia Demjén, Andrew Hardie, Sheila Payne and Paul Rayson

Routledge
Taylor & Francis Group
NEW YORK AND LONDON

First published 2018
by Routledge
711 Third Avenue, New York, NY 10017

and by Routledge
2 Park Square, Milton Park, Abingdon, Oxon OX14 4RN

Routledge is an imprint of the Taylor & Francis Group, an informa business

Library of Congress Cataloguing-in-Publication Data
A catalog record for this book has been requested

ISBN: 978-1-138-64265-2 (hbk)
ISBN: 978-1-315-62983-4 (ebk)

Typeset in Sabon
by Apex CoVantage, LLC

Contents

Acknowledgements

The research presented in this book was supported by the UK's Economic and Social Research Council (ESRC grant number: ES/J007927/1).

We are grateful to: Jane Demmen and Veronika Koller for their contributions to the project on which this book is based; Stephen Wattam for designing the database described in Chapter 3; Andrew Kehoe and Matt Gee (Birmingham City University) for modifying their online tool eMargin to accommodate our needs; Lorna Holden and David Stutt for helping us as short-term interns at different points in the course of the project; and the healthcare professionals who kindly agreed to be interviewed as part of our study.

In this book, we draw from parts of the following previous publications by our team, which were all published under a CC BY license:

Demjén, Z. (2016). Laughing at cancer: Humour, empowerment, solidarity and coping online. *Journal of Pragmatics*, *101*, 18–30.

Demjén, Z., Semino, E., and Koller, V. (2016). Metaphors for 'good' and 'bad' deaths: A health professional view, *Metaphor and the Social World*, 6, 1–19.

Demmen, J., Semino, E., Demjén, Z., Koller, V., Hardie, H., Rayson, P., and Payne, S. (2015). A computer-assisted study of the use of Violence metaphors for cancer and end of life by patients, family carers and health professionals, *International Journal of Corpus Linguistics*, *20*(2), 205–231.

Semino, E., Demjén, Z., and Demmen, J. (2016, advance access). An integrated approach to metaphor and framing in cognition, discourse and practice, with an application to metaphors for cancer. *Applied Linguistics*.

Semino, E., Demjén, Z., Demmen, J., Koller, V., Payne, S., Hardie, A., and Rayson, P. (2017). The online use of Violence and Journey metaphors by patients with cancer, as compared with health professionals: A mixed methods study, *BMJ Supportive and Palliative Care*, 7, 60–66.

1 Introduction

1.1 What This Book Is About

This book presents the methodology, findings and implications of a large-scale corpus-based study of the metaphors used to talk about cancer and the end of life (including care at the end of life) in the UK.[1]

Our topic, rationale and approach are best introduced by means of an example. The extract in Example 1.1 is taken from a contribution to a UK-based online forum dedicated to cancer, from January 2008.[2] Contributors to this forum include people who have cancer and people who look after (or have looked after) someone with cancer, such as a partner, spouse or parent. The author of this particular forum post is a man whose wife recently died of cancer. For the purposes of our discussion, we will call him Peter. In the post, Peter responds to a woman who has asked for advice about the problems that her own illness is causing in her relationships with friends and family, and particularly her husband. As is often the case in peer-to-peer online communication about illness (Harvey and Koteyko 2013: 163–211), Peter provides advice and encouragement on the basis of his own personal experiences (NB: throughout this book, original spellings are retained in quotations from the online data).

Example 1.1

I don't quite know where to start with any comment about your situation, but I have been where your hubby currently is and I have run the whole gambit of emotions. I have been at an all time low, wishing somehow it could be me, not my wife, going through the ordeal. Then I have been secretly glad that it wasn't me that was ill, because I am the world's worst patient and would have been more trouble to my wife than her illness ever was. We had days when the situation kicked our lives to pieces, and we had some days that gave us moments of extreme delight. Cancer is a journey, some people have similar experiences to others on that journey, but by and large the journey has many twists and turns that means no two people go

> the exact same route. I think it is like trying to drive a coach and horses uphill with no back wheels on the coach. You do need to stop occasionally and rest the horses, review the situation with your husband. Its his time to step up to the plate. [. . .] My wife when she was diagnosed wanted me to divorce her. Can you imagine that. We had been happily married for 40 years but she tried for several months to make me leave her. When we eventually talked it through, I discovered it was because she loved me so and did not want me to endure her suffering. [. . .] Naturally, being kind of stubborn, I refused to go, I worked on the basis that this was an enemy attacking my loved one and it had picked a fight with me as well. I wish I could say that we won all the battles, and that she is alive and well and cancer free. We did however win a significant number of the skirmishes to make me proud to have been worthy to be by my darling's side. [. . .] The other thing that is very true is the emotions you are both rollercoasting along with have all been experienced by so many on this site that you will be flooded with kindly warm support. I am a praying soul so shall be adding you to my list. Wishing you the very best with all you face kindest Regards

In this extract, Peter discusses the two main topics that we are concerned with in this book: the experience of being affected by cancer; and the experience of the end of life and care at the end of life. More specifically, Peter's post addresses the consequences that caring for someone with incurable cancer can have for one's emotions, perceptions of oneself and others, relationships and so on. Although these consequences are mostly negative, they can also be positive, as in the 'moments of extreme delight' mentioned by Peter.

In this book, we are particularly concerned with the metaphors that are used to talk about these topics and experiences. The post above is a good example of why metaphor is an important phenomenon to consider in relation to cancer and the end of life. Peter writes metaphorically about the experience of cancer as a 'journey' and as a 'fight', and about the contrast between positive and negative emotions in terms of the opposition between up and down (e.g. 'I have been at an all time low', 'the emotions you are both rollercoasting along with'). These metaphors do not just make it possible to verbalise experiences that could not easily be expressed using literal language. They also reveal Peter's own specific and sometimes conflicting perceptions, views, attitudes and challenges.

For example, several metaphors in Example 1.1 emphasise Peter's sense of vulnerability, difficulty and lack of control while his wife was ill, such as 'days when the situation kicked our life to pieces' and the simile 'like trying to drive a coach and horses uphill with no back wheels on the coach'.[3] Other metaphors, in contrast, present him as determined, active and resilient, such as 'I worked on the basis that this was an enemy attacking my loved one and it had picked a fight with me as well'. As we explain in more detail later, metaphors have a 'framing' function: different metaphors can both reflect and facilitate different ways of making sense of and evaluating a particular topic or experience (e.g. Lakoff and Johnson 1980; Ritchie 2013; Semino et al. 2016). The Fight[4] metaphor makes cancer into an enemy to be confronted, while the Journey metaphor does not involve an opponent, but rather impediments to moving forward.

Military metaphors for cancer in particular have often been criticised (e.g. Sontag 1979; Miller 2010) because they tend to frame the relationship between the sick person and the illness as a battle, and the person him- or herself as 'losing the battle' if they do not get better. Later in this book, we show how this and other types of metaphors can indeed have harmful implications, for example by leading to negative self-perceptions, and/or by contributing to a sense of disempowerment. However, in Example 1.1 Peter's own Military metaphor emphasises his pride at being with his wife throughout her illness, even though she ultimately died of it (cf. 'to make me proud to have been worthy to be by my darling's side'). This begins to suggest a point that we will provide evidence for throughout the book: the framing effects of metaphors are a *context- and usage-dependent phenomenon*. Different people may use the same broad kind of metaphor in different ways at different points in time. It is important to consider variation across groups, individuals and contexts, from the perspective of both research on metaphor and research and practice in healthcare. We will look particularly at the metaphorical language used by members of three different participant groups in healthcare: people diagnosed with advanced cancer, unpaid family carers looking after someone who has cancer, and healthcare professionals.

In order to study systematically the metaphors used by the members of these three groups to talk about cancer and the end of life, we adopted the methods of corpus linguistics (see McEnery and Hardie 2011)—a branch of linguistics that exploits computer-aided methods to study a variety of linguistic phenomena in large digital collections of texts known as 'corpora' (singular, 'corpus'). We built a 1.5-million-word corpus consisting of interviews with and online forum posts by people diagnosed with advanced cancer, family carers and healthcare professionals (see Chapter 3 for more detail). We then used a combination of qualitative analysis and corpus linguistic methods to identify and analyse the metaphors used in the corpus to talk about cancer and the end of life, including care at the end of life.[5] In the course of the book, we present a range of qualitative and quantitative findings that have implications for different fields, including particularly: metaphor theory and analysis; corpus linguistic and computational approaches to metaphor; and training and practice in cancer, hospice, palliative and end-of-life care. This book has therefore been written to cater for audiences from these different fields.

In the next section, we provide a brief overview of the background to this book, i.e.: language, illness and healthcare (section 1.2.1), metaphor (section 1.2.2) and corpus linguistics (section 1.2.3). More detail on each of these areas is provided in Chapter 2. In section 1.3, we spell out the contribution of this book, particularly for metaphor studies, corpus linguistics and healthcare research and practice. In section 1.4 we provide a chapter-by-chapter overview of the book, and some suggestions for how readers from different disciplinary backgrounds might approach the different chapters.

1.2 Background to This Book

1.2.1 Language, Illness and Healthcare

Language is central to the practice and provision of healthcare, and mediates the ways that we experience illness. It can both facilitate and obstruct positive experiences and good quality care. When it works well, language improves information provision, diagnosis, support, self-management and self-esteem, resulting in the overall empowerment of both patients and healthcare professionals. However, language can also cause misunderstandings, misdiagnoses, frustration, anxiety and stigma, resulting in overall disempowerment. In particular, people with serious and potentially life-limiting illnesses such as cancer need to (be helped to) understand the nature of their condition and its likely consequences. Their interactions with healthcare professionals may involve a new diagnosis, a change in the illness trajectory or a transition from curative-oriented therapy to supportive and palliative care. These difficult interactions often have to happen in clinical environments that are noisy, busy and time-pressured, and hence not usually conducive to good communication. Professionals may also be reluctant to initiate conversations with patients because they lack skills, are uncertain about the patient's prognosis or may not have an established relationship. They may be uncomfortable with the emotions that can be generated in addressing difficult topics and may withdraw particularly from interacting with terminally ill patients, offer inappropriately optimistic information or change the focus to 'safer' topics.

Communication in doctor-patient encounters has received considerable scholarly attention, particularly with regard to issues such as power imbalances and sources of misunderstanding (e.g. Ong et al. 1995; Harvey and Koteyko 2013: 7–38). There is also evidence that communication skills training programmes can improve clinicians' ability to talk with patients with serious illness, and cancer in particular (Gysels et al. 2004; Moore et al. 2013). In addition, a growing body of work has started to show the important insights that can be gained from studying how illness and healthcare are talked about outside doctor-patient interactions, such as in first-person accounts by patients and in media reporting on serious and/or infectious diseases. This broader focus on different types of communication about illness can lead to a better understanding of the subjective experience of illness, including cancer (e.g. Appleton and Flynn 2014), and also shed light on socio-cultural views of illness that can influence self-perceptions, social relations, preventative behaviours and compliance with treatment (e.g. Hanne and Hawken 2007). These insights can in turn be used to facilitate sensitive and effective communication in institutional healthcare settings (e.g. Charon 2006; Carel 2013). For example, it has been shown that being exposed to patients' narratives makes a positive contribution to the learning and communication skills of medical students (Easton 2016; Snow et al. 2016). Indeed, a 2016 World Health Organization report on 'The Cultural Contexts of Health' (Greenhalgh 2016: ii) significantly concludes that research on narratives of health and illness can 'convey the individual experience of illness and well-being, thereby complementing (and sometimes challenging) epidemiological and public health evidence'.

In this context, attention to language in communication about illness is paramount. This does not just mean focusing on *what* people say, but also paying detailed and systematic attention to *how* they say what they say (e.g. Sarangi 2004; Hunt and Carter 2012). For example, we have suggested that *how* Peter uses metaphors in Example 1.1 gives us insights into aspects of his experiences that he does not state explicitly, such as an alternation between a sense of helplessness and feelings of defiance and pride. It is in fact well-known that metaphors are particularly important in the communication and experience of illness (see 1.2.2 and 2.5.1; see also Demjén and Semino 2017 for an overview). However, there is also awareness that metaphors can be, as Czechmeister (1994: 1227) puts it in relation to cancer, a 'two-edged sword'. When they work well, they can help people express, understand and cope with the experience of illness. When they work badly, they can cause misunderstandings and negative emotions.

By exploring systematically the metaphors used by patients, family carers and healthcare professionals in the context of cancer and the end of life, we hope to increase healthcare professionals' awareness of their own and others' uses of language, so that they can adopt more sensitive and effective communication strategies with patients and their families.

1.2.2 Metaphor

Definition

Metaphor in verbal communication involves talking and, potentially, thinking about one thing in terms of another, where the two things are different, but some form of similarity can be perceived between them.

For example, in the extract above, Peter talks about cancer in terms of an 'enemy' who had 'attack[ed]' his wife and therefore 'pick[ed] a fight' with him too. Illnesses such as cancer and physical attacks by an enemy are different kinds of experiences, but they can be perceived as similar: both are unwelcome; both have negative and potentially fatal consequences; both require some kind of action; and so on. We describe these similarities as 'perceived' because they are not objectively given or constrained in an absolute sense. Rather, they are at least in part created in the production and interpretation of the metaphor itself. In the terms we used in the previous section, they are part of the *framing* that a particular use of metaphor imposes on its topic. In addition, each choice of metaphor facilitates further inferences, evaluations, emotional reactions and so on. Peter's Fight metaphor does not just evaluate the illness negatively, but also presents the relationship between the couple and the illness as an antagonistic one, and suggests that their role is to find every possible way to treat the effects of the cancer, even though it could not be cured.

Given our definition, metaphor in language includes striking and creative uses of language (such as Peter's 'skirmishes' with cancer), as well as expressions that have very conventional metaphorical meanings (such as Peter's use of 'going through' to refer to coping with a difficult experience, rather than to physical movement). More generally, metaphor in language can take many different forms. These include not just 'A is B' statements (e.g. 'Cancer is a journey') and 'similes' (e.g. 'like trying to drive a coach and horses uphill with no back wheels on the coach'), but a wide variety of expressions involving different structures and types of words (e.g. the use of 'flooded', 'warm' and 'support' in: 'you will be flooded with kindly warm support').

In some cases, a particular word works metaphorically on its own in a particular textual context, such as Peter's use of 'low' to indicate extremely negative emotions, rather than a physical position. In other cases, several words are used together to express the same metaphorical comparison, resulting in what is traditionally known as 'extended metaphor'. This applies to Peter's Journey and Fight metaphors in Example 1.1. In our analysis, we consider the whole range of possible linguistic manifestations of metaphor and discuss, where relevant, the consequences that different choices may have on the meanings and framings communicated. In Chapter 3, we will describe in more detail our approach to identifying and quantifying metaphor.

Metaphor and (Dis)Empowerment

In this book, we are particularly concerned with how different uses of metaphor frame the roles and mutual relationships of members of different participant groups in healthcare, and with the empowering or disempowering effects of these framings. The notions of *power* and *empowerment* in healthcare have been approached in different ways from different disciplinary perspectives (see Collins 2015 for an overview). We see (dis)empowerment in language as the process through which linguistic choices reflect, facilitate and/or undermine different kinds and degrees of agency, validation, evaluation and control, with implications for identities, emotions and relationships.

For the specific purposes of our metaphor analysis, we define empowerment and disempowerment as, respectively, an increase or decrease in the degree of agency that someone has, or is perceived to have, within the metaphorical framing suggested by the text. Agency, in this sense, is the (perceived) ability to control or freely react to events for one's own benefit, where this ability is desired by the person and not externally imposed. Following van Leeuwen (2008: 23), we allow for different ways in which agency can be realised in language, and specifically in linguistic structures that include metaphorical expressions. For example, the expressions 'I am battling with cancer' and 'my fight against terminal cancer' (from our patient online data) both have the patient in the role of agent within the metaphorical scenarios suggested by 'battling' and 'fight'. This is signalled in different ways, however, i.e. through the choice of grammatical subject for the verb 'battle' ('I') and through the possessive expression preceding the noun 'fight' ('my') (see Collins 2015 for a similar approach to (dis)empowerment in healthcare communication). We will return to agency and (dis)empowerment in metaphor use in the discussion of our findings.

Conceptual Metaphor Theory

Metaphor has been the focus of scholarship since classical antiquity, in fields as diverse as rhetoric, philosophy, ethics, politics, philology, linguistics, literary and cultural criticism, psychology, cognitive science and, more recently, computer science. Despite disciplinary and paradigmatic differences, it is widely recognised as a crucial tool for communication and reasoning. This is precisely because it can be used, as we have started to show, to express complex meanings and subjective experiences vividly and concisely—and, potentially, to explain, evaluate, persuade, entertain and so on.

Over the last four decades, research on metaphor in a variety of fields has been influenced by Conceptual Metaphor Theory (CMT), which was initially proposed in Lakoff and Johnson's (1980) book *Metaphors We Live By* (see also Lakoff 1993; Lakoff and Johnson 1999; Kövecses 2010). CMT focuses on patterns of related and conventionalised metaphorical expressions, such as the following:

> He got a head start in life. He's without direction in his life. I'm where I want to be in life. I'm at a crossroads in my life. He'll go

places in life. He's never let anyone get in his way. He's gone through a lot in life.

(Lakoff 1993: 223)

All these sentences refer to some aspect of life in terms of movement or travel. In terms of CMT, they are evidence of the conceptual metaphor LIFE IS A JOURNEY,[6] which is claimed to be shared by speakers of English. Conceptual metaphors are described as conventionalised metaphorical ways of understanding a 'target' conceptual domain (e.g. LIFE) in terms of a 'source' conceptual domain (e.g. JOURNEY). Conceptual metaphors consist of systematic sets of correspondences, or mappings, across the two domains in conceptual structure. In the LIFE IS A JOURNEY conceptual metaphor, the person living the life corresponds to a traveller; purposes correspond to destinations; difficulties correspond to obstacles on a journey; and so on. The choice of source domain highlights some aspects of the target domain and hides others, resulting in what we have called a particular 'framing' of the topic of the metaphor (Lakoff and Johnson 1980: 163). For example, the JOURNEY source domain highlights the importance of achieving one's purposes in life (which corresponds to reaching one's destinations), and backgrounds the role of reflection, contemplation or even failure in life.

Typically, target domains are complex, abstract, subjective, diffuse and/or sensitive experiences (such as illness, the emotions and death), whereas source domains are simpler, more concrete and/or less subjective (such as movement or position in space) (see also Dancygier and Sweetser 2014: 62–71). More specifically, within CMT it is claimed that many conventional conceptual metaphors are 'embodied'; i.e. their source domains are physical experiences such as movement in space or physical contact with another person. For example, in CMT's terms, Peter's use of 'low' in 'I have been at an all time low' is a linguistic realisation of the conceptual metaphor SAD IS DOWN. According to Lakoff and Johnson (1980: 15), this metaphor has its 'physical basis' in the fact that a '[d]rooping posture typically goes along with sadness and depression'.

While CMT initially focused on highly conventional metaphorical expressions in language (e.g. someone's 'direction' in life), it was also developed to provide an account of novel or creative uses of metaphor (Lakoff and Turner 1989; see also Semino 2008, 2011). Much creativity, it is argued, involves novel uses of conventional conceptual metaphors. For example, Peter's Journey metaphor is consistent with a conventional conceptual metaphor ILLNESS/CANCER IS A JOURNEY, which can in turn be seen as part of the more general LIFE IS A JOURNEY metaphor. At the same time, the expression 'drive a coach and horses uphill with no back wheels on the coach' is not conventional in English, and describes difficulty in terms of a very specific type of problem on a journey. More radical creativity, in contrast, involves the creation of original metaphorical mappings between domains, such as Hurley's (2014) striking description of her own cancer cells as refugee children:

> I saw my cancer not as an invader, not an enemy to be fought, but as refugee children who had lost their way. The little refugee cells were hungry, dirty, tired, sullen, and needed care: to be fed, cleaned up and comforted before being resettled into a new and better life, elsewhere, where both they and I would be safe.
>
> (Hurley 2014: 312)

Although some of its main tenets had been suggested before (e.g. Jäkel 1999), CMT caused a major paradigm shift. It placed metaphor centre stage in many disciplines as a crucial cognitive tool, and as pervasive in both verbal and non-verbal communication. Subsequent studies have applied CMT to different languages and cultures (e.g. Kövecses 2005) and provided some empirical evidence for its claims (e.g. Gibbs 1994; Thibodeau and Boroditsky 2011). On the other hand, the theory has been extensively criticised, particularly for lacking a rigorous method for postulating conceptual metaphors from linguistic evidence, and for disregarding variation in metaphor use across different types of texts and contexts (e.g. Murphy 1996; Vervaeke and Kennedy 1996; Steen 1999; Deignan et al. 2013; Deignan 2017).

Current Research on Metaphor Relevant to This Book

Our approach to metaphor in this book is influenced by CMT in two main respects: we regard metaphor in language as related to metaphor in thought, and we attribute to metaphor an important framing function, which is particularly relevant to the context of serious illnesses such as cancer and (care at) the end of life. However, we primarily build on, and aim to contribute to, more recent work on metaphor that relies on the systematic analysis of *authentic* or *attested* linguistic data, to make claims about the role of metaphor in both discourse and cognition.

A wide range of studies have been carried out on the use of metaphor in different genres and domains of communication, such as politics (e.g. Musolff 2016), economics (e.g. Koller 2004), education (e.g. Cameron 2003), science (e.g. Brown 2003), psychotherapy (e.g. Tay 2013) and reconciliation (e.g. Cameron 2011). This work often relies on a combination of qualitative analysis and quantitative corpus-based methods (e.g. Koller 2004; Charteris-Black 2004). More importantly, this large body of work shows that metaphors in language vary considerably in form and function depending, broadly speaking, on the *context* of use. Important factors in the context include: the genre/type of the text; the preceding 'co-text', i.e. what has been previously said or written in the particular instance of communication; the roles, identities and goals of participants in the communication; the discourse communities to which participants belong; the historical period and cultural background; the institutional setting; and so on (e.g. Semino 2008; Steen et al. 2010; Deignan et al. 2013).

From this perspective, metaphor use in context is seen as the result of the dynamic interaction of this variety of factors (e.g. Gibbs and Cameron 2008; Gibbs 2017), and explanations tend to be provided in terms of more specific kinds of conceptual structures than the broad source and target domains of CMT, such as the notion of particular *scenarios* (e.g. Musolff 2006, 2016). For example, Peter's Journey metaphor in Example 1.1 involves a very specific travel scenario, and is best explained as emerging from an interaction of factors, including: conventional conceptual metaphors for illness and cancer involving the JOURNEY source domain; Peter's own personal experience of living with his wife while she was ill; his experiences after she died; the online forum environment; Peter's previous interactions on the forum; the post to which Peter is responding; and the incremental textual context of the post itself.

In this book, we rely on these recent developments to do justice to both general tendencies and individual/contextual specificities in how metaphor is used in our data to perform a variety of functions, such as conveying views, emotions and attitudes; negotiating relationships; and building both individual and group identities (see also Demmen et al. 2015; Semino et al. 2016; Semino et al. 2017).

1.2.3 Corpus Linguistics

Given the series in which this book appears, it might seem unnecessary to point out the usefulness of corpus methods for a systematic study of metaphor use in large datasets. However, this is likely to be unknown territory for readers who are not specialists in linguistics. We will therefore provide a brief introduction here, before going into more detail in Chapters 2 and 3.

The value of corpus linguistics is perhaps best introduced by considering the issue of characterising the meaning of some particular word in a particular language. Competent speakers of that language might approach this by relying on their own intuitive knowledge, sitting back and thinking about the word's definition and its potential different meanings. They might think about how they use the word and the ways they have seen it used in different kinds of texts, insofar as they can remember them. But there are many aspects of how words are used that are not easily accessible to this kind of reflection. What is the core meaning of the word, and what phrases or idioms can it contribute to? Does the word carry any specific associations or evaluations? Does the word have any specific meanings in particular domains? Is it part of a technical vocabulary or regional dialect that many people know nothing about? How has the meaning of the word changed over time? To answer some of these questions, one might go beyond one's own knowledge and experience by consulting other people or a dictionary. However, dictionary entries are inevitably limited in the amount of detail they provide, and lexicographers themselves are faced professionally with the same kinds of questions about word meanings, uses and evidence. Ultimately, a scientific approach to word meanings requires the analysis of a large number of real language examples, in order to see what patterns there are. Some of the language evidence will fit speakers' intuitions, but there will also be patterns that are only revealed when considering systematically a large number of instances. Indeed, dictionaries of English and other languages increasingly rely on evidence from corpora for the definition of words and the exemplification of meanings.

In the extract quoted at the beginning of the chapter, for example, Peter uses the expression 'pick a fight with' as follows:

> I worked on the basis that this was an enemy attacking my loved one and it had picked a fight with me as well.

From a CMT perspective, this would be seen as a linguistic realisation of a conceptual metaphor such as ILLNESS/CANCER IS A WAR. In our own analysis of Example 1.1, we have also talked generally about Peter's use of a Fight metaphor, and made a connection with Military metaphors more generally. However, does this do full justice to the implications of Peter's specific choice of words? In Figure 1.1, we provide an extract from a *concordance* of the expression 'picked a fight with' in the Oxford English Corpus, which contains 2.5 billion words of contemporary English from around the world. A concordance provides all instances of

workshop and I , uppity loudmouthed campus activist that I was ,	picked a fight with	him ? I think that 's why he likes me so much , actually . </p>
alcoholists . As usuall Mr T drunk himself under the table twice and	picked a fight with	someone else since he was so drunk he could hardly walk . And
everything we all know about crabs in a barrel , David Poland has	picked a fight with	his fellow online movie and celebrity bottom feeder , Roger
excellence and urbane sophistication , The New Yorker magazine , has	picked a fight with	down-to-earth Scranton . </p><p> Yes , it 's true . Scranton
chili . </p><p> It 's a good day for chili . </p><p> Brad DeLong	picked a fight with	Jonah Goldberg last week , criticizing a Goldberg column about
Torah , and then wrote it all down so thet the Orthodox you just	picked a fight with	can bore you for hours on the subject . It 's called the Talmud
interest , and penalties the IRS claims the church owes . Who	picked a fight with	whom has fueled a significant portion of the dialogue to date
found , and therefore it didn't matter the issue on which you	picked a fight with	the Administration , in the end that fight was justified .
with the rest of BOS , this is all about the money . When you	picked a fight with	these warriors you made a bet on the outcome . If you win you
showing neither respect for nor fear of his older playmate ,	picked a fight with	him and was sent away from the Palace to live with relatives
all good . </p><p> Gig from Hell ! : Bogalusa , La - Drunk local	picked a fight with	singer and duked it out on the dance floor while band kept
discovered yet by a certain A-List social software expert who I 've	picked a fight with	before ;-)) . </p><p> Janet - thanks for your kind words .
Adoration Quota) missing . When I went to bed last night , Uni	picked a fight with	Nefreet so that when I opened the door to intervene , he could
Now , she was determined to have her say and she deliberately	picked a fight with	him . He was indifferent , however . The closer he was to Jane
Fitz had a fight yesterday . No , that 's not quite right . She	picked a fight with	Fitz and he had no idea what it was about . But I found out
he was impotent . </p><p> One fine night , he went drinking and	picked a fight with	me when he was back . In his drunken state , he hit me and
come unstuck in time . He 's more than four minutes off . He	picked a fight with	a woman who neglected to be frightened . </p><p> First published
's independence movement in 1848 , ruled autocratically and	picked a fight with	Serbia that was the proximate cause of World War I (and their
the desire to start a fight " , the report says . </p><p> " I	picked a fight with	someone on the street . They were the first people I come across
council , said : " I do sympathise . But Mr Fitzmaurice has	picked a fight with	the wrong people . His argument is with the Labour government

Figure 1.1 Extract From Concordance of 'Picked a Fight With' From the Oxford English Corpus

a word or expression in the corpus, with the immediately preceding and following text.

The concordance shows that, when the expression 'picked a fight with' is used literally, it tends to refer to unmotivated, unprovoked and often mindless physical aggression aimed at an innocent individual, as in 'he went drinking and picked a fight with me when he was back. In his drunken state, he hit me'. When the expression is used metaphorically to refer to arguments or disputes, these associations[7] seem to persist, as in 'The New Yorker magazine has picked a fight with down-to-earth Scranton'. These very brief observations can help provide a more nuanced account of Peter's choice of words: one of the ways in which he seems to perceive his wife's cancer is in terms of unprovoked aggression against him personally, which required an immediate response on his part.

This example begins to show how using a large, principled collection of naturally occurring language (that is, a *corpus*) makes it possible to test—and therefore to validate or to reject—hypotheses about the way that language works, and to refine an understanding of the potential implications of specific linguistic choices. Because a corpus is *large*, it is possible to uncover and quantify examples of low frequency language features. Because a corpus is *principled* in its design—that is, it is designed to be representative of one or more varying forms of a language in a balanced way—it is possible to take into account a much wider variety of language data than we would have access to via individual intuition. Corpora therefore facilitate the empirical examination of linguistic phenomena (not just metaphor) across a number of topics (not just illness and healthcare). Corpora are, moreover, often designed to support the *comparison* of language in different settings or contexts of use. As we have mentioned, in this book we work with a corpus that contains sub-components representing the usage of members of three different participant groups in healthcare in two different communicative settings (interviews and online fora). Using methods devised in corpus linguistics and natural language processing (of which more in Chapter 2), one can pursue questions in language description or linguistic theory; but it is also possible to gain deep insights into the use of language *in society* for a variety of communicative purposes.

Corpus methods are necessarily computer-assisted since they entail dealing with large amounts of machine-readable data. In our case, we have both re-used existing tools (e.g. Wmatrix, Rayson 2009; and AntConc, Anthony 2014) and designed new software in order to collect online forum data, to process interview transcripts and to assist the process of our analysis (e.g. the database introduced in Chapter 3, section 3.5.3). Part of our data has been *manually* analysed using annotation/editing tools (e.g. eMargin), but we have also exploited other software that applies linguistic annotation *automatically* (e.g. the UCREL Semantic Analysis System, or USAS; Rayson 2009). Finally, as we have just briefly shown, we have made use of a type of retrieval software called *concordancers*. These tools for corpus analysis permit searching for examples in context (concordances), but often support other techniques such as comparison of subsets of the data (keyness) or extraction of co-occurrence patterns between different words (collocation). In Chapters 2 and 3, we will provide more details on the general and specific methods that we have used in our analyses.

The application of corpus linguistic methods to the study of communication about health and illness is a relatively recent but extremely timely development. Greenhalgh's (2016) World Health Organization report on 'The Cultural Contexts of Health' emphasises the importance of 'appropriate and rigorous methods' if qualitative research on narratives of health and illness is to be accepted alongside more established, quantitative epidemiological approaches in the health sector. Corpus linguistics makes it possible to combine qualitative and quantitative analysis in an explicit and rigorous manner, and is therefore ideally suited to bridge the methodological divide in healthcare research that Greenhalgh identifies.

1.3 The Contribution of This Book

This book presents what is, to the best of our knowledge, the largest-scale study to date of metaphor in the experience of cancer and (care at) the end of life. As such, it makes contributions to (applied) linguistics, discourse analysis and medical/health humanities, as well as specific contributions to metaphor studies, corpus linguistics and healthcare research and practice.

With respect to *metaphor studies*, this book contributes to a growing body of research that brings together discourse analysis, cognitive linguistics and corpus linguistics to shed light on the role of metaphor in different types of communication. More specifically:

- It demonstrates an innovative, eclectic approach to the use of corpus linguistic methods for the study of metaphor in large datasets;
- It presents in both depth and breadth the frequencies, forms and functions of the metaphors that are used to talk about a range of sensitive topics (including particularly illness, death and the emotions) and shows how these are dependent on who is speaking/writing and in what genre;
- It explains how the findings of the analysis relate to recent developments in research on metaphor, including particularly work on framing, metaphor scenarios and accounts of metaphor based on Dynamical Systems Theory (e.g. Ritchie 2013; Musolff 2016; Gibbs 2017);
- It provides a concrete example of the potential real-world applications of research on metaphor.

With respect to *corpus linguistics* (and computational linguistics more generally), this book shows how a range of methods can be deployed in the identification and analysis of metaphor in large datasets. More specifically:

- It presents a systematic and rigorous approach to the construction of a corpus that includes online forum data, and spells out how to manage and downsample this kind of data;
- It shows how corpus methods can be used to scale up from the manual analysis of metaphorical expressions in a small data sample to a systematic analysis of metaphorical expressions in a large corpus;
- It demonstrates the use of keyness analysis combined with lexical and automatic semantic tagging to identify potential metaphorical expressions (or *metaphor candidates*) in a corpus, and to compare metaphor frequencies and use in different sections of the corpus.

With respect to *healthcare research and practice*, this book shows what insights can be gained by noticing and 'unpacking' the metaphors used by different participants in healthcare to talk about cancer and (care at) the end of life. More specifically:

- It shows what metaphors are commonly used by members of the three participant groups, and points out both differences and similarities across the groups;
- It reveals the possible effects and functions of different patterns of metaphor use, for example to engender a sense of community among cancer patients communicating in a peer-to-peer online forum;
- It argues that there are no inherently 'good' or 'bad' metaphors in communication about illness, but rather that different *uses* of metaphor may be more or less (dis)empowering, depending on how they reflect and reinforce different emotions, self-perceptions and degrees of agency and control;
- It shows healthcare professionals how to recognise and interpret metaphors in their own language, in the language used by patients and family carers, and in written documents produced by governments, hospices, hospitals and charitable organisations;
- It identifies potential power relations embedded within language and played out in clinical contexts, and highlights opportunities for empowerment;
- It has implications for how to engage with the metaphors used by patients and family carers in clinical contexts, and generally for how to employ metaphors sensitively and effectively in healthcare communications.

Our datasets are drawn from English-language sources collected in the United Kingdom, which means that we are not able to make claims about how metaphors are used in other languages or other countries. However, we hope that our methods and findings will be relevant to other contexts, and that international readers may be inspired to examine the use of metaphor in other parts of the world and other languages (see also Potts and Semino 2017 for an initial comparison of our professional online data with a similar US corpus).

1.4 The Contents of This Book and How to Read It

In the rest of this book, we present the background to our project (Chapter 2), our data and methodology (Chapter 3), our findings (Chapters 4 to 10) and our conclusions (Chapter 11). In writing the book, we have aimed to cater for three main audiences: metaphor scholars, corpus linguists and healthcare researchers and practitioners. As a result, the introductions to metaphor and corpus linguistics in this chapter and in Chapter 2 do not assume any previous knowledge. The chapters in which we present our findings (Chapters 4 to 10) include detailed summaries of our main points at the beginning and the end, and keep to a minimum the use of technical terms from corpus linguistics and metaphor research. The conclusions (Chapter 11) are structured according to the likely interests of different readerships, and a glossary at the end of the book provides definitions of the main technical terms we employ. Nonetheless, different sections and chapters are particularly accessible or relevant to different audiences, as we explain in more detail later.

Chapter 2 provides an overview of the interdisciplinary background to the research we present in this book: (a) healthcare communication, and particularly work on communication about cancer and the end of life; (b) corpus linguistics and its methods; and (c) metaphor, with a focus on research on metaphor in discourse and recent methodological and theoretical developments. After introducing each area in turn, we draw the three separate threads together by discussing corpus-based and computational approaches to metaphor, and previous research on metaphors in communication about illness/cancer and dying. While the whole chapter aims to be accessible to all our audiences, the overviews of corpus linguistics and metaphor are detailed and extensive, and may be less relevant to readers who are primarily interested in our findings.

Chapter 3 introduces our data and methods, and is particularly relevant to (corpus) linguists, or to anyone interested in employing a similar approach. We begin with an introduction to our data and our rationale for the selection of our respective sources. We then describe in detail how the data was collected and compiled into our 1.5-million-word corpus. We then introduce our main method for identifying metaphors in language and discuss our initial manual intensive (qualitative) analysis of a 92,000-word sample from our corpus. Finally, we outline the automated quantitative analysis of our complete corpus, including how it was informed by the initial manual sample analysis.

Chapters 4–10 present our results, and combine quantitative and qualitative analyses of our data. Several of these chapters begin with further methodological details which are relevant to (corpus) linguists but are not essential for understanding the significance of our findings. Chapters 4–6 focus on particular types and patterns of metaphors, while Chapters 7–10 focus on specific topics of special significance to one or more groups of people.

Chapter 4 provides a general overview of our findings, starting with an analysis of key words and key semantic domains in each section of the corpus, and showing the main differences in vocabulary and topics among the three participant groups and the two genres that we studied. We then consider the main types of metaphors identified in the corpus, i.e. metaphors drawing from the semantic domains of: Animals, Journey, Machines, Obstacles, Openness, Religion and Magic, Restraint, Sports and Games, Violence and Wholeness. This general analysis enabled us to identify some specific patterns in the corpus that receive more detailed consideration in the rest of the book, namely:

- The two most frequent types of metaphors: Violence metaphors and Journey metaphors (Chapters 5 and 6);
- Three important topic areas that are often expressed metaphorically: the relationship between patients and healthcare professionals; the notions of a 'good' and a 'bad' death; and the emotions of bereaved family carers (Chapters 7–9);
- A striking and relevant phenomenon in the patient data, namely humour in metaphor use (Chapter 10).

Chapter 5 presents a quantitative and qualitative analysis of Violence metaphors in the corpus, including what, in previous work on metaphors for illness, are variously called 'fight', 'battle', 'war' or 'military' metaphors. We begin by showing differences in the frequencies of these metaphors in different sections of the corpus, and then consider three main topics that the members of our three participant groups express in terms of Violence metaphors: the relationship with the disease; the effects of illness, treatment and death; and the relationship with the healthcare system. We show that, while there is considerable evidence that Violence metaphors can be harmful, they can clearly be empowering for some patients in particular, when they are used to express personal determination and/or mutual solidarity.

Chapter 6 is concerned with the use of 'cancer journey' and other Journey metaphors in our corpus. As with Chapter 5, we begin by comparing the frequencies of Journey metaphors in the different sections of our corpus. In order to make sense of these differences, we then present a detailed analysis of the use of Journey metaphors to talk about two specific topics: the experience of illness (including the end of life) and treatment options. We show how, as in the case of Violence metaphors, Journey metaphors can be used in a variety of different ways, including to express both positive and negative views and emotions, and to suggest different degrees of (dis)empowerment on the part of patients. We finish by reconsidering the opposition between Journey and Violence metaphors by focusing on the individuals in our online data who use both types of metaphors, whether in combination or separately.

Chapter 7 discusses the metaphors that are used by patients on the one hand and healthcare professionals on the other to describe their mutual relationships. More specifically, we consider three broad topic areas where metaphors play a role in both datasets, but where differences between the two groups are important: descriptions of members of the other group; descriptions of what healthcare professionals do for patients; and descriptions of particularly sensitive aspects of the relationship, i.e. interactions with healthcare professionals in the patient data, and emotional involvement with patients in the healthcare professionals' data. We show how these metaphors are often evaluative, and we highlight issues to do with agency, power and control from the different perspectives of the members of the two groups.

In Chapters 8, 9 and 10, we take each group of participants and investigate the metaphors they use for a particularly salient aspect of their experience or for a particular communicative function. Chapter 8 is devoted to healthcare professionals, Chapter 9 to family carers and Chapter 10 to patients.

Chapter 8 focuses on the metaphors that healthcare professionals in our data use to describe a 'good' or a 'bad' death. We show that the difference between good and bad deaths is partly expressed via different frequencies of contrasting metaphors, such as 'peacefulness' and 'openness' as opposed to 'struggle' and 'pushing away' professional help. Such metaphors are used to: evaluate deaths and the dying; justify those evaluations; present a remarkably consistent view of different types of deaths; and promote a particular 'framing' of a good death, which is closely linked with the dominant socio-cultural and professional contexts that healthcare professionals operate in.

Chapter 9 discusses the variety of metaphors that bereaved carers use in our online data to talk about their emotional experiences following the death of the person they cared for. We begin by considering metaphors for the individual felt experience of grief, and then go on to discuss metaphors for the social implications of bereavement. We finish by reflecting on the implications of our findings for, on the one hand, studying metaphors for emotions and, on the other hand, understanding the challenges and needs of the bereaved carers represented in our data.

Chapter 10 is concerned with how and why patients on one particular thread on the online forum use humorous metaphors. We examine three specific types of humorous metaphors: (a) personifications of cancer and treatment paraphernalia, (b) participants' figurative references to one another, and (c) co-created metaphorical fantasy scenarios. We discuss how these humorous metaphors are used to talk about embarrassing or taboo topics, facilitate a sense of empowerment and strengthen the social bonds among contributors to the online forum.

Finally, Chapter 11 spells out the main conclusions and implications of our study, with separate sections dedicated to methodology, metaphor theory and practical applications in healthcare.

Notes

1. The research presented in this book was supported by the UK's Economic and Social Research Council (ESRC grant number: ES/J007927/1). Ethical approval for all aspects of the study was granted by Lancaster University's Research Ethics Committee.
2. The owners of the online forum were contacted to inform them about our data collection, and they expressed no objection. Any information that can identify contributors, including nicknames and electronic handles, is either omitted or changed.
3. As we explain in Chapter 3, we regard similes as one of the different manifestations of metaphor in language.
4. In this book, we use words with an initial capital to group metaphorical expressions that draw from the same area of experience or semantic field.
5. We define end-of-life care as care in the last two years of life.
6. In CMT, small capitals are typically used to refer to conceptual metaphors and conceptual domains.
7. These associations may in fact be due to the fact that 'picked' suggests a deliberate action on the part of an individual. 'Picked' is itself used metaphorically in relation to both physical and non-physical fights.

References

Anthony, L. (2014). *AntConc* (Version 3.4.3) [Computer Software]. Tokyo, Japan: Waseda University. Retrieved from www.laurenceanthony.net/

Appleton, L., and Flynn, M. (2014). Searching for the new normal: Exploring the role of language and metaphors in becoming a cancer survivor. *European Journal of Oncology Nursing*, *18*(4), 378–384.

Brown, T. L. (2003). *Making truth: Metaphor in science*. Urbana, IL: University of Illinois Press.

Cameron, L. (2003). *Metaphor in educational discourse*. London: Continuum.

Cameron, L. (2011). *Metaphor and reconciliation*. New York: Routledge.

Carel, H. (2013). *Illness* (2nd ed.). Stocksfield: Acumen Publishing Limited.

Charon, R. (2006). *Narrative medicine: Honoring the stories of illness*. Oxford: Oxford University Press.

Charteris-Black, J. (2004). *Corpus approaches to critical metaphor analysis*. Basingstoke: Palgrave Macmillan.

Collins, L. (2015). *Language, corpus and empowerment: Applications to deaf education, healthcare and online discourse*. London: Routledge.

Czechmeister, C. A. (1994). Metaphor in illness and nursing: A two-edged sword. *Journal of Advanced Nursing*, *19*(6), 1226–1233.

Dancygier, B., and Sweetser, E. (2014). *Figurative language*. Cambridge: Cambridge University Press.

Deignan, A. (2017). From linguistic to conceptual metaphors. In E. Semino and Z. Demjén (Eds.), *The Routledge handbook of metaphor and language* (pp. 102–116). London and New York: Routledge.

Deignan, A., Littlemore, J., and Semino, E. (2013). *Figurative language, genre and register*. Cambridge: Cambridge University Press.

Demjén, Z., and Semino, E. (2017). Using metaphor in healthcare: Physical health. In E. Semino and Z. Demjén (Eds.), *The Routledge handbook of metaphor and language* (pp. 385–399). London and New York: Routledge.

Demmen, J., Semino, E., Demjén, Z., Koller, V., Hardie, H., Rayson, P., and Payne, S. (2015). A computer-assisted study of the use of Violence metaphors for cancer and end of life by patients, family carers and health professionals. *International Journal of Corpus Linguistics*, *22*(2), 205–231.

Easton, G. (2016). How medical teachers use narratives in lectures: A qualitative study. *BMC Medical Education*, *16*(3).

Gibbs, R., and Cameron, L. (2008). The social-cognitive dynamics of metaphor performance. *Journal of Cognitive Systems Research*, *9*(1–2), 64–75.

Gibbs, R. W., Jr. (1994). *The poetics of mind: Figurative thought, language, and understanding*. Cambridge: Cambridge University Press.

Gibbs, R. W., Jr. (2017). Metaphor, language and dynamical systems. In E. Semino and Z. Demjén (Eds.), *The Routledge handbook of metaphor and language* (pp. 56–70). London and New York: Routledge.

Greenhalgh, T. (2016). *Cultural contexts of health: The use of narrative research in the health sector* (Health Evidence Network (HEN) synthesis report 49). Copenhagen: WHO Regional Office for Europe.

Gysels, M., Richardson, A., and Higginson, I. J. (2004). Communication training for health professionals who are for patients with cancer: A systematic review of effectiveness. *Supportive Care in Cancer*, *12*(10), 692–700.

Hanne, M., and Hawken, S. J. (2007). Metaphors for illness in contemporary media. *Medical Humanities*, *33*(2), 93–99.

Harvey, K., and Koteyko, N. (2013). *Exploring health communication: Language in action*. London: Routledge.

Hunt, D., and Carter, R. (2012). Seeing through the bell jar: Investigating linguistic patterns of psychological disorder. *Journal of Medical Humanities*, *33*(1), 27–39.

Hurley, K. E. (2014). To fight, or not to fight: A cancer psychotherapist with cancer confronts the battle metaphor. *Women & Therapy*, *37*(3–4), 311–318.

Jäkel, O. (1999). Kant, Blumenberg, Weinrich: Some forgotten contributions to the cognitive theory of metaphor. In R. W. Gibbs, Jr. and G. J. Steen (Eds.), *Metaphor in cognitive linguistics* (pp. 9–27). Amsterdam: John Benjamins.

Koller, V. (2004). *Metaphor and gender in business media discourse: A critical cognitive Study*. Basingstoke: Palgrave Macmillan.

Kövecses, Z. (2005). *Metaphor in culture: Universality and variation.* Cambridge: Cambridge University Press.

Kövecses, Z. (2010). *Metaphor: A practical introduction* (2nd ed.). Oxford and New York: Oxford University Press.

Lakoff, G. (1993). The contemporary theory of metaphor. In A. Ortony (Ed.), *Metaphor and thought* (pp. 202–251). Cambridge and New York: Cambridge University Press.

Lakoff, G., and Johnson, M. (1980). *Metaphors we live by.* Chicago: University of Chicago Press.

Lakoff, G., and Johnson, M. (1999). *Philosophy in the flesh: The embodied mind and its challenge to western thought.* New York: Basic Books.

Lakoff, G., and Turner, M. (1989). *More than cool reason: A field guide to poetic metaphor.* Chicago: University of Chicago Press.

McEnery, T., and Hardie, A. (2011). *Corpus linguistics: Methods, theory and practice.* Cambridge: Cambridge University Press.

Miller, R. S. (2010). Speak up: 8 words & phrases to ban in oncology! *Oncology Times*, *32*(12), 20.

Moore, P., Wilkinson, S., and Rivera Mercado, S. (2013). Communication skills training for health care professionals working with cancer patients, their families and/or carers. *Cochrane Database of Systematic Reviews*, (3), Art. No.: CD003751.

Murphy, G. L. (1996). On metaphoric representation. *Cognition*, *60*(2), 173–204.

Musolff, A. (2006). Metaphor scenarios in public discourse. *Metaphor and Symbol*, *21*(1), 23–38.

Musolff, A. (2016). *Political metaphor analysis: Discourse and scenarios.* London: Bloomsbury.

Ong, L. M., de Haes, J. C., Hoos, A. M., and Lammes, F. B. (1995). Doctor-patient communication: A review of the literature. *Social Science & Medicine*, *40*(7), 903–918.

Potts, A., and Semino, E. (2017). Healthcare professionals' online use of Violence metaphors for care at the end of life in the US: A corpus-based comparison with the UK. *Corpora*, *12*(1), 55–84.

Rayson, P. (2009). *Wmatrix: A web-based corpus processing environment.* School of Computing and Communications, Lancaster University. Retrieved from http://ucrel.lancs.ac.uk/wmatrix/

Ritchie, D. (2013). *Metaphor.* Cambridge: Cambridge University Press.

Sarangi, S. (2004). Towards a communicative mentality in medical and healthcare practice. *Communication & Medicine*, *1*(1), 1–11.

Semino, E. (2008). *Metaphor in discourse.* Cambridge: Cambridge University Press.

Semino, E. (2011). Metaphor, creativity, and the experience of pain across genres. In J. Swann, R. Carter, and R. Pope (Eds.), *Creativity in language: The state of the art.* Basingstoke: Palgrave Macmillan.

Semino, E., Demjén, Z., and Demmen, J. (2016 advance access). An integrated approach to metaphor and framing in cognition, discourse and practice, with an application to metaphors for cancer. *Applied Linguistics.*

Semino, E., Demjén, Z., Demmen, J., Koller, V., Payne, S., Hardie, H., and Rayson, P. (2017). The online use of "Violence" and "Journey" metaphors by cancer patients, as compared with health professionals: A mixed methods study. *BMJ Supportive and Palliative Care*, *7*(1), 60–66.

Snow, R., Crocker, J., Talbot, K., Moore, J., and Salisbury, H. (2016). Does hearing the patient perspective improve consultation skills in examinations? An exploratory randomized controlled trial in medical undergraduate education. *Medical Teacher*, *38*(12), 1229–1235.

Sontag, S. (1979). *Illness as metaphor*. London: Allen Lane.

Steen, G. (1999). From linguistic to conceptual metaphor in five steps. In R. W. Gibbs, Jr. and G. J. Steen (Eds.), *Metaphor in cognitive linguistics* (pp. 57–77). Amsterdam: John Benjamins.

Steen, G. J., Dorst, A. G., Herrmann, J. B., Kaal, A. A., Krennmayr, T., and Pasma, T. (2010). *A method for linguistic metaphor identification: From MIP to MIPVU*. Amsterdam: John Benjamins.

Tay, D. (2013). *Metaphor in psychotherapy: A descriptive and prescriptive analysis*. Amsterdam and Philadelphia, PA: John Benjamins.

Thibodeau, P. H., and Boroditsky, L. (2011). Metaphors we think with: The role of metaphor in reasoning. *PLoS ONE*, *6*(2), e16782.

van Leeuwen, T. (2008). *Discourse and practice: New tools for critical discourse analysis*. Oxford: Oxford University Press.

Vervaeke, J., and Kennedy, J. (1996). Metaphor in language and thought: Falsification and multiple meanings. *Metaphor and Symbol*, *11*(4), 273–284.

2 Background

Metaphor, Corpus Linguistics and Communication About Cancer and the End of Life

2.1 Introduction

This chapter outlines the interdisciplinary background to the research we present in this book. Because our research operates at the intersection of three (sub-)disciplinary concerns—the study of metaphor; the methods of corpus linguistics; and the study of healthcare communication, especially as linked to cancer and end-of-life care—we initially introduce some of the background for each of these three areas separately. As the driving motivation for our study, the *why* of our study, is understanding and improving communication about cancer and the end of life, in section 2.2 we begin by looking at research into healthcare communication from outside the field of linguistics: what we know and why it is important. In section 2.3, we then explore the basic principles and methods of corpus linguistics, thereby outlining the background to the *how* of our study. The *what* is introduced in section 2.4, where we outline the background of recent relevant research into metaphor. Throughout these sections, we revisit and extend some of the concepts we introduced in Chapter 1.

Finally, in sections 2.5 and 2.6, we pull the seemingly separate threads together, addressing what role metaphors tend to play in communication around illness, cancer and dying, and how the study of metaphor has drawn on corpus-based and computational methods (we will outline the difference between the latter two in section 2.6). The chapter aims to be accessible to all our audiences, and does not assume any prior knowledge of the areas we have mentioned. However, the overviews of corpus linguistics and metaphor are detailed and extensive, and may be less relevant to those primarily interested in our findings.

2.2 Why This Topic Matters: Practice-Based Research Into Healthcare Communication

The study of communication has never been the sole preserve of linguists. Like many other scholars, healthcare researchers have, over the years, inquired into many aspects of communication in their own disciplinary and practice contexts. And in those contexts, understanding and improving communication really matters. It is therefore unsurprising that an extensive literature exists on healthcare communication as its own discipline, independent of linguistics as a field. We will, therefore, briefly consider the ways in which communication has been studied in this more practice-oriented discipline, as well as the healthcare practices (especially related to cancer and end-of-life contexts) that have informed and been informed by such studies.

Despite the significant attention paid by such practice-oriented healthcare communication research to language and communication, the importance of language as a symbolic artefact, and the ways it can express underlying meanings and implicit facets of emotions and cognition (for example through metaphor) are perhaps under-recognised. Although some research has been directed at the communicative experiences of patients and carers, arguably most effort in this field has been devoted to exploring the practices of physicians and other professionals providing healthcare, including particularly cancer and hospice nurses. This reflects an awareness of the need to improve healthcare communication that has grown since the 1980s, as well as the specific recognition that successful information provision (which is often seen as the purpose of such communication), alongside other aspects of what might be evaluated as good communication in cancer care, is fundamental to facilitating medical decision-making, reducing psychopathology and improving patient experiences. Fallowfield et al. (2002) identified major deficits in interaction between cancer patients and their medical professionals: professionals would concentrate on pathology and neglect expressions of empathy and attention to patient cues. Fallowfield et al. argued that these could be reduced through focused training. This and similar studies led to the development of a range of communication skills training programmes for cancer care professionals, such as 'Connected', a mandatory course for oncology staff in direct contact with patients in the UK (for an evaluation of this course see Turner et al. 2011).

In practical terms, there are three important components of the practice of healthcare communication: information provision, medical decision-making and advance care planning. These three aspects form a logical sequence, in that, in order to make treatment decisions in the short term or to engage in planning for future medical scenarios, patients need to have access to both sufficient information and the ability to conceptualise different outcomes—even undesirable ones, like dying.

Information provision could imply a one-way provision of advice from medical staff to patients, but in reality it is much more complex. Information provision can involve two-party (dyadic) exchanges between professionals (doctors, nurses and other health or social care professionals)—with or without patients or family members/carers—but is by no means limited to such exchanges. It also includes the difficult exchanges (both verbal and in writing) between teams of professionals from the same or other disciplines, and the information provided to and by the general public and news media. It is critical here to distinguish among the different types of information that may be communicated, which may have very different levels of emotional sensitivity. Disclosing distressing information, for example, is known to be difficult for both patients and doctors (e.g. Schofield et al. 2006).

Specifically in the case of cancer, the main categories of information conveyed to patients are the likelihood of cure or spread of the disease and treatment options. However, while doctors tend to concentrate on the medical details of the disease process, there is evidence that patients find it more important to discuss the impact of cancer on daily life and how to obtain support in managing their disease (Corner et al. 2007). This suggests that not only is there a difference between linguistic and practice-based approaches to health communication, but there might also be a difference between how doctors see 'good' communication and what patients perceive to qualify as 'good' communication. Little is known in the non-linguistic literature about how metaphor influences or is used in various types of information-provision exchanges—or indeed how metaphor is used to represent cancer in public health messages, in appeals for funding or in policy guidelines.

Medical decision-making is required once a cancer diagnosis has been made and disclosed to a patient. There is evidence that most cancer patients prefer either shared decision-making or delegation of the responsibility to doctors, rather than taking a primary role in decision-making about treatment options (Beaver and Booth 2007), although there are potential variations related to the patient's age and educational attainment. Once again, little is known about the role of metaphor in treatment representations—for example describing chemotherapy as the 'big guns' or radiotherapy as 'burning out the enemy'—and the choices made by patients, although we review what *is* known in section 2.5. Some patients will decline active treatment or opt for what is described euphemistically as 'watchful waiting'. However, very few patients decline all forms of medical care, especially comfort measures such as pain and symptom control (Radley and Payne 2009).

Advance care planning is the process of reviewing life goals and preferences concerning medical treatment and care, discussing these goals or preferences with relatives and healthcare providers, and recording them if appropriate. Since 2008, following the launch of the End of Life Care Strategy for England and Wales (Department of Health 2008), healthcare professionals are expected to sensitively facilitate planning ahead at the same time as managing uncertainty. This process typically involves a number of discussions between the patient and a healthcare professional or trained facilitator, during which patients are encouraged to express their preferences for the type of care they wish to receive near the end of life. Advance care planning requires patients to imagine scenarios such as dying or being mentally incompetent, which may be profoundly distressing. Therefore, perhaps not surprisingly, both patients and doctors struggle to have these conversations, and patients may delay documenting their preferences until it is too late. These types of interactions would also benefit from a better understanding of the role metaphor can play in helping or hindering sensitive communication.

Much of the research described so far, and skills training based on it, takes a somewhat simplistically quantitative approach to language—for example by counting 'cues' or utterances which are claimed to 'block' effective communication. There is little acknowledgement of the representational or relational functions of language, or of the use of metaphors, analogies and other linguistic features which can provide insight into the meanings underlying speech and text (Wilkinson 1999). It is only more recently that a systematic review of research using conversation and discourse analytic approaches to communication in advanced disease has provided some evidence of the more nuanced strategies that facilitate better communication (Parry et al. 2014).

Research specifically into metaphorical understandings within healthcare communication has proceeded along similarly functional lines. For example, Froggatt (1998) investigated the metaphors associated with nurses' emotion-work, as part of a larger study of British hospice nurses' professional and personal experiences of death. She argued that two pervasive ways to understand emotion were the metaphors of 'body as a container' and 'emotions as energy', and that this finding could be used to show nurses how to manage the emotional labour that is inevitably part of close encounters with dying patients and their families. Looking at another environment where death is commonly encountered, namely residential nursing homes for older people, Moss et al. (2003) described how the metaphor of 'family' could be used to explain the engagement of nursing staff with older residents nearing the end of life, including the impact of the eventual deaths.

There have also been some studies of patients' use of metaphor in palliative care contexts. Southall (2013) identified and reviewed 14 such empirical papers, concluding that metaphorical communication is often seen as offering potential benefits to patients by facilitating new ways of understanding their condition and perhaps helping them to adopt new coping strategies. There was little evidence of potential harm arising from specific metaphors, possibly due to inadequately critical research. There also appears to be little evidence of how family carers use metaphors to relate their experiences of caregiving or of witnessing the impact of cancer on close relationships.

Some of the descriptions and understandings of metaphor summarised here are consistent with the linguistic view; others less so. This is partly because metaphor itself is defined differently in different fields, and partly because of the different methods and objectives of practice-based health communication research compared to research in linguistics. Nevertheless, the settings this research has investigated represent at least part of the context within which some of our interview participants and forum contributors work, and so our outline of this area provides an overview (albeit brief) of the healthcare communication context within which we situate this book. In fact, the practical needs of those working in healthcare, and the practical applicability of our findings and recommendations, are central to our interest in language use—specifically metaphor. We will propose practical implications and applications of our various findings throughout the course of the book, and particularly in the conclusions (Chapter 11).

In the sections that follow, we move from the context of practice-based healthcare research to outlining the specifically *linguistic* contexts for our study.

2.3 How We Can Study It: A Brief Overview of Corpus Linguistics and Its Methods

Turning first to the background of our primary methodology, an explanation of the *how* of this study, in this section we introduce the basic ideas and analytic techniques of *corpus linguistics*.

Corpus linguistics is a branch of linguistics defined by the methods that it uses. While there are many of these methods, all of them involve studying language by looking at very large samples of naturally occurring language in use, that is, the collections of texts that we call *corpora* (the plural of *corpus*). This is in contrast to other linguistic methods, which are based either on relatively small samples of language usage or on other kinds of data altogether. Because of the large size of language corpora—even the smallest tend to be roughly the same length as a novel, and the biggest are thousands or millions of times larger—it is impractical, if not impossible, to analyse them with traditional hand-and-eye, qualitative language research methods. Corpus linguistics is devoted to developing and applying the methods needed to approach these very large datasets. For this reason, corpus linguistics is often described as a methodology that can be applied across many different areas of linguistics (see McEnery and Wilson 2001: 2; McEnery et al. 2006: 7–8).

The large size of language corpora has several important consequences. The first is that the only way to analyse a corpus in a realistic time frame is with the aid of a computer. Hence, corpora are almost universally stored digitally, as *machine-readable text*, and the computer is the key tool for searching and sifting the data in the corpus. The second consequence is that we cannot look in detail at every single bit of language in the corpus; there is too much of it. Often we cannot even look in detail at all examples of the phenomenon we are interested in. For this reason, methods for statistically summarising the data in a large body of digital text are central to corpus linguistics. As a result, corpus linguistics has a reputation as being oriented towards quantitative data and primarily interested in different forms of number crunching. But this is not an accurate picture. In fact, corpus linguistics is inextricably both qualitative and quantitative. Many corpus methods do generate statistical outputs, but interpreting these—understanding what they are telling us about the nature of the language and how it is used—always requires the linguist to engage with actual examples from the corpus and the meanings that the language-in-use expresses. Other methods generate example sets as their primary output, which the analyst then assesses in a qualitative manner—but a quantitative characterisation of those judgements across the example set is nearly always necessary. Thus, both qualitative and quantitative modes of analysis are essential to corpus linguistics (Biber et al. 1998: 4).

Corpus linguistics in its modern form dates from the early 1960s, and has grown in scope and popularity over the last 50 years alongside the expansion of computer technology from a highly specialised niche interest to an indispensable everyday tool. Early corpora of general English were used mostly to look at issues of grammar; recent 'standard' descriptive grammars of the English language rely heavily on corpus analysis. Subsequently, from the 1980s, corpora began to be applied in lexicography, and today all serious dictionary development is built around corpus data. In the period between about 1995 and 2010, however, there emerged a new trend of using large corpora to analyse patterns in meaning and discourse—that is, using corpus methods to research common or socially important ways of talking (and thinking) about different topics (e.g. Baker 2006).

The study of metaphor in use in the corpus data has become an important part of this. Corpus data and methods are particularly suited to this enterprise because patterns of discourse meaning, including metaphor use, are established incrementally via the accumulation of multiple individual instances of use. In concrete terms, if we have one example of a person, such as Peter from Chapter 1, talking about an illness as a metaphorical 'enemy attacking my loved one', then that is interesting as an example, but does not tell us anything about wider patterns. But if we find the same or similar metaphorical treatment of illness repeatedly in a million-word corpus containing texts from different writers or speakers, then this gives us an insight into a widespread and conventional way of *talking* about this topic, which in turn potentially tells us something about typical ways people (or, collectively, societies) *think* about this topic, or even make decisions in that topic area. We will return to this point in the next section.

As might be expected after a five-decade history, corpus linguists have come up with a very large array of techniques that can be used to identify and analyse patterns in corpus data. But all are rooted in the two basic things that we can ask a computer to do with a large body of digital text. The computer cannot actually read the text for meaning the way a human analyst can. But it *can* (a) find all the examples in a corpus of some query defined by a human user, and present them for analysis; and (b) count all the instances of some specified phenomenon, and present a summary of their frequencies to the user (see McEnery and Hardie 2012: 2). These most basic methods are often applied at the level of the words in the corpus. We can ask the computer to search the corpus for some word-form we are interested in, such as 'enemy', and present a table of all examples of that word together with some preceding and some following context: this is called a *concordance* (an example of a concordance is given in Figure 1.1 in Chapter 1). Similarly, we can ask the computer to count how many instances there are of each different word-form in the corpus: this is called a *frequency list*. These methods can, however, also be applied at the level of *tags* or *annotation*.

Tags are layers of analysis that are overlaid onto the raw text of a corpus, often assigning the words of the corpus into categories in some schema (see McEnery and Hardie 2012: 29–35). For example, we can classify all the words grammatically, labelling each one according to whether it is a noun, a verb, an adjective and so on. This is called *part-of-speech tagging*, and often looks something like the following extract from Example 1.1, where 'PPIS1' stands for a first-person singular pronoun, 'VVD' stands for a past-tense verb, and so on:[1]

> I_PPIS1 refused_VVD to_TO go_VVI, I_PPIS1 worked_VVD on_II the_AT basis_NN1 that_CST this_DD1 was_VBDZ an_AT1 enemy_NN1 attacking_VVG my_APPGE loved_JJ one_PN1 and_CC it_PPH1 had_VHD picked_VVN a_AT1 fight_NN1 with_IW me_PPIO1 as_RR21 well_RR22.

A similar analysis that classifies words according to their meaning is called *semantic tagging* (Rayson 2009); this technique will be central to much of the analysis presented later in this book (and is introduced in more detail in Chapter 3). Once tagging has been added to a corpus, we can generate concordances based on a tag rather than for a word-form, and we can generate frequency lists for tags representing grammatical or semantic categories.

Two further basic methods, collocation and keyness, are based on looking at unusual features of concordance and frequency list data. *Collocation* refers to the tendency of words (or tags) to repeatedly co-occur with particular other words (or tags) (McEnery et al. 2006: 82–85). The collocates of a word, that is, the items that occur nearby to it in a concordance more often than would be expected statistically, are an essential aspect of its meaning. Similarly, when we compare frequency lists for two corpora, we can identify *key* items from these lists (*keywords* or *key tags*): items which are more frequent in one corpus than we would expect, statistically, on the basis of the other corpus. Again, the keyness method will be illustrated in detail later in this book.

In summary, then, the various tools of corpus linguistics enable us to analyse our large corpus systematically and thoroughly. It simply would not be possible to work through 1.5 million running words of text without them. We will rely on the methods discussed so far and, where necessary, more complex tools throughout this book. In Chapter 3, and in the methods sections of subsequent analysis chapters, we will outline the specific tools that we use and the ways in which we do so.

We now turn to the underpinnings of our study in terms of metaphor research. First we outline in more detail two key aspects of metaphor that make it particularly important for our study; this is followed by an overview of the literature on metaphor and illness and death.

2.4 What We Will Focus On: Metaphor

In this section we provide more detail on two issues central to our approach to metaphor in this book: the framing function of metaphor, and the contextual nature of metaphor use. We briefly introduced these in Chapter 1.

As we described in Chapter 1, metaphor is a way of talking, and potentially thinking, about one thing as if it was something else, where a similarity can be perceived between the two entities (Semino 2008). Usually, the thing we want to express or think about (the 'topic' or 'target') is abstract, subjective, complex and/or sensitive in some way, while the thing we use to describe it (the 'vehicle' or 'source') is often more concrete, physical and tangible. Illness, death and the emotions associated with them are among the experiences that are typically talked about metaphorically, precisely because of their sensitive and subjective nature. This is why our study uses metaphor as a window onto the experiences of cancer and the end of life.

But metaphor is important to consider for other reasons too. It conveys meanings compactly, efficiently and vividly, and can bridge the gap between the fluidity and continuity of life, on the one hand, and the discreteness of language as a set of symbols used to represent it, on the other (Ortony 1975). Among the meanings it conveys—indirectly or implicitly—is often some attitude, evaluation or stance. The perceived similarity between two entities that is captured by metaphor also inevitably provides a particular take on the topic at hand; it highlights some aspects (the similarities that can be established between the two) and backgrounds others (things that are different or irrelevant for the comparison). This helps to communicate the aforementioned evaluation, and can facilitate some inferences while making others more unlikely.

Together, the foregrounding and backgrounding of different aspects of the topic contribute to what we describe as 'framing'.

In fact, although metaphor has multiple functions, this capacity to indirectly add an evaluative dimension to what is said is among its most important functions (e.g. Lakoff and Johnson 1980; Lakoff 1996; Goatly 2007; Semino et al. 2016). For instance, Peter's use of 'picked a fight' in the example discussed in Chapter 1 suggests a stark contrast between his and his wife's innocence and the maliciousness of the disease—thereby communicating a particularly negative perception of it. Summarising the literature, Deignan (2010) discusses four ways in which metaphors can evaluate:

- By creating entailments or implications;
- By triggering 'scenarios' or 'mini-narratives' (cf. Musolff 2006), suggesting how things (should) work or how situations (should) play themselves out;
- By aligning the speaker with a particular social, political or ideological group through the choice of a source domain that indexes that group;
- By exploiting the connotations of literal meanings.

The indirect or off-record nature of metaphorical evaluations (i.e. the fact that praise or condemnation tends to be implicit in the metaphor rather than baldly stated) can be particularly useful in interactive situations, especially those concerning vulnerable individuals or sensitive topics, where it can be difficult or inappropriate to evaluate directly. In Semino et al. (2014), for example, we noted how healthcare professionals in our data sometimes used metaphor and narratives to attribute bad deaths to patients' personalities or ways of life. We return to this point in Chapter 8.

All that said, the choice of any particular metaphor, or indeed of patterns of metaphor, cannot be properly explained without taking into consideration its contextual nature. This is partly what the discourse-based approaches we introduced in Chapter 1 have begun to do. However, the increasing evidence that metaphor varies depending on multiple aspects of the context of use highlights the need for a more inclusive theoretical approach to metaphor—one that is capable of accounting for the multitude of variables at play.

In this vein, an important recent development is the application of *Dynamical Systems Theory* to the study of metaphor (e.g. Gibbs and Cameron 2008; Cameron et al. 2010). In mathematics, Dynamical Systems Theory aims to model the behaviour of complex systems that evolve over time depending on an interaction between their present state and multiple rules or factors. The theory has been extended and applied to the study of other phenomena, including language learning, cognitive development and the use of metaphor in discourse. Gibbs and Cameron (2008) argue, for example, that metaphor use in any interaction is influenced by many different variables, including at least:

- Enduring metaphorical concepts, such as conventional conceptual metaphors;
- What has been said or written before;
- Body movements and gesture at the time of speaking;
- Occupation and interests, which influence what might be familiar to a speaker;
- The degree of intimacy and social distance between speakers;
- Conventions and norms in the specific socio-cultural group;
- Linguistic and cultural norms.

Because it was designed to cope with the idea of an indefinite number of variables, the dynamical systems approach is able to integrate multiple theoretical views of metaphor, and encourages scholars to recognise, and to account in their interpretations for, multiple factors that might influence metaphor use (Gibbs 2017).

An example of this is the difference between accounting for contextually specific uses of metaphor and making claims about general patterns. We hinted at this distinction in Chapter 1, when we discussed Peter's specific use of the Military metaphor as different from the more general 'Battle' metaphor for cancer, as critiqued for example by Sontag (1979) and Granger (2014). Peter's Military metaphor not only has a specific linguistic form, but also has its own emotional and interpersonal meanings, which express something about his relationship with his wife. But the form in which these meanings are expressed is also partly determined by the specific context: his understanding of who he is on the online forum where he writes, and what others have said on the forum before him. Interestingly, this kind of context-specific use develops not just at an individual level, but also at the level of 'discourse communities'—people who share texts and communicative practices (Barton 2007; Deignan et al. 2013). To characterise this phenomenon, Gibbs and Cameron (2008) and Cameron and Deignan (2006) propose the term *metaphoreme* to refer to:

> a bundle of stabilized but flexible word-meaning links that incorporate particular affective and pragmatic values with particular lexicogrammatical forms and cultural preferences, and seem to work as emergent attractors in the dynamics of speech community talk.
>
> (Gibbs and Cameron 2008: 73)

Metaphoremes can be generally shared by the speakers of a particular (variety of a) language (e.g. the metaphorical uses of emotional 'baggage' in English) or can emerge as 'in group' usages within more restricted discourse communities (e.g. the expression 'lollipop trees' to indicate childlike drawings in a primary school classroom) (Cameron and Deignan 2006). This notion is particularly useful for describing and explaining some of the potential idiosyncrasies of metaphor use in our datasets, and their framing effects. We will return to it at various points, including particularly in Chapter 10 (see also Semino et al. 2016).

In the following section, we move on to review metaphor research more directly related to our topic of study—that is, earlier work that has addressed the issue of metaphorical language in relation to illness and/or death.

2.5 Metaphor in the Context of Illness and Death

2.5.1 Metaphor and Illness

It is appropriate to begin a discussion of metaphor and illness with reference to Susan Sontag's classic treatises on metaphors and cancer, tuberculosis and AIDS (Sontag 1979, 1989), which we already mentioned in the previous chapter. Sontag (1979) argued that Military metaphors around cancer in particular (such as 'invasive', 'aggressive' or 'colonisation') encourage a punitive view of the illness, constructing the patient as a victim and the disease as the culprit. Her proposed solution to the shortcomings of these metaphors was their complete elimination from communication around health and illness, and their replacement by literal language only. While this position came to be seen as both unrealistic and unnecessarily critical (including by Sontag (1989) herself), the advantages and disadvantages of metaphor in general and specific metaphors in particular in the context of illness have continued to be debated ever since. The results that we will outline in Chapters 5 and 6 will serve as, among other things, our contribution to these debates.

The now large and varied literature on metaphor use in relation to physical illness includes work on public communication about illness, such as news reports (e.g. Koteyko et al. 2008) and adverts (e.g. Reisfield and Wilson 2004), as well as on the 'lived experience' of illness and health(care). The latter body of research often focuses on specific groups of people (e.g. patients, general practitioners) or specific conditions, such as cancer (e.g. Gibbs and Franks 2002), epileptic seizures (e.g. Schwabe et al. 2008) or motor-neuron disease (e.g. Locock et al. 2012). A range of different aspects of the experience of illness are considered, such as physical symptoms, emotions and patients' views of themselves and their lives. There is also some recent research on metaphor as a facilitating tool in communication about health and illness, for example to improve general well-being (Taylor and McLaughlin 2011) or increase understanding of the illness itself and of management regimes (Naik et al. 2011). We have already touched on studies in this final category in sections 2.1 and

2.2. Our review of the metaphor literature in the following will therefore focus specifically on cancer and dying, as well as considering studies involving different groups of individuals.

Among the linguistic studies that have investigated the use of metaphor by cancer patients, Gibbs and Franks (2002) provided one of the most comprehensive accounts using a Conceptual Metaphor Theory framework (CMT; introduced in Chapter 1). They studied metaphors used in interviews with six women who had survived breast cancer, and noted that all interviewees used very conventional metaphors based in ordinary embodied experiences. These linguistic metaphors related to conceptual mappings such as CANCER IS AN OBSTACLE ON LIFE'S JOURNEY, CANCER IS A FLUID WITHIN THE SELF/CONTAINER, CANCER AND ITS TREATMENT IS A GAME and CANCER CLEARS VISION AND ALLOWS FOR NEW UNDERSTANDINGS. These metaphors allowed the women to express emotions, to integrate the illness into their lives and to highlight the experience's potential to stimulate intellectual and emotional growth. Analysing focus group discussions with 18 people who had recently been treated for cancer, Appleton and Flynn (2014) similarly emphasised the multiple functions that metaphors can have in the experience of illness. They pointed out ways in which people had different responses to common metaphorical expressions such as cancer 'journey' or cancer 'survivor', but showed that metaphors appeared to be consistently central to how participants managed their emotions and identities during and after cancer treatment. In a secondary analysis of 46 interviews with people affected by motor-neurone disease, Locock et al. (2012) also noted the importance of metaphor in communicating emotions (see also Charteris-Black and Seale 2010). Both Appleton and Flynn (2014) and Locock et al. (2012) concluded that attention to patients' metaphor use would facilitate more meaningful exchanges between them and healthcare professionals. While studies specifically investigating metaphors of emotion in healthcare contexts are rare, the repeated mention of emotions and their communication in the preceding studies (and in section 2.2) is not incidental. Emotions, as part of our interior worlds, are a very typical example of the aspects of our experience that are subjective and intangible, and therefore often expressed via metaphor. We address this topic, with a specific focus on carer emotions, in Chapter 9.

In addition to studies exploring the 'lived experience' of specific illnesses, there are also studies that focus on the variation between different groups of individuals involved in the healthcare process. For example, Skelton et al. (2002) compared the metaphor use of general practitioners (GPs) and patients in a corpus of 373 GP consultations in the UK. They found that war-related metaphors in relation to illnesses (e.g. 'battle' and 'attack') were commonly used by both groups. However, doctors also tended to use machinery-related metaphors, particularly in explanations (see also Krieger et al. 2010) and self-descriptions; they characterised themselves as 'problem-solvers' and 'controllers of disease'. The authors suggest that this reflects doctors' need to present themselves as authoritative, and their attempts to reinterpret patients' descriptions as familiar and comprehensible accounts. This may be reassuring to patients, who instead primarily used metaphors to describe their symptoms and emotional or psychological states. Reisfield and Wilson (2004), reviewing other studies, also noted the dominance of what they call the 'martial metaphor' for cancer, not just among doctors and patients, but also in the advertising of chemotherapy drugs and the promotion of cancer support fora. At the same time, they pointed out that there *are* other metaphors—and patients, in particular, often 'devise their own metaphors based on things they know and value' (Reisfield and Wilson 2004: 4026). We have already indicated the importance of war-related metaphors, and we will return to these in Chapter 5. We will also outline the variety of metaphors used in our data in Chapter 4. For now, it is simply worth noting that there is an emerging consensus in the literature on metaphor and illness that individual variation needs to be recognised when introducing and responding to metaphors in interaction with patients.

2.5.2 Metaphor and Death/Dying

There has also been research into metaphors for death and dying, mostly within the tradition of CMT. These studies tend to be based on decontextualised or literary examples, and to focus on conventional conceptual metaphors, such as DEATH IS SLEEP, DEATH IS DARK, DEATH IS A REAPER, DEATH IS A JOURNEY, DEATH IS DEPARTURE, DEATH IS THE END OF THE JOURNEY, DEATH IS AN ADVERSARY or DEATH IS REST (e.g. Lakoff and Turner 1989; Lakoff 2008; Ritchie 2013). These conceptual metaphors capture death as an event or state, rather than a process with a period of time leading up to it. Needless to say, they also all evaluate death categorically as negative. In Chapter 8, we will discuss the shortcomings of this research in relation to the end of life as an extended period and to dying as a potentially prolonged process.

Research in healthcare and hospice contexts specifically has tended to discuss metaphor only implicitly in relation to quality of death (e.g. Steinhauser et al. 2000; Vig et al. 2002; Zimmermann 2012). Such studies often advocate a conscious and sensitive use of metaphor, especially on the part of professionals interacting with patients (e.g. Canter 1988; Czechmeister 1994; Reisfield and Wilson 2004), as we noted in section 2.2. A notable exception is Vivat's (2008) ethnographic exploration of spiritual care in a Scottish hospice, which found that most workers conceptualised life as being 'here' and death as being 'somewhere else'. This is consistent with the typical conceptual metaphors of death, but Vivat (2008) noted that in this particular hospice these metaphors were physically realised—since people did not die or even discuss death in the public spaces of the establishment, but were moved somewhere else. Moreover, the process of dying was referred to most frequently as 'going down' and 'going downhill'. Vivat (2008) noted the link with the conceptual metaphor BAD IS DOWN, and suggested that because of these negative connotations, hospice staff often attempted to 'cheer patients up'. This of course is consistent with the framing function of metaphor, and also suggests that different metaphors for dying might have led to different actions on the part of hospice staff. In contrast, Langley-Evans and Payne (1997) found that patients in a palliative care context openly talked among themselves about death and dying, including using metaphors (e.g. 'looked death in the face many times') and humour. We discuss the use of humour and metaphor in our online patient data in Chapter 10.

This brings to a close our overview of prior research on metaphors for illness, cancer and death: the intersection point between metaphor research and the field of healthcare communication studies. In the next section, we move on to another intersection point among the three primary topics of this book—that between metaphor research and the insights of corpus and computational linguistics.

2.6 Automated Methods and Metaphor Analysis

Metaphor scholars increasingly exploit, in a variety of ways and for a variety of purposes, the computer-aided methods developed within corpus linguistics (see section 2.3) and computational linguistics (see section 2.6.2) (more on this distinction later). Generally speaking, the study of any linguistic phenomenon can benefit from that phenomenon being systematically analysed in large quantities of naturally occurring data, i.e. from the kind of analysis that corpus methods make possible. This applies particularly to phenomena that are claimed to be frequent in language, and that are given centre stage in theory-making at least in part *because* of their frequency, such as conceptual metaphors in CMT. The study of metaphor therefore benefits from the scope and systematicity of corpus methods. However, as we discuss in section 2.6.2 (and in Chapter 3), automating the identification and interpretation of metaphor is far from straightforward. We begin this section by outlining some key insights that systematic, corpus-based approaches to metaphor have already contributed, before exploring the computational complexities that still prevent fully automated metaphor analysis.

2.6.1 Corpus Methods and Metaphor

The methods of corpus linguistics have been used to contribute to metaphor theory and analysis in several different ways. As we briefly mentioned in Chapter 1, they have been used to test claims about frequency and conventionality made within CMT, resulting in both further evidence and challenges for the theory (e.g. Stefanowitsch 2006). Other corpus-based studies have advanced the study of variation in metaphor use over time, across languages, in different types of texts, and by different speakers and discourse communities. The latter type of work is particularly relevant here, since we will be considering two types of texts and three different groups of participants (see Chapter 3).

A large number of studies have used corpus methods to study the forms and functions of metaphor in different text types and by different speakers. These studies often address questions that pertain to those particular text types and their contexts of use, rather than (or in addition to) contributing to metaphor theory. For example, Koller (2004) showed how Sports and War metaphors dominate in reports about the economy and reflect a sexist bias. Charteris-Black (2012) used corpus methods to study the use of metaphor in a corpus of interviews with people with depression. Among other things, he showed that men and women tended to use similar metaphors, but suggested that the few differences that do emerge may be relevant in therapeutic processes. Although our own analyses do not touch on gender issues, the studies of Koller and Charteris-Black are relevant to our work because both point to the potential pitfalls of making generalisations about metaphor in language and cognition without taking into account variation at the level of speakers/writers, genres and discourses (see also O'Halloran 2007; Deignan et al. 2013).

Corpus-based studies have also shown that particular functions of metaphor may be a result of systematic variation that needs to be accounted for. For example, L'Hôte (2014) illustrated the ways in which metaphor is used to project a political party's revised identity in a corpus of New Labour texts in the UK from 1997 to 2007. Partington et al. (2013: 131ff) examined concordances of tuning devices (i.e. words or phrases that signal a metaphor) in a corpus of reviews in British broadsheet newspapers to show the ways in which creative, humorous metaphors and similes can be used to entertain the reader. Similarly, Veale's (2012: 121) study of similes on the World Wide web revealed, among other things, how certain simile structures, e.g. 'about as . . . as. . . ', tended to be used creatively and humorously, especially when the adjective following the first *as* was positive: e.g. 'about as useful as a chocolate fireguard'.

However, corpus-based techniques are not the only computer-assisted methodology that has been brought to bear on the analysis of metaphor. As we will see in the following more specialised section, the related but distinct approach of *computational linguistics/natural language processing* has also made substantial contributions.

2.6.2 *Computational Approaches to Metaphor Identification*

Alongside research on metaphor using corpus linguistic methods, there has been a growing interest in the area from researchers in computational linguistics (or natural language processing; NLP), who are beginning to realise the importance of metaphor for the automatic analysis of language in a number of areas and applications. While corpus linguistics is oriented towards the use of computer-based methods to analyse and understand language structure and usage, NLP is concerned with using linguistic data resources—including corpora—to develop and analyse computational systems and applications that can process and to some degree 'comprehend' human language. The two disciplines have worked closely together for many years, for example to develop the part-of-speech and semantic taggers that we referred to in section 2.3.

Knowledge about particular aspects of language from corpora and linguistic theories (such as the grammatical or semantic categories within which words can be classified) are embedded in dictionaries, rules and probabilistic language models. These knowledge-based resources are then employed by the computational tagging software to replicate, automatically and on a larger scale, the manual annotation of a corpus. Developing and training taggers (and other language processing software) is not a straightforward task. However, in state-of-the-art NLP, both part-of-speech and semantic tagging, as well as many other fundamental processes, can be replicated with high accuracy (above 90%) by computer software. Other types of language analysis, however, can be more difficult to carry out automatically. This is usually because they require (a) more complex distinctions among the items being analysed, (b) longer or more varied stretches of text to be 'understood', or (c) elements of world (i.e. contextual) knowledge outside of the text itself. Unfortunately for us, the automatic detection and interpretation of metaphor is among these more challenging NLP tasks. In the remainder of this section, we outline some of the studies that are starting to enable the automated analysis of metaphor, and that therefore form the NLP backdrop of our own methods as outlined in Chapter 3.

Despite its challenges, computational researchers have long been tackling the problem of metaphor detection and interpretation, and impressive gains in accuracy have recently been achieved. This can be seen, for instance, in the recent international workshops on Metaphor in NLP, 2013–2016, or in Dunn's (2013) review of the performance of four state-of-the-art detection systems on the Vrije University Amsterdam Metaphor Corpus (VUAMC). A variety of approaches have been taken so far, with systems focusing on features of individual words, such as semantic similarity (Sporleder and Li 2009) or abstractness (Turney et al. 2011); on exploiting source-to-target domain mappings (Shutova et al. 2013); or on linking domains at a sentence level (Dunn 2013). Some computational approaches restrict their application to specific domains, genres or parts of speech to limit the scope of the task. For example, Pasanek and Sculley (2008) investigated the extraction of figurative expressions across multiple genres, but they only considered metaphors for one target domain: the mind.

In terms of the information about language and the world that is encoded in computer systems designed for metaphor identification and analysis, many approaches use features such as *concreteness* ('How concrete is this word?') and/or *imageability* ('How readily does this word bring an image to mind?') (Turney et al. 2011). Although these two concepts are closely linked (concrete entities being typically the easiest to visualise mentally), Dellantonio et al. (2014) argued that imageability involves internal sensory experience as well as external sensory information, whereas concreteness involves external sensory information only. This is evidenced by entire classes of words where imageability behaves quite differently to concreteness. In line with Dellantonio et al.'s results, Gargett and Barnden (2015) have developed an approach employing fine-grained measures of affective meanings (drawn from Warriner et al. 2013). These measures are used to model the task of detecting words used metaphorically, in part, as the search for an optimal combination of sentiment scores with concreteness and imageability measures as well as other linguistic information. Combining different measurable factors that may hint at metaphorical usage in this way significantly boosts detection performance, up to around 80%.

While approaches to detecting metaphor computationally are increasingly common, work on interpreting them automatically is somewhat rarer. Previous computational research on finding the meanings of metaphors includes: work which takes the approach of querying a database of known metaphors (Martin 1988); studies deploying automated systems able to reason about source- and target-domain information to determine metaphorical content (Barnden 2009; Ovchinnikova et al. 2014); and research into the use of automatic paraphrasing to find synonymous literal expressions (Shutova 2010). Among the problems being tackled by current computational research is the need to tailor automatic approaches to specific genres, registers and discourse communities—given the systematic variation these involve, as we have outlined in the preceding.

Overall, then, while there are clear advantages to using the systematic methods of corpus linguistics, and the insights of NLP that permit at least semi-automated metaphor analysis, there is clearly still much room for development. In this book, we primarily use the software tool Wmatrix (Rayson 2009) to identify potential metaphorical expressions, or metaphor candidates, in our corpus. This tool implements some of the recent insights and advances we have introduced in this section. In Chapter 3, we outline in more detail the combination of methods that we harnessed to make the most of the current state of knowledge, and the ways in which we have contributed to this body of work.

2.7 Summary

In this chapter, we have set out the key background of our study in the three main fields that inform our research: health communication, corpus methods and metaphor studies. These fields broadly inform, respectively, why we felt our study was important, how we approached it and what we specifically investigated in language.

First, we introduced the relevant literature in practice-oriented healthcare communication—noting the efforts made in that field to address practical issues of communication practices and their impact on the standard of care that is provided to patients. As we argued, this practical dimension is the most urgent reason why the research in this book can be said to matter. Second, we introduced our methodological perspective, namely corpus linguistics: the study of language via computer-assisted analysis of very large bodies of text. Third, we introduced our analytic perspective of metaphor, outlining some of the key developments and previous work underpinning the research in this book within the field of metaphor studies. All of these fields are rich and varied in themselves, so our very brief overviews here are not in any way meant to represent the breadth and complexities involved. Rather, our summaries should serve to signal to the reader the variety of approaches and insights that we draw on throughout this book.

In the second part of the chapter, we explored intersections among the three key perspectives. At the intersection of metaphor and healthcare communication, we outlined work investigating metaphors used for illness and death, as well as metaphorical language in communicative contexts involving patients, caregivers and/or healthcare professionals. At the intersection of metaphor and corpus linguistics, we saw how corpus-based methods have enriched the study of metaphorical language in natural discourse, especially with regard to systematic variation, as well as how computational (or NLP) methods have made it possible to automate the identification of metaphors in corpora, albeit not perfectly.

What we have not explored—since, prior to our study, it did not exist—is work linking all three of these primary perspectives. To put it informally, this is where this book comes in. That is, our study commences here, building on the work reviewed in this chapter by operating at the intersection, not only of healthcare and metaphor, nor only of metaphor and corpus, but of all three: looking at metaphor in healthcare communication (specifically in the context of cancer and end-of-life care) via the methods of corpus and computational linguistics. This three-sided perspective is the unique and novel contribution of this book.

We now turn in the next chapter to a detailed discussion of the data and methods on which the analyses in the remainder of the book are based.

Note

1. The tagset used in this example is CLAWS7, which is provided automatically with Wmatrix (Rayson 2009), the corpus analysis tool that we use most extensively in our analyses in this book. The full tagset is available here: http://ucrel.lancs.ac.uk/claws7tags.html

References

Appleton, L., and Flynn, M. (2014). Searching for the new normal: Exploring the role of language and metaphors in becoming a cancer survivor. *European Journal of Oncology Nursing*, *18*(4), 378–384.

Baker, P. (2006). *Using corpora in discourse analysis*. London: Continuum.

Barnden, J. A. (2009). Metaphor and context: A perspective from artificial intelligence. In A. Musolff and J. Zinken (Eds.), *Metaphor and discourse* (pp. 79–94). Basingstoke: Palgrave.

Barton, D. (2007). *Literacy: An introduction to the ecology of written language*. Oxford: Blackwell.

Beaver, K., and Booth, K. (2007). Information needs and decision-making preferences: Comparing findings for gynaecological, breast and colorectal cancer. *European Journal of Oncology Nursing*, *11*(5), 409–416.

Biber, D., Conrad, S., and Reppen, R. (1998). *Corpus linguistics: Investigating language structure and use*. Cambridge: Cambridge University Press.

Cameron, L., and Deignan, A. (2006). The emergence of metaphor in discourse. *Applied Linguistics*, 27(4), 671–690.

Cameron, L., Maslen, R., and Low, G. (2010). Finding systematicity in metaphor use. In L. Cameron and R. Maslen (Eds.), *Metaphor analysis*. London: Equinox.

Canter, D. (1988). How do we know that it works? Therapeutic outcome as negotiation. *Complementary Medical Research*, 2, 98–106.

Charteris-Black, J. (2012) Shattering the bell jar: Metaphor, gender and depression. *Metaphor and Symbol*, 27(3), 199–216.

Charteris-Black, J., and Seale, C. (2010). *Gender and the language of illness*. Basingstoke: Palgrave.

Corner, J., Wright, D., Hopkinson, J., Gunaratnam, Y., McDonald, J. W., and Foster, C. (2007). The research priorities of patients attending UK cancer treatment centres: Findings from a modified nominal group study. *British Journal of Cancer*, *96*, 875–881.

Czechmeister, C. A. (1994). Metaphor in illness and nursing: A two-edged sword: A discussion of the social use of metaphor in everyday language, and implications of nursing and nursing education. *Journal of Advanced Nursing*, *19*(6), 1226–1233.

Deignan, A. (2010). The evaluative properties of metaphors. In Z. Todd, A. Deignan, & L. Cameron (Eds.), *Researching and applying metaphor in use* (pp. 357–373). Amsterdam/Philadelphia: John Benjamins.

Deignan, A., Littlemore, J., and Semino, E. (2013). *Figurative language, genre and register*. Cambridge: Cambridge University Press.

Dellantonio, S., Mulatti, C., Pastore, L., and Job, R. (2014). Measuring inconsistencies can lead you forward: The case of imageability and concreteness ratings. *Language Sciences*, *5*, 708.

Department of Health. (2008). *End of life care strategy promoting high quality care for all adults at the end of life.* London: DH. Retrieved April 2017, from www.gov.uk/government/uploads/system/uploads/attachment_data/file/136431/End_of_life_strategy.pdf

Dunn, J. (2013). Evaluating the premises and results of four metaphor identification systems. In A. Gelbukh (Ed.), *Proceedings of CICLing 2013, LNCS 7816*, Springer Heidelberg, pp. 471–486.

Fallowfield, L., Jenkins, V., Farewell, V., Saul, J., Duffy, A., and Eves, R. (2002). Efficacy of a cancer research UK communication skills training model for oncologists: A randomised controlled study. *The Lancet*, *359*, 650–656.

Froggatt, K. (1998). The place of metaphor and language in exploring nurses' emotional work. *Journal of Advanced Nursing*, *28*(2), 332–338.

Gargett, A., and Barnden, J. (2015). Modeling the interaction between sensory and affective meanings for detecting metaphor. In *Proceedings of the Third Workshop on Metaphor in NLP, NAACL 2015*, Denver, CO, pp. 21–30.

Gibbs, R. W. (2017). Metaphor, language and dynamical systems. In E. Semino and Z. Demjén (Eds.), *The Routledge handbook of metaphor and language.* Abingdon: Routledge.

Gibbs, R. W., and Cameron, L. (2008). The social-cognitive dynamics of metaphor performance. *Cognitive Systems Research*, *9*(1–2), 64–75.

Gibbs, R. W., and Franks, H. (2002). Embodied metaphor in women's narratives about their experiences with cancer. *Health Communication*, *14*(2), 139–165.

Goatly, A. (2007). *Washing the brain: Metaphor and hidden ideology.* Amsterdam: John Benjamins.

Granger, K. (2014). Having cancer is not a fight or a battle. *The Guardian* (http://www.theguardian.com/society/2014/apr/25/having-cancer-not-fight-or-battle, accessed June 2015).

Koller, V. (2004). *Metaphor and gender in business media discourse.* Basingstoke, UK: Palgrave.

Koteyko, N., Brown, B., and Crawford, P. (2008). The dead parrot and the dying swan: The role of metaphor scenarios in UK Press coverage of Avian Flu in the UK in 2005–2006. *Metaphor and Symbol*, *23*, 242–261.

Krieger, J.L., Parrott, R.L., and Nussbaum, J.F. (2010). Metaphor use and health literacy: A pilot study of strategies to explain randomization in cancer clinical trials. *Journal of Health Communication: International Perspectives*, 16: 3–16.

Lakoff, G. (1996). *Moral politics: What conservatives know that liberals don't.* Chicago: University of Chicago Press.

Lakoff, G. (2008). *The political mind: Why you can't understand 21st-century politics with an 18th-century brain.* New York: Viking.

Lakoff, G. and Johnson, M. (1980). *Metaphors we live by*, Chicago: University of Chicago Press.

Lakoff, G., and Turner, M. (1989). *More than cool reason: A field guide to poetic metaphor.* Chicago: University of Chicago Press.

Langley-Evans, A., and Payne, S. (1997). Light-hearted death talk in a palliative day care context. *Journal of Advanced Nursing*, *26*(6), 1091–1097.

L'Hôte, E. (2014). *Identity, narrative and metaphor: A corpus-based cognitive analysis of new labour discourse.* Basingstoke: Palgrave Macmillan.

Locock, L., Mazanderani, F., and Powell, J. (2012). Metaphoric language and the articulation of emotions by people affected by motor neurone disease. *Chronic Illness*, *8*, 201–215.

Martin, J. H. (1988). *A computational theory of metaphor*. Technical report, University of California, Berkeley, CA.
McEnery, T., and Hardie, A. (2012). *Corpus linguistics: Method, theory and practice*. Cambridge: Cambridge University Press.
McEnery, T., and Wilson, A. (2001). *Corpus linguistics* (2nd ed.). Edinburgh: Edinburgh University Press.
McEnery, T., Xiao, R. Z., and Tono, Y. (2006). *Corpus-based language studies: An advanced resource book*. London: Routledge.
Moss, M. S., Moss, S. Z., Rubinstein, R. L., and Black, H. K. (2003). The metaphor of 'family' in staff communication about dying and death. *Journal of Gerontology*, *58B*(5), S290–S296.
Musolff, A. (2006). Metaphor scenarios in public discourse. *Metaphor and Symbol*, *21*(1), 23–38.
Naik, A. D., Teal, C. R., Rodriguez, E., and Haidet, P. (2011). Knowing the ABCs: A comparative effectiveness study of two methods of diabetes education. *Patient Education and Counseling*, *85*(3), 383–389.
O'Halloran, K. (2007). Critical discourse analysis and the corpus-informed interpretation of metaphor at the register level. *Applied Linguistics*, 28(1), 1–24.
Ortony, A. (1975). Why metaphors are necessary and not just nice. *Educational Theory*, *25*(1), 45–53.
Ovchinnikova, E., Israel, R., Wertheim, S., Zaytsev, V., Montazeri, N., and Hobbs, J. (2014). Abductive inference for interpretation of metaphors. In *Proceedings of the Second Workshop on Metaphor in NLP, ACL 2014*, Baltimore, MD, pp. 33–41.
Parry, R., Land, V., and Seymour, J. (2014). How to communicate with patients about future illness progression and end of life: A systematic review. *BMJ Supportive and Palliative Care*, *4*, 331–341.
Partington, A., Duguid, A., and Taylor, C. (2013). *Patterns and meanings in discourse: Theory and practice in corpus-assisted discourse studies*. Amsterdam: John Benjamins.
Pasanek, B., and Sculley, D. (2008). Mining millions of metaphors. *Literary and Linguistic Computing*, *23*(3), 345–360.
Radley, A., and Payne, S. (2009). A sociological commentary on the refusal of treatment by patients with cancer. *Mortality*, *14*(4), 309–324.
Rayson, P. (2009). *Wmatrix: A web-based corpus processing environment*. School of Computing and Communications, Lancaster University. Retrieved from http://ucrel.lancs.ac.uk/wmatrix/
Reisfield, G. M., and Wilson, G. R. (2004). Use of metaphor in the discourse on cancer. *Journal of Clinical Oncology*, *22*(19), 4024–4027.
Ritchie, L. D. (2013). *Metaphor*. Cambridge and New York: Cambridge University Press.
Schofield, P., Carey, M., Love, A., Nehill, C., and Wein, S. (2006). Would you like to talk about your future treatment options? Discussing the transition from curative cancer treatment to palliative. *Palliative Medicine*, *20*(4), 397–406.
Schwabe, M., Reuber, M., Schöndienst, M., and Gülich, E. (2008). Listening to people with seizures: How can linguistic analysis help in the differential diagnosis of seizure disorders? *Communication and Medicine*, *5*(1), 59–72.

Semino, E. (2008). *Metaphor in discourse*. Cambridge: Cambridge University Press.

Semino, E., Demjén, Z., and Demmen, J. (2016, advance access). An integrated approach to metaphor and framing in cognition, discourse and practice, with an application to metaphors for cancer. *Applied Linguistics*.

Semino, E., Demjén, Z. and Koller, V. (2014). '"Good" and "bad" deaths: Narratives and professional identities in interviews with hospice managers'. *Discourse Studies*, 16: 667–685.

Shutova, E. (2010). Automatic metaphor interpretation as a paraphrasing task. In *Human Language Technologies, NAACL*, pp. 1029–1037.

Shutova, E., Teufel, S., and Korhonen, A. (2013). Statistical metaphor processing. *Computational Linguistics*, *39*(2), 301–353.

Skelton, J. R., Wearn, A. M., and Hobbs, F. D. R. (2002). A concordance-based study of metaphoric expressions used by general practitioners and patients in consultation. *British Journal of General Practice*, *52*, 114–118.

Sontag, S. (1979). *Illness as metaphor*. London: Allen Lane.

Sontag, S. (1991 [1979, 1989]). *Illness as metaphor and AIDS and its metaphors*. London: Penguin.

Southall, D. (2013). The patient's use of metaphor within a palliative care setting: Theory, function and efficacy. A narrative literature review. *Palliative Medicine*, *27*(4), 304–313.

Sporleder, C., and Li, L. (2009). Contextual idiom detection without labelled data. In P. Koehn and R. Mihalcea (Eds.), *Proceedings of EMNLP-09, ACL*, Stroudsburg, PA, pp. 680–690.

Stefanowitsch, A. (2006). Corpus-based approaches to metaphor and metonymy. In A. Stefanowitsch and S. T. Gries (Eds.), *Corpus-based approaches to metaphor and metonymy*. Berlin: Mouton de Gruyter.

Steinhauser, K. E., Clipp, E. C., Mcneilly, M., Christakis, N. A., Mcintyre, L. M., and Tulsky, J. A. (2000). In search of a good death: Observations of patients, families, and providers. *Annals of Internal Medicine*, *132*(10), 825–832.

Taylor, R., and Mclaughlin, K. (2011). Terror and intimacy: Unlocking secrets at the end of life. *Journal of Holistic Healthcare*, *8*, 12–17.

Turner, M., Payne, S., and O'Brien, T. (2011). Mandatory communication skills training for cancer and palliative care staff: Does one size fit all? *European Journal of Oncology Nursing*, *15*, 398–403.

Turney, P. D., Neuman, Y., Assaf, D., and Cohen, Y. (2011). Literal and metaphorical sense identification through concrete and abstract context. In *Proceedings of the 2011 Conference on the Empirical Methods in Natural Language Processing*, pp 680–690.

Veale, T. (2012). *Exploding the creativity myth: The computational foundations of linguistic creativity*. London: Bloomsbury.

Vig, E. K., Davenport, N. A., and Pearlman, R. A. (2002). Good deaths, bad deaths, and preferences for the end of life: A qualitative study of geriatric outpatients. *Journal of the American Geriatrics Society*, *50*(9), 1541–1548.

Vivat, B. (2008). "Going down" and "getting deeper": Physical and metaphorical location and movement in relation to death and spiritual care in a Scottish hospice. *Mortality*, *13*(1), 42–64.

Warriner, A. B., Kuperman, V., and Brysbaert, V. (2013). Norms of valence, arousal, and dominance for 13,915 English lemmas. *Behavior Research Methods*, *45*, 1191–1207.

Wilkinson, S. (1999). A longitudinal evaluation of a communication skills programme. *Palliative Medicine*, *13*, 341–348.
Zimmermann, C. (2012). Acceptance of dying: A discourse analysis of palliative care literature. *Social Science and Medicine*, *75*(1), 217–224.

3 Data and General Methodology

3.1 Introduction

In the previous chapter, we introduced the theoretical underpinnings of the study that this book is based on. In this chapter, we provide a detailed account of our data and methods. The first part of the chapter (sections 3.2, 3.3 and 3.4) provides an overview of our data, the rationale for the selection of our respective sources, and a detailed description of how the data was collected and compiled into our corpus. The second half of the chapter (section 3.5) focuses on our methods of data analysis. We describe our processes and procedures for identifying relevant metaphors, and then discuss our initial intensive manual (qualitative) analysis of a 92,000-word sample. Finally, we outline the automated quantitative analysis of our complete corpus, demonstrating how it was informed by the initial manual sample analysis.

Much of this chapter will go into some technical detail on metaphor analysis and corpus analysis. We therefore expect that different sections will be relevant to some of our readers but not to others. We have aimed to label sections clearly enough that readers can quickly find the parts that suit their interests.

This chapter covers our *main* methods—those used systematically for all the analyses we discuss in subsequent chapters. What we do not cover in this chapter are the specific adjustments or expansions that were necessary for particular analyses, or the individual methods we used to supplement our main approach in specific cases. These are always discussed in the relevant analysis chapters (Chapters 5 to 10).

3.2 Three Groups of Participants

The Metaphor in End-of-Life Care (MELC) project that this book is based on was concerned with how different groups of people talk about their experiences of cancer and (care at) the end of life. We focused on three groups in particular, which we refer to as 'participant groups' (some might call them '(key) stakeholders' in healthcare):

1. Patients, i.e. people with cancer;
2. Unpaid carers for someone with cancer, i.e. 'lay people in a close supportive role who share in the illness experience of the patient and who undertake vital care work and emotional management' (NICE 2004: 155);
3. Healthcare professionals.

For each participant group, we focused on two broad types, or *genres*, of data:

1. Semi-structured interviews;
2. Contributions to online fora and blogs.

More specifically, what we will call the 'MELC corpus' includes semi-structured interviews with:

- 29 patients with a diagnosis of advanced cancer, or what is often described as 'terminal' cancer (collected in a previous study; Payne et al. 2008);
- 17 unpaid carers looking after family members who have a diagnosis of advanced cancer (collected in a previous study; Payne et al. 2009);
- 16 senior healthcare professionals working in hospice or palliative care.

The corpus also includes online writing produced in the period 2007–2012 by:

- 56 patients and 56 carers, all of whom contributed to various threads on one particular UK-based online forum dedicated to cancer;
- 307 healthcare professionals, writing about death and dying in online fora, blogs or comments on blog posts.

The patients whose contributions we selected for inclusion either self-declared as having advanced cancer or wrote about death, dying, terminal illness and palliative care generally. Similarly, we selected carers who posted frequently on threads to do with death, dying and terminal illness and who declared themselves as caring, or having cared, for individuals affected by these experiences. Together with healthcare professionals, these three groups of participants represent key players in the network of care, although of course they do not include everyone that is part of this network (e.g. paid carers). By contrast, the two types of data are mutually complementary, in that each balances out the drawbacks of the other as the basis for a study of this kind.

It is perhaps not necessary to justify the inclusion of patients in our study: they are arguably the focus of healthcare, including palliative and end-of-life care, and they are also ostensibly positioned at the centre of governmental policy and decision-making. Their care and support needs are potentially relevant to every member of society, as anyone may find themselves experiencing these needs and consequently using healthcare services at some point in their life. We use the term 'patient', rather than 'service-user', for example, because it applies more accurately to our dataset: while our interviewees were all users of healthcare services, this is not something we are able to claim with certainty about the online contributors. In addition, at least some of the unpaid family carers represented in our corpus are *also* users of services, so we felt that using the term 'patient' allowed us to best capture who we actually mean.

Family carers are often regarded as a neglected group (Grande et al. 2009). Yet they make enormous contributions to and sacrifices for the care of people with long-term or advanced illnesses. As such, we felt that it was particularly important to include their voices as equal participants in our study. The carers in our data may or may not actually be related to the people they care for, although they are mostly their spouse or child. The defining characteristic of these carers is that they are not trained or paid for their caring duties. We should also say that the specific carers in our data are not linked to the specific patients in our data: the selection of representative individuals for each participant group was entirely independent. Approaching the selection of data in this way made it more likely that a wider variety of views would be present within the texts we analysed.

Our group of healthcare professionals is perhaps more internally diverse than our groups of patients and carers. Professionals are defined by the fact that they have had medical or healthcare training and are paid for the care they provide. However, while for patients and carers we can assume a degree of homogeneity across our interviews and online data, the same cannot be said for our healthcare professional data. For our semi-structured interviews, we specifically sought out 16 professionals in hospice or palliative care who held some kind of leadership role; i.e. they were managers or team leaders. We felt that hospice/palliative care professionals in leadership roles would be able to provide a more complete perspective, reflecting not only on their own views, but also on the perspectives of other kinds of healthcare professionals working alongside them. In compiling our subcorpus of online healthcare professional data, we were not able to be so specific. This was, on the one hand, because there were fewer healthcare professional contributions openly available online than we expected (see later discussion) and, on the other hand, because healthcare professionals writing online were less likely to declare details of their work such as their specialism. Therefore, for the online section of our healthcare professional data, we simply selected contributors who wrote about death, dying and terminal illness online. Where the writers mentioned a specific illness, we found this to be predominantly cancer. Overall, we felt that, as long as we bore these differences mind in when drawing conclusions, this diversity actually improved the quality of our data by representing a wider range of voices.

By systematically analysing the metaphors used by these three groups to talk about cancer, the end of life and end-of-life care, we gain a better understanding of the phenomenology or 'lived experience' of illness, dying and healthcare, and the different ways in which they can impact three key groups of people.

3.3 Two Genres

It is well-recognised that people tailor their language use to the contexts, purposes and modes within which they are communicating at any particular moment (e.g. Biber and Conrad 2009). Recent studies have shown that this also applies to metaphor use: it can vary considerably depending on text type, and this variation has both theoretical and practical implications (Deignan et al. 2013). A proper account of this variation is particularly important when the communication under study involves sensitive topics such as cancer and the end of life. Moreover, this accounting for variation is even more critical when the choice of particular metaphors is controversial, as is the case with Violence metaphors in relation to illness and dying. For these reasons, the MELC corpus includes data drawn from two rather different types of texts (semi-structured interviews and online forum and blog contributions), representing the spoken and written modes respectively. We refer to these two text types as different 'genres' because they have different structural characteristics and communicative purposes, and involve different 'discourse communities'—groups of people who 'have texts and practices in common' (Barton 2007: 75; see also Swales 1990; Biber and Conrad 2009).

Semi-structured interviews and online contributions complement each other in other ways too (for a detailed discussion see Seale et al. 2010). In the former, interviewers are able to guide the discussion towards topics of particular interest and to explore these in greater depth with follow-up questions. There is a certain degree of uniformity across a collection of such interviews, leading to data that easily permits comparisons across individuals, and researchers will often have access to rich demographic information about interviewees. In semi-structured settings, interviewees are allowed enough flexibility to express themselves freely in response to open-ended questions in a relaxed atmosphere (Dörnyei 2007). On the other hand, conducting interviews is time-intensive and potentially precludes interviewees from discussing issues of particular relevance to them that happen not to form part of the pre-selected questions. Working with online data, we would typically not encounter these obstacles, but this genre brings challenges of its own.

Broadly speaking, online environments offer relative anonymity, reduced inhibition (Suler 2004), as well as round-the-clock availability and accessibility, irrespective of geographical or physical constraints (see also Herring 2007; Seale et al. 2010). This means that people can contribute from within their preferred environments, whenever they want, and without having to provide their real names. Contributions to an online forum count as spontaneous and undirected (although recent research has begun to question the dichotomy between 'elicited' and 'spontaneous' story-telling; Koven 2011), and while in interviews people are generally asked to recall past states, online participants tend to write about their current or very recent experiences. Thus, patients in particular tend to be 'doing their illness here and now' rather than retelling it, and are therefore more likely to discuss sensitive or taboo subjects (Seale et al. 2010: 600). Such data provides insights into 'an experience as it is lived rather than as it is enacted in the researcher-constructed environment of the interview' (Seale et al. 2010: 600). There is also increasing evidence of the importance of peer-to-peer online interactions about illness for the formation of social bonds and support networks, as well as for the management of long-term conditions (e.g. Prestin and Chou 2014; Stommel and Lamerichs 2014; Allen et al. 2016; Zhang et al. 2017). From the researcher's perspective as well, online data has advantages. It is available in large quantities and is easily and quickly accessible. Although the ethical issues involved in research on online communication are complex and still the subject of debate, there is some consensus that anything a person posts to a forum that is open to public view on the web can be used as research material without seeking informed consent from the individual contributor, as long as anonymity is fully preserved. This is because it is already wholly in the public sphere, and the contributor can be assumed to have known this when they posted it (see, for example, Androutsopoulos 2008 and Seale et al. 2010).

At the same time, of course, some of these advantages are also the disadvantages of online data. Firstly, this kind of data only represents people who have access to the Internet and are comfortable with writing about their experiences online. Secondly, the anonymity afforded by online environments means that we often have very little demographic or background information on those who contribute, and we cannot always trust the information that is volunteered. Finally, researchers have no control over what does or does not get discussed and elaborated within an online discourse, and the contributors' interests may not match those of the researcher. However, it is precisely these disadvantages that are balanced out by combining online data with semi-structured interviews.

The following section provides more detail on exactly how data was collected and compiled into our corpus.

3.4 Collecting the Data

The decisions outlined in the preceding sections implied a six-part design for the construction of the corpus: three participant groups for each of two genres. In this section, we describe in detail the approach we took to the collection of each part of the corpus.

The original target size for our corpus design was 100,000 words of interviews and 400,000 words of online data for each group, for a total of 1.5 million words. Table 3.1 provides an overview of the corpus we actually built, with word counts for each of its six sections, as well as totals for each participant group and each genre. As the table shows, the overall word count is 1,525,924 words, which is consistent with our target. However, the figures for several sections of the corpus differ from the target figures due to the degree of availability of the different types of data we aimed to include in our corpus. For the online part of the corpus, while patient and carer data was readily available, professionals' data was extremely scarce. We therefore collected approximately 500,000 words for each of the online patient and carer sections, and 250,000 words for the online professional section. In the carer and healthcare professional interviews, we had a slight (but far from methodologically compromising) shortfall relative to our original target, simply as a result of what was and was not suitable for our purposes in the datasets that we re-used and collected.

One notable point about the corpus is that the online section is roughly 82% of the whole. We will take this into account as relevant in reporting our findings.

We now provide more detail on the construction of each section of the corpus.

Table 3.1 Composition of the MELC Corpus, With Word Counts for Each Section

	Patients	*Carers*	*Healthcare Professionals*	*Totals*
Interviews	100,859	81,564	89,943	272,366
Online fora and blogs	500,134	500,256	253,168	1,253,558
Totals	600,993	581,820	343,111	1,525,924

3.4.1 Interviews

Each of these six sections of the MELC corpus required a distinct approach. As we have already suggested, with the patient and carer online data, we were able to access massive amounts of relevant data, and the main problem was *narrowing down* what we collected to a suitable subset for analysis. With the interview data, the difficulties were precisely opposite: the process of contacting potential interviewees, conducting the interviews and transcribing the resulting recordings is extremely labour-intensive and time-consuming. Therefore, in order to get the largest possible set of interview data, we decided to begin by considering existing datasets, and to focus our own efforts on what we needed to *add* to those datasets to reach our goal in terms of corpus size—that is, in the region of 100,000 running words for each participant group.

The existing data which we used came from two earlier studies led by one of the present authors (Payne), one involving interviews with patients (Payne et al. 2008), the other interviews with carers (Payne et al. 2009). Our own collection therefore focused on healthcare professionals. It might be argued that this approach undermines the comparability of the three participant groups (and the advantages of using interviews in the first place), since we obviously could not design the interview questions used in these earlier projects. However, in terms of the interview design, the interviews of the three groups would have been different even if we had done them all afresh—the questions that can be asked of a patient, a carer and a healthcare professional will inevitably be different. Moreover, all the interviews were *semi-structured*; i.e. the interviewer had a standard set of questions from which to begin discussion, but conversation was allowed to flow freely from there. Thus, the open-ended nature of the discussion created the opportunity for the natural, unprompted production of metaphorical expressions. As such, the questions, different though they were for each group, served to make sure that the overall subject of discourse was relevant to cancer (care), palliative care or the end of life (and end-of-life care), and thus that most metaphorical expressions produced would be likely to refer to one of these topic areas.

The patient data was originally collected for the Ethnicity and Cancer Care project, funded by Dimbleby Cancer Care (Payne et al. 2008). From this project's data, we selected 29 interviews with patients with advanced cancer, conducted in their homes or in hospice day-care settings. The original project surveyed and contrasted two ethnic groups, people of (i) white English and (ii) Chinese origin; we only sampled from the patients in the former group, since the specific and particular experience of the UK Chinese immigrant community was not our concern. These patients had been recruited via cancer support centres and hospice day-care centres. The interviews we selected for inclusion in the corpus were balanced for gender and age of the patient, as far as possible (albeit most were, in the end, older people), and were between 40 and 70 minutes in length. Moreover, we only included interviews where the participant had made use of hospice or palliative care services at some point. For carer interviews, we re-used data originally collected by Payne et al. (2009) in a project for Help the Hospices. These 17 interviews with unpaid family carers of terminally ill patients lasted between 20 and 75 minutes. Eleven were face-to-face interviews conducted in the carers' homes, and six were telephone interviews.

The interviews with both patients and carers contained sections that were less relevant to our purposes, as they focused on the interviewee's life in general before the onset of their own illness or the illness of the person they cared for. For our purposes, we only kept those parts of the interviews that focused on the interviewee's life subsequent to the cancer diagnosis. This resulted in the carer corpus being somewhat smaller than intended, as can be seen in Table 3.1 (81,564 words of interviews with carers, as opposed to 100,859 for patients).

Finally, in our own data collection, in 2012 we conducted 16 interviews with healthcare professionals in leadership positions working in hospice or palliative care. We recruited participants via Lancaster University's postgraduate degree schemes for hospice leaders, via an advertisement in the *Help the Hospices* newsletter and via personal contacts. Each interview lasted approximately 30 to 45 minutes. The total size of the professional interviews is 89,943 words. The interview questions for all three sets of interviews can be found in Appendix 1.[1] For ease of readability, in the course of the book we lay out our extracts from the interviews as continuous text and use orthographic marks to provide minimal information about intonation contours: a full stop indicates falling or final intonation; a comma indicates continuing intonation, whether within or across clause boundaries; and three full stops indicate a significant pause.

3.4.2 *Online Fora*

The online forum data for carers and patients was collected from various threads of one UK-based online forum, run by a charity dedicated to cancer. Despite the public-sphere status of contributions posted to publicly accessible online fora, as already explained, we nevertheless considered it wise, from the perspective of research ethics, to inform the organisation hosting the forum of our plans; we met with no objections. This covers the ethics of our *study* of the data, but not our *reproduction* of the data (as excerpts in this book and other academic publications); as noted in Chapter 1, we have addressed the latter ethical issue by anonymising all excerpts of the data to ensure that these posts—while already in the public sphere—do not become more widely distributed, to the potential detriment of an identifiable participant.

Table 3.2 Size Metrics for the Patient/Carer Online Forum

Metric	*Size of Forum*
Users	23,561
Threads	30,221
Posts	400,108
Words	50,208,214

Table 3.2 summarises the total amount of text we were able to collect from a single online forum for cancer patients and their carers.

We collected discussions posted on this very large forum over a period from 2007 to 2012. Most of the corresponding data from healthcare professionals was collected from a separate publicly accessible online forum for medical professionals. After identifying relevant parts of this data, as discussed later, we did not have a large enough corpus to meet our target for this participant group. We therefore supplemented these contributions with relevant posts from UK-based doctors' blogs, and online comments from medical professionals on *British Medical Journal* articles addressing end-of-life/palliative care issues.

3.4.3 Managing and Downsampling Online Forum Data

In this section, we address some technical issues relating to the construction of the online sections of our corpus.

In contrast to the interviews, collecting more online forum data for patients and carers than we actually needed was not difficult. The challenge was organising and managing the data, including its internal structure: we had to identify (at least some of) the internal differentiating factors within the many million words of text we downloaded, and thus 'zero in' on the right parts to include in our main corpus.

This challenge is linked to a broader issue regarding corpus data from the web. Generally, automatically collected web corpora tend to lack structure. For instance, the WaC (Web-as-Corpus) project (Baroni et al. 2009) has collected a number of very large corpora using web spider software to automatically download webpages; the resulting corpora lack internal structure (i.e. they do not contain information about how individual texts belong to larger groupings), and can thus be described as 'flat'. However, not all data crawled from the web is necessarily flat in this way. It is quite possible for web data from a particular source to have a rich internal structure in terms of the experience of users who viewed it in its original online context. This is certainly true of online fora. The discussions hosted in these fora are structured into threads, i.e. individual discussions, each made up of a set of chronologically sequential posts. A 'flat' download of a web forum would neglect the structure of threads/

posts, and merely collect pages—that is, individually rendered views of the forum. One thread frequently extends across many different pages, once it has too many posts for them all to be displayed simultaneously. This situation is illustrated in Figure 3.1, with the 'flat' structure (concrete downloadable pages) shown at the bottom, and the more complex, hierarchical conceptual structure (posts within threads within a forum) at the top.

The general question then is how we should approach the problem of maintaining a rich conceptual structure, rather than a flat structure, in data collected from the web. Once this is accomplished, the problem we mentioned—efficiently identifying suitable sub-samples for analysis—becomes, if not trivial, then at least highly tractable.

We accomplished actual downloading of the fora using bespoke web spider programs, which, in the process of downloading various pages, organised the download into the conceptual structure of threads. These same programs then processed the data from the HTML markup format used for web display into the XML format typically used for corpus analysis, with each XML document corresponding to a thread, and separate posts within the thread explicitly marked up using XML tags. In the construction of 'flat' web corpora, a webpage's HTML is typically just stripped out, along with 'boilerplate' text (page headers and footers, side menus and other incidental material surrounding the actual page content). Critically, our customised programs instead interpreted the HTML surrounding individual forum posts to extract key metadata on the posts, such as the username of the contributor who wrote it, and the date/time of posting. This metadata was recorded in the output XML markup.

To actually access all this information on the internal structure of the downloaded data, we transferred the metadata for posts and threads in the corpus to a relational database, whose structure is presented in

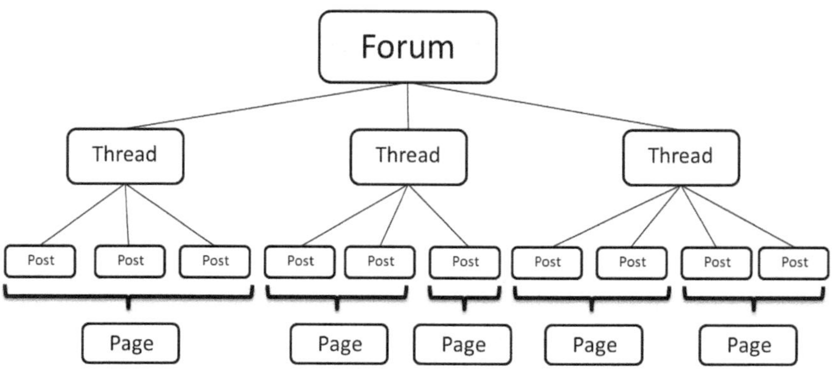

Figure 3.1 The Hierarchical Conceptual Structure of an Online Forum, Compared to How It Is Concretised in Downloadable Pages

Figure 3.2. A relational database typically includes multiple data tables, where each table represents one particular type of data object. The primary data objects in this case were the 'thread' and the 'post'; however, the fact that we recorded the author of each post meant that the forum 'user' was also a data object. Moreover, since we downloaded data from multiple fora, the threads from a given forum were all grouped as a single corpus. Figure 3.2 shows, for each data object, what items of data were held. Each object has an 'id', which is a unique ID number (or 'key' in database terminology). These ID numbers could then be referenced, where necessary, by other types of object. Hence, one attribute of a post is the ID of the thread in which it occurs. These links between key fields (where one object has an attribute which refers to the key of another object) are shown by arrows in Figure 3.2. Moreover, the database contains disk-file references to the actual XML text of the corpus (the 'byte offset' attribute of the post) so that the underlying text of every post or thread can be accessed.

Finally, we created a web interface to this database and the XML documents underlying it, which allowed us to explore the network of links—viewing many different 'slices' of the data, for instance a single thread, or all the posts by a particular user, or their first or last post (chronologically speaking).

One of the first things that this interface allowed us to discover was that there was a strong 'long tail' effect in the main forum we downloaded.

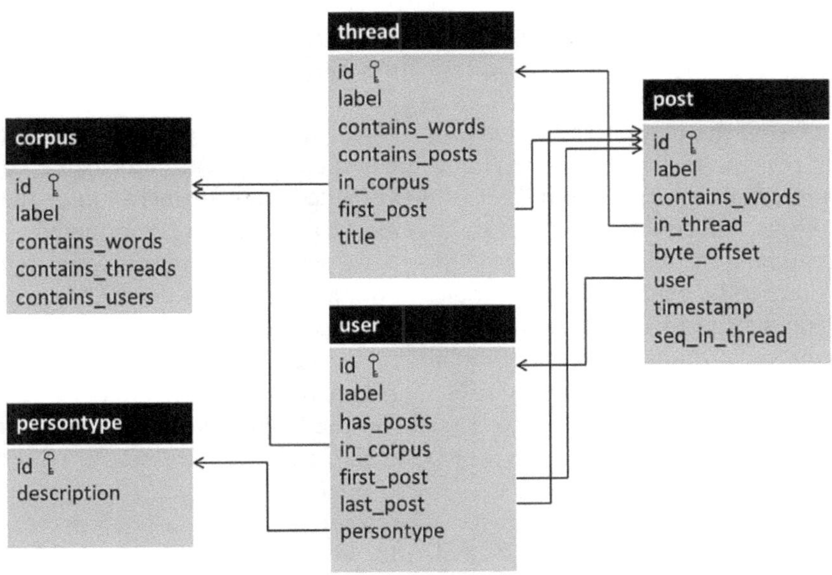

Figure 3.2 Database Structure for the Forum Data

Although there were around 24,000 users (see Table 3.2), nearly all of them authored very few posts—often just one—whereas a much smaller number of users were responsible for a large number of posts. This gave us a clue regarding how we should focus our analysis on a manageable subset of the downloaded data, or, to use a term common in corpus linguistics, how we should 'downsample' it. Clearly, the discourse of an online forum is better typified by the linguistic behaviour of habitual users than by one-off contributions from passers-by. A minimum of 1,000 words per user was adopted as a threshold for possible inclusion in the corpus.

Since the forum was used by both cancer patients and carers for cancer patients, we also needed to separate out different types of user to fit our corpus design (so that posts by patients and carers could be sampled for the corresponding sections of the corpus). The web interface allowed us to annotate users with their 'person type'—the final database object—which included 'patient' and 'carer', as well as other person types not relevant for our purposes (e.g. 'non-carer relative/friend'). This classification was done manually by examining how users identify themselves in their initial posts to the forum. This process was feasible because the database structure made it possible for us to classify solely the small set of high-volume contributors who accounted for most of the forum's discourse, around 700 users in total; a manual classification of all 23,561 users was out of the question. The criteria for labelling participants were as follows: a user was labelled as a 'patient' if they self-identify as such—most of these users also state or imply that they have advanced cancer specifically, as we explained earlier; a user was labelled as a 'carer' if they self-identify as caring for someone with advanced cancer, or for someone who has recently died following terminal cancer.

Using this classification system, for both participant types, a selection of relevant posts concerning end-of-life and palliative care was identified and extracted from the full set of downloaded data for inclusion in the corpus. Which threads and posts counted as 'relevant' was determined by searching the text of the threads for a small set of search terms which we found to be diagnostic of the topics in question, namely 'death', 'dying', 'end of', 'hospice', 'palliative', 'life' and 'support'; this set of search terms emerged from the process of defining our much smaller sample corpus, which we will discuss in section 3.5.2. Thus, the selection of data for the corpus is determined *both* by a focus on the language of the most prolific forum users *and* by the topic(s) of the stretches of discourse under consideration.

The same interface was used to extract relevant posts by professionals from the respective downloads, which, as already noted, came from a number of different sites. Although the online sources we used for all three participant groups were UK-based, we cannot be certain that all users were native speakers of English, and we did not have access to their demographic details. However, our observations indicate that the vast majority were UK-based and fluent speakers of English.

Common misspellings and abbreviations (e.g. 'recieve', 'ur') were corrected throughout the corpus, as the corpus software we used (see section 3.5.4) is more accurate with text in standard orthographic spelling. However, we retain original spellings when quoting from the online data in the course of the book.

Having described the collection of our data and the composition of our corpus, it is now time to turn to our method for identifying metaphor in general, as well as for our target topic specifically.

3.5 Analysing and Quantifying Metaphor

Our starting point for identifying metaphorical expressions in our data through manual analysis was the well-established Metaphor Identification Procedure (MIP) described in Pragglejaz Group (2007). According to this procedure, an expression is regarded as metaphorically used when (a) its 'contextual meaning' contrasts with a 'basic meaning' that is more physical and concrete (although not necessarily more frequent), and (b) where the contextual meaning can be understood via a comparison with the basic meaning.

The full procedure is as follows:

1. Read the entire text-discourse to establish a general understanding of the meaning.
2. Determine the lexical units in the text-discourse.
    a. For each lexical unit in the text, establish its meaning in context, that is, how it applies to an entity, relation, or attribute in the situation evoked by the text (contextual meaning). Take into account what comes before and after the lexical unit.
    b. For each lexical unit, determine if it has a more basic contemporary meaning in other contexts than the one in the given context. For our purposes, basic meanings tend to be
        i. More concrete [what they evoke is easier to imagine, see, hear, feel, smell, and taste];
        ii. Related to bodily action;
        iii. More precise (as opposed to vague);
        iv. Historically older;

    Basic meanings are not necessarily the most frequent meanings of the lexical unit.

3. If the lexical unit has a more basic current-contemporary meaning in other contexts than the given context, decide whether the contextual meaning contrasts with the basic meaning but can be understood in comparison with it.
4. If yes, mark the lexical unit as metaphorical.

(Pragglejaz Group 2007: 3)

Consider, for example, the use of the word 'veteran' in the following example, from the online patient section of the MELC corpus:

Example 3.1

I would also be more than happy for any of you to contact me for a chat or a moan. I am fast becoming a chemo <u>veteran</u> as I am on my third lot just now.

The contextual meaning of 'veteran' in the extract could be expressed as 'someone who has a lot of experience of chemotherapy'. This meaning is different from the main and most basic meaning of this word in English, which is characterised by the *Macmillan Online Dictionary*, for example, as 'someone who was in the armed forces, especially during a war' (Macmillan Dictionary Online 2017). According to the MIP, this meaning is more basic in that it is historically older, more closely related to bodily action and, arguably, more concrete. Crucially, the contextual meaning can be understood by comparison with the basic meaning: someone with a lot of experience of chemotherapy can help and advise other people with cancer in the same way as someone with a lot of experience of war can advise people who have less experience. In addition, the experience of chemotherapy can be compared to the experience of war in that it is difficult, traumatic and potentially dangerous, and can therefore deeply change people both physically and emotionally.[2]

MIP also requires analysts to make explicit additional components of their analysis: the dictionary they use for reference, what they consider to be the unit of analysis and whether there are any significant *a priori* exclusions. Taking these in order:

- We used the *Macmillan Online Dictionary* as a point of reference for basic meanings, as it is recent and corpus-based, and therefore a reliable source of information on current usage.
- Generally, an individual word is taken as one lexical unit for the purposes of metaphor analysis; i.e. the word was our unit of analysis. There were, however, two main exceptions to this rule: proper nouns and phrasal verbs (e.g. 'go through' in the sense of experiencing something bad). Although these may consist of more than one word, they often form a type of 'inseparable unit', and we therefore

considered them to constitute one lexical unit. Phrasal verbs were identified based on their labelling as such in the Macmillan dictionary.

- In the process of identifying relevant basic meanings, we followed the decision made in Pragglejaz Group (2007) to cross part-of-speech boundaries in searching for basic meanings where the different parts of speech share the same base form. This applies, for example, to the use of 'key' in 'I think the patients, families and health professionals should make the key decisions' (from the online professional section of the corpus). The Macmillan dictionary classifies 'key' in this kind of use as an adjective, with the meaning of 'very important'. If we only consider 'key' as an adjective for the purposes of our analysis, there is no contrast between the basic meaning of the adjective and its contextual meanings in our example. However, 'key' as an adjective shares the same base form as 'key' as a noun, which has the basic meaning of a small metal object used for opening locks. We therefore considered the meaning of the noun as a relevant basic meaning for the purposes of our analysis. As a result, 'key' in the example we have quoted was analysed as a metaphorical expression. This contrasts with cases such as the adverb 'openly' and the adjective 'open', which are related by derivation and do not share a base form. In such cases, we did not consider the basic meaning of the adjective when analysing the adverb for metaphoricity (but see Steen et al. 2010 for a different view on this issue).
- For the purposes of our analysis, we considered potential metaphoricity in 'open class words' (nouns, verbs, adjectives and adverbs) and prepositions. In addition, we excluded some common words and expressions from our metaphor identification process. These were the prepositions 'for', 'of', 'with' and 'about'; 'to' as an infinitive marker; and the verbs 'have', 'be', 'get', 'make' and 'do', as well as 'go' when it is used as a semi-auxiliary (e.g. 'I kind of wake up wondering if she's going to be alive'). These were excluded because they are 'delexicalised' to a considerable extent; that is, they lack sufficient semantic content for an analyst to be able to establish and distinguish basic and contextual meanings with enough precision. There are also some data-specific words or terms that have been excluded, for example technical terms such as 'power of attorney' and 'end of life' and some exclamations (e.g. 'what the hell').

Our approach to the analysis of metaphoricity in our corpus was further refined and extended by drawing on some aspects of MIPVU—a development of the MIP that was produced at the Vrije Universiteit in Amsterdam (Steen et al. 2010). We followed MIPVU in downgrading the criterion that basic meanings of lexical units should be historically older than contextual meanings. This is because evidence from the *Oxford English Dictionary* and other sources is not always detailed or reliable enough to apply this criterion consistently. In practice, the MIP criteria concerning concreteness, precision and relatedness to bodily action were sufficient to make decisions, and those decisions were broadly consistent with historical information where this was available.

More importantly, we followed MIPVU in including within our analysis similes and other explicit figurative comparisons that are beyond the scope of the original MIP. This applies to cases such as 'it [cancer] is like trying to drive a coach and horses uphill with no back wheels on the coach', from the opening example in Chapter 1. The travel-related words in this simile are used in their basic meanings, and would not therefore be identified as metaphorical through the MIP. However, the whole scenario that follows the preposition 'like' is being used to describe an aspect of living with cancer. As such, similes and other explicit comparisons between unlike things fall within the general definition of metaphoricity in language we provided in Chapter 1 (section 1.2.2).[3]

Steen et al. (2010) make a relevant distinction between two different ways in which the cross-domain mappings of Conceptual Metaphor Theory (CMT) can be realised linguistically, namely through:

a. Language that is used 'indirectly', i.e. metaphorical expressions involving a contrast between basic and contextual meanings, such as 'veteran' in Example 3.1;
b. Language that is used 'directly', i.e. with no contrast between basic and contextual meanings; this applies to similes and other 'explicit invitations for comparison' (Steen et al. 2010: 11), such as 'if you can think of this chapter in your life as a reluctant journey', from our online patient data.

Steen et al. capture both 'direct' and 'indirect' metaphoricity in language by means of the label 'metaphor-related words'. In this book, we distinguish among metaphorical expressions, similes, etc., whenever appropriate. However, we also use the general terms 'linguistic metaphor' or simply 'metaphor' to capture the wide variety of ways in which metaphoricity is realised in our corpus.

Because of the approach we have adopted, the linguistic metaphors we discuss vary considerably in their degree of conventionality in English. For example, the metaphorical use of 'veteran' in 'a chemo veteran' is a specific case of a conventional metaphorical use of the noun, which the Macmillan dictionary captures as 'someone who has a lot of experience doing a particular activity' (Macmillan Dictionary Online 2017). This contrasts with, for example, the use of 'skirmishes' in our opening example in Chapter 1: 'we did, however, win a significant number of skirmishes'. This metaphorical use of 'skirmishes' to refer to moments or aspects in the attempt to recover from cancer is not one of the conventional uses of the noun, and can therefore be described as a relatively more creative or novel case of metaphoricity, even though it relies on the conventional view of cancer as an enemy to be fought (Lakoff and Turner 1989).

The final restriction on our analysis of metaphor concerns the topics that we were interested in, or *target domains*, in terms of CMT. Because we were specifically investigating metaphor use around cancer and end-of-life care, we were not interested in *all* metaphors in our data, but only in those relevant to our, admittedly very broad, set of topics. We therefore restricted our analysis to metaphors that related to a person's whole experience of cancer, the end of life and end-of-life care. This included their conversations with others, their emotions and any practical aspects they mentioned. We also included all metaphors to do with death and dying. As we outlined earlier, the relevance of examples to our topics of interest was partly ensured by our data selection process. We excluded, however, metaphors that related to patients' or carers' lives prior to the onset of the illness, as well as highly conventional metaphors that did not capture relevant aspects of the experience of cancer and the end of life, such as the use of spatial metaphors in relation to time (e.g. 'as time passes').

Having described our metaphor identification procedure, in the next section we introduce the intensive, qualitative manual analysis of a representative sample from our corpus which we then used to inform our subsequent quantitative explorations in the complete MELC corpus.

3.5.1 Manual Analysis of a Sample From the Corpus

As there does not yet exist any fully automated corpus-based method for identifying or analysing metaphor, analyses of large datasets often begin with a qualitative analysis of a sample of the data. We therefore extracted an approximately 15,000-word sample from each section of the corpus and conducted a manual analysis of linguistic metaphors in this sample that would then inform a computer-aided analysis of the whole corpus.

When all six sections were combined together, the sample corpus was composed of 92,105 words, as shown in Table 3.3.

3.5.2 Sample Construction

Our sampling processes were slightly different for the interviews and the online forum contributions, reflecting the differences between these genres, as discussed earlier in the chapter (and resulting in a sample slightly over the target 90,000 words). The sample interviews were selected based on:

a. Their relevance to our topic (cancer, end of life and end-of-life care);
b. The degree to which respondents focused on their own experience and emotions (as opposed to discussing practical arrangements, for example);
c. The prevalence of metaphorical expressions based on a first reading.

Table 3.3 Composition of the Sample Corpus, With Word Counts for Each Section

	Patients	*Unpaid Family Carers*	*Healthcare Professionals*	*Totals*
Semi-structured interviews	16,768	14,164	16,743	47,675
Contributions to online fora	15,235	15,010	14,185	44,430
Totals	32,003	29,174	30,928	92,105

These three criteria ensured that our manual analysis encompassed the most relevant and metaphorically rich data, yielding the best starting point for the subsequent semi-automated analysis.

In the case of healthcare professionals, the first criterion was met by all interviewees, as the interview questions were designed by the MELC team and focused on the experience of end-of-life care. As such, for this participant group the more important criteria for inclusion in the sample were (b) and (c). In the case of patients and unpaid family carers, all three criteria were important. Where possible, we tried to achieve a gender balance in the sample, but less than a quarter of patients, and 40% of carers, were men. For family carers and healthcare professionals, the sample consisted of three interviews each, while for patients, because the interviews were shorter, we needed four interviews to reach the required number of words.

A similar manual technique was employed to extract a sample of the carer and patient online data. The posts of some of the most prolific contributors were cross-referenced with the threads that were identified as relevant to our topic (by means of the online interface described in section 3.4.3). The posts of those who had contributed to relevant threads were downloaded from the online interface as plain text files. This rather substantial amount of data was then manually explored (using a simple 'find text' tool) for the expressions 'death', 'dying', 'end of', 'hospice' and 'palliative'. All posts that included these words were read, and if the post indeed proved relevant to our topic, its text was copied into a new 'Sample' document, specific to the contributor. For carers, the additional search terms of 'life' and 'support' were added, as the original terms did not yield enough results.

Sample selection for the online professional data proceeded in a slightly different way. As outlined in section 3.4.3, it was more difficult and time-consuming to collect sufficient data for the whole online professional corpus. The sample therefore needed to be constructed and manually analysed before the whole online professional corpus was complete. We used the blog and forum sections of the host site where the majority of our online professional corpus came from, and ran manual searches for the terms 'end-of-life care', 'hospice', 'palliative care', 'end of life', 'death' and 'dying'. These terms differ slightly from the search terms for carers and patients because we wanted to obtain comparable results to the patient and carer online data, which began with the criterion that they had contributed to a relevant thread. Since the complete online professional corpus was not ready at that time, we replicated this criterion by including extra search terms. The original forum site presented its search results in order of relevance, and we focused on those posts, comments or blogs where the title or first section included the search terms. We selected our sample from these by prioritising posts that had at least one response and that contained some relevant metaphors. These were collected into a 'Sample' document, as with the carer and patient samples. This modified procedure for the professionals' data resulted in a differently organised sample, as the distinct method allowed us to select entire threads, rather than posts by individual users. This means that, while all interviews, as well as online contributions by patients and family carers, are organised by interviewee or contributor in the sample corpus, the sample online contributions by professionals are organised by thread. The sample consists of seven threads altogether.

3.5.3 Sample Analysis

Once the sample was selected, we used our modified MIP as already detailed to identify metaphorical expressions and similes relevant to the experience of cancer and the end of life. This process involved three members of the project team checking and discussing the analysis. We therefore needed a tool for manual annotation that allowed multiple-user access to the data. We opted for eMargin, a collaborative text annotation tool developed at Birmingham City University (http://emargin.bcu.ac.uk/). eMargin's online interface allows multiple users to annotate a text simultaneously. Three types of annotation can be added: highlighting in various colours, comments and tags. The annotations can be added to individual words or to larger sections of a text.

We used highlighting to mark linguistic metaphors, and subsequently used tags to assign these expressions to semantic domains corresponding to their literal meanings. This was done in a data-driven fashion, using labels—such as Violence (or Military), Movement (or Journey), Restraint, Animal, Openness, Sport/Games, Magic, Religion, Obstacle, Wholeness and Machines—that were as close as possible to the actual language in the data (cf. Cameron and Maslen 2010); an example of this labelling process can be seen in Figure 3.3. The resulting semantic categories will be discussed in detail in Chapter 4.

In borderline cases of metaphoricity, our criterion of last resort was 'When-in-Doubt-Leave-It-In' (cf. Steen et al. 2010), expressed as a

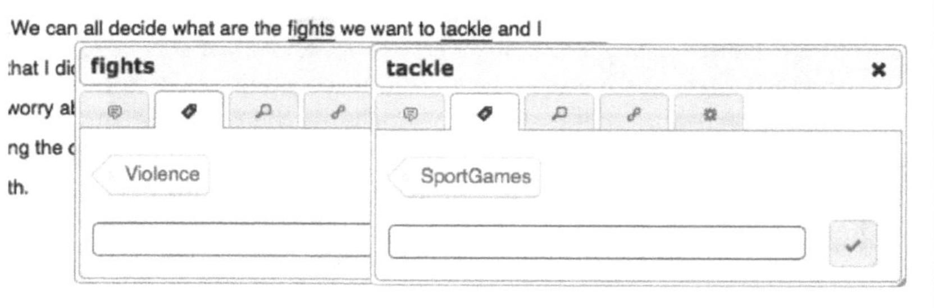

Figure 3.3 Example of Annotation of the Sample Corpus in eMargin Software

'WIDLI' tag. Once all the relevant metaphors had been identified and subsumed under semantic fields corresponding to potential source domains, it was time to scale up the analysis to the entire corpus. That process is the topic of the next part of this chapter.

3.5.4 Scaling Up

As we noted earlier, state-of-the-art automatic computational methods for locating metaphors in text are not yet capable of matching humans at identifying a wide range of metaphor types. We therefore had to find another way of approaching our research. The method we adopted relies on the automatic semantic tagging built into our main corpus tool, Wmatrix (Rayson 2008). Our working hypothesis was that semantic categories assigned by the semantic tagging software (described later) would be useful as part of a procedure for investigating, in CMT terms, source and target domains in the corpus. We will now provide a little more detail about the semantic tagging system, before showing how it was successfully exploited to scale up the manual approach in the sample corpus—generating queries to run against the complete corpus.

The USAS Semantic Tagger

The UCREL Semantic Analysis System (USAS) is a tagging program designed to assign a semantic category label (or semantic tag) automatically to every word or phrase in a corpus. The USAS category scheme consists of 232 tags that represent coarse-grained semantic fields. These are arranged in a hierarchical taxonomy, with 21 major discourse domains at the top level, as shown in Figure 3.4. This taxonomy originates in lexicographic research, from a system of semantic tags employed in the *Longman Lexicon of Contemporary English* (McArthur 1981); these were adapted and extended during the creation of USAS. In contrast

A: General and abstract terms
B: The body and the individual
C: Arts and crafts
E: Emotional actions, states and processes
F: Food and farming
G: Government and the public domain
H: Architecture, buildings, houses and the home
I: Money and commerce
K: Entertainment, sports and games
L: Life and living things
M: Movement, location, travel and transport
N: Numbers and measurement
O: Substances, materials, objects and equipment
P: Education
Q: Linguistic actions, states and processes
S: Social actions, states and processes
T: Time
W: The world and our environment
X: Psychological actions, states and processes
Y: Science and technology
Z: Names and grammatical words

Figure 3.4 The 21 Major Domains at the Top of the USAS Taxonomy

to other types of content analysis system such as Linguistic Inquiry and Word Count (LIWC) (Tausczik and Pennebaker 2010), the USAS tagger attempts to assign a contextually appropriate tag by taking into account the meaning of a word or phrase in the wider sentence or discourse context. To do this, it relies on a large dictionary of words and phrases, each with a list of potential tags, created manually by linguists over a period of 27 years. For example, the word 'bank' would be tagged as I1 (Money generally) for senses relating to a financial institution or a building containing a branch of such a bank, but as W3 (Geographical terms) if the context indicates that the particular example is related to river banks. Moreover, the system is sensitive to part-of-speech distinctions. USAS will assign one of the I1 or W3 tags to instances of 'bank' as noun, but for instances of 'bank' identified as a verb, the system will instead choose between I1 (Money generally), for the act of banking money, and M1 (Moving, coming and going) for turning an aircraft. The semantic tagger attempts to choose the correct tag in context from the dictionary list using a number of disambiguation methods which we do not need to explain in detail here (further explanation of this process can be found in Rayson et al. 2004). The key point here is that the tagger puts the most likely tag for each word or phrase at the start of the list of tags applied to that word or phrase, while the other, less likely tags are retained lower down in that list. If we look solely at this first-choice tag for all words and phrases in a text, then the tagger is accurate around 91% of the time (Rayson et al. 2004).

It should be noted that the semantic tagger itself was not designed to be used for metaphor analysis. However, as we have shown in the previous chapters, metaphors are regularly employed in language, and hence they are an important feature for automatic semantic analysis to consider. The dictionary embedded in the tagger does contain both literal and figurative (including metaphorical) senses for many of the words and phrases it knows, but unfortunately for our work here, the tagger itself does not differentiate between these types of senses, other than to try to assign the correct meaning in context. During the application of the tagger in this research, we have piloted ways to work with the output of the tagger for metaphor analysis, as explained later. In the future, the tagger itself will be improved in this respect using computational methods being developed in the natural language processing community, for example measures of concreteness and imageability, as outlined in Chapter 2.

One important aspect of the tagger's contextual disambiguation is its ability to mark phrases or multiword expressions (MWEs) with single tags. Many different types of MWEs are marked in this way: phrasal verbs (e.g. 'lift up'), noun phrases (e.g. 'football shirt'), proper names (e.g. 'Milton Keynes') and idiomatic expressions (e.g. 'living the life of Riley'). In some cases, these formulaic sequences can be discontinuous, especially in the case of phrasal verbs. MWE tagging is especially important to avoid assigning incorrect senses to the separate words within the instances of MWEs found in a text.

Having provided an overview of the inner workings of the semantic tagger, we can now return to see how it was exploited for metaphor research in our project.

Using the USAS Semantic Tagger for Metaphor Analysis

The manually analysed and tagged files from the Sample corpus were exported in XML format from the eMargin tool and imported into a database (called MELCdb) that was specially designed for the MELC project by Dr Stephen Wattam at Lancaster University. The MELCdb system also incorporated an interface tailored to make it possible for us to search for the metaphor groups that had been manually marked up in the text, alongside the automatically inserted semantic tags from USAS. This enabled us to extract a list of words for each eMargin metaphor group label, together with their most likely USAS tags. Taking the example of the manually applied Violence tag from eMargin, this database allowed us to identify the following seven USAS tags assigned automatically to the example metaphorical expressions shown here:

- G3 (Warfare): e.g. 'battle', 'fight' as a verb;
- A1.1.1 (General actions, making): e.g. 'blast', 'confront';
- A1.1.2 (Damaging and destroying): e.g. 'destroy', 'shatter';
- E3– (Violent/angry): e.g. 'hit', 'attack';
- S8+ (Helping): e.g. 'defend', 'protect';
- S8– (Hindering): e.g. 'fight' as a noun;
- X8+ (Trying hard): e.g. 'struggle'.

This process of matching manual labels to automatic tags resulted in a list of semantic tags that we could use to search the complete corpus—since the full corpus had also been automatically tagged with USAS. Of course, the process is not perfect, since not all instances of words and phrases assigned these seven tags will be metaphorical: many examples will be retrieved in such a search that will need to be subsequently discarded from a detailed analysis. Moreover, in some cases the manually tagged metaphors pointed towards some large and quite generic USAS categories. This was particularly the case with items manually tagged in the sample analysis as Movement or Journey metaphors. USAS placed these items in various 'M' categories (Movement, location, travel and transport). Rather than attempt to extract concordances for entire domains such as M, however, we began by concordancing specific words selected from the USAS domains M1, M3, M6 and M7 (which the database indicated as the most likely prospects for finding similar items to those manually tagged as metaphorical in the sample corpus). These were: 'journey*', 'path*', 'road*', 'step*', 'route*', 'way* through', 'go*/com* through', 'forward*', 'backward*', 'run*', 'move*', 'travel*', 'turn*', 'direction*' and 'place*' (NB: here the asterisk functions as a wildcard; i.e. it stands for any sequence of zero or more characters). This more selective approach enabled us to manage the data more easily and efficiently. Despite its imperfections, this method proved to be a very fruitful first pass for us to filter down the results.

The next step in our method was to use the Wmatrix software (Rayson 2008). Wmatrix is a web-based concordancer which implements all the main methods in corpus linguistics that we briefly introduced in Chapter 2: concordances, frequency lists, collocation and keyness. Wmatrix also applies the USAS semantic tagger to any text loaded into the system, so that semantic tags as well as words can be analysed.

As we mentioned in Chapter 2, the keyness method involves comparing frequency lists for two corpora and identifying items which are more frequent than expected in one corpus than in the other 'reference' corpus, to a statistically significant extent. Typically, this analysis is carried out at the word level. However, Wmatrix also makes it possible to apply the keyness method to semantic tags. This was an invaluable additional tool for cross checking which semantic tags might be worthy of further consideration. For each file loaded into the system, Wmatrix prepares a frequency list of the semantic tags present in the tagged file, which can be compared to a semantic frequency list from a larger reference corpus to generate a list of key semantic tags. This list of key semantic tags can be sorted by a variety of statistical measures, and tags which are highly key are those which appear significantly more frequently relative to the reference corpus. The tags at the head of the sorted list could then be examined via concordances, to triangulate against analyses arising from the list of tags generated by mapping from the manual eMargin tags.

Examples and results of this key semantic tag approach will be described in Chapter 4 to highlight the main differences in vocabulary and topics among the six different parts of our corpus.

As well as using Wmatrix's existing affordances for corpus analysis, we also specially adapted the software for the MELC project. The main adaptation was to enable what we termed 'broadsweep' searching. As noted earlier, USAS assigns a list of semantic tags to each given word or phrase, in order of likely relevance in context. Normally, however, searches in Wmatrix (and other tools) are limited to the first-choice semantic tag for each word or phrase. This can be a limitation when trying to identify metaphors belonging to a particular source domain, as the first-choice semantic tag assigned by USAS for conventional metaphorical expressions could well correspond to the target domain, i.e. to the meaning of the word/phrase in context. In a broadsweep search for some semantic tag, that tag is searched for anywhere on the list of possible tags, rather than just in the first-choice tags. This is advantageous for the purposes of identifying metaphorical expressions. For example, we found that the Sport/Games tag manually assigned in the analysis of the sample corpus in eMargin correlated well with the USAS tags K5.1 (Sports) and K5.2 (Games). A normal search for these semantic tags retrieved concordances for words such as 'exercise', 'game', 'race' and 'ride'. However, when we expanded this using a broadsweep search, we could also extract concordances for other potentially interesting high frequency words such as 'play' and 'fight', i.e. words where K5.1 and/or K5.2 is a possible analysis, but was not judged most likely in context by USAS.

Bringing all of these methods together, we were able to use the combination of eMargin manually tagged data, mapped to USAS semantic tags, to search the complete corpus, along with other search terms of potential interest identified using a key semantic tag list and results from the broadsweep search. Finally, armed with data from these three approaches, we extracted concordances for the selected semantic tags and analysed them manually to identify which examples were actually used metaphorically and were of relevance to our study's focus on cancer and (care at) the end of life. This more comprehensive approach to using semantic tags therefore enabled us to identify a greater diversity of metaphors than would otherwise have been possible based only on restricted word searches. Allowing the corpus data to guide us was important because we wanted to explore the full range of metaphors that patients, carers and professionals use to talk about our topics of interest, beyond what has also been described in the literature and what we saw from the smaller scale manual analysis in our 92,000-word representative Sample corpus. The results of these methods will be presented over the course of the next several chapters.

3.6 Summary

In this chapter, we began by presenting our rationale for selecting, as a focus for our study, three participant groups (patients, unpaid family carers and healthcare professionals) and two genres (interviews and online forum posts or blogs). We described in detail the process of constructing the MELC corpus and provided details of its final composition. We then introduced our approach to analysing metaphors in the corpus. This involved clarifying our metaphor identification method, describing the construction and manual analysis of a sample from our larger corpus and explaining how we used the software tools in Wmatrix to scale up our sample analysis to the complete corpus. We hope that, by describing these processes in detail, we have made it possible for others to replicate our approach, and also provided the necessary background for the findings we report in the rest of this book.

Notes

1. Individual consent was obtained from all interviewees, and ethical approval was obtained at Lancaster University.
2. The focus on comparison in this approach to metaphor identification makes it possible to distinguish cases such as 'veteran' from the use of expressions such as 'white coat' to refer to a doctor. The latter phenomenon is known as metonymy and relies on some form of association or contiguity between what is said and what is meant, such as the association between doctors and the wearing of white coats.
3. For the purposes of quantification, the words used in similes were approached in the same way as for metaphorical expressions; i.e. we counted open class words and prepositions, with the exclusions mentioned earlier.

References

Allen, C., Vassilev, I., Kennedy, A., and Rogers, A. (2016). Long-term condition self-management support in online communities: A meta-synthesis of qualitative papers. *Journal of Medical Internet Research*, *18*(3), e61.

Androutsopoulos, J. (2008). Potentials and limitations of discourse-centred online ethnography. *Language@Internet*, 5. Retrieved from www.languageatinternet.org/articles/2008/1610

Baroni, M., Bernardini, S., Ferraresi, A., and Zanchetta, E. (2009). The WaCky Wide Web: A collection of very large linguistically processed web-crawled corpora. *Language Resources and Evaluation*, *43*(3), 209–226.

Barton, D. (2007). *Literacy: An introduction to the ecology of written language*. Oxford: Blackwell.

Biber, D., and Conrad, S. (2009). *Register, genre, and style*. New York: Cambridge University Press.

Cameron, L. and Maslen, R. (Eds.) (2010). *Metaphor analysis: Research practice in applied linguistics, social sciences and the humanities*. London: Equinox.

Deignan, A., Littlemore, J., and Semino, E. (2013). *Figurative language, genre and register*. Cambridge: Cambridge University Press.

Dörnyei, Z. (2007). *Research methods in applied linguistics: Quantitative, qualitative and mixed methodologies*. Oxford: Oxford University Press.

Grande, G., Stajduhar, K., Aoun, S., Toye, C., Funk, L., Addington-Hall, J., Payne, S., and Todd, C. (2009). Supporting lay carers in end of life care: Current gaps and future priorities. *Palliative Medicine*, *23*(4), 339–344.

Herring, S.C. (2007). A faceted classification scheme for computer-mediated discourse. *Language@Internet* 4 article 1.

Koven, M. (2011). Comparing stories told in interviews and spontaneous conversation. *Language in Society*, *40*(1), 75–89.

Lakoff, G., and Turner, M. (1989). *More than cool reason: A field guide to poetic metaphor*. Chicago: Chicago University Press.

Macmillan Dictionary Online. [online]. Available at: http://www.macmillandictionary.com/ [Accessed 29 Sep. 2017]

McArthur, T. (1981). *Longman lexicon of contemporary English*. London: Longman.

National Institute for Clinical Excellence (NICE). (2004). *Improving supportive and palliative care for adults with cancer: A manual*. London: NICE.

Payne, S., Chapman, A., Froggatt, K., Gott, M., and Chung, M. (2008). *Ethnicity and cancer: Examining psychosocial transitions for older people*. Final report, Dimbleby Cancer Care, September 2008. Retrieved from www.dimblebycancercare.org/upload/Payne%20FINAL%20report%20Aug%2008.pdf

Payne, S., Ingleton, C., Nolan, M., and O'Brien, T. (2009). *Evaluation of the help the hospices major grants programme for carers of those who are terminally ill*. Final report, Help the Hospices, July 2009.

Pragglejaz Group. (2007). MIP: A method for identifying metaphorically used words in discourse. *Metaphor and Symbol*, *22*(1), 1–39.

Prestin, A., and Chou, W. S. (2014). Web 2.0 and the changing health communication environment. In H. Hamilton and W. S. Chou (Eds.), *The Routledge handbook of language and health communication* (pp. 184–197). London and New York: Routledge.

Rayson, P. (2008). From key words to key semantic domains. *International Journal of Corpus Linguistics*, *13*(4), 519–549.

Rayson, P., Archer, D., Piao, S. L., and McEnery, T. (2004). The UCREL semantic analysis system. In *Proceedings of the Workshop on Beyond Named Entity Recognition Semantic Labelling for NLP tasks in association with 4th International Conference on Language Resources and Evaluation (LREC 2004)*, May 25, Lisbon, Portugal, pp. 7–12.

Seale, C., Charteris-Black, J., MacFarlane, A., and McPherson, A. (2010). Interviews and internet forums: A comparison of two sources of qualitative data. *Qualitative Health Research*, *20*(5), 595–606.

Steen, G. J., Dorst, A. G., Herrmann, B. J., Kaal, A. A., Krennmayr, T., and Pasma, T. (2010). *A method for linguistic metaphor identification: From MIP to MIPVU*. Amsterdam: John Benjamins.

Stommel, W., and Lamerichs, J. (2014). Interaction in online support groups: Advice and beyond. In H. Hamilton and W. S. Chou (Eds.), *The Routledge handbook of language and health communication* (pp. 198–211). London and New York: Routledge.

Suler, J. (2004). The online disinhibition effect. *CyberPsychology & Behavior*, 7(3), 321–326.
Swales, J. (1990). *Genre analysis*. Cambridge: Cambridge University Press.
Tausczik, Y. R., and Pennebaker, J. W. (2010). The psychological meaning of words: LIWC and computerized text analysis methods. *Journal of Language and Social Psychology*, *29*, 24–54.
Zhang, S., O'Carroll, E. B., Owen, J., Bakken, S., Elhadad, N. (2017). Online cancer communities as informatics intervention for social support: Conceptualization, characterization, and impact. *Journal of the American Informatics Association*, 24(2), 451–459.

Websites

eMargin. Retrieved April 2017, from http://emargin.bcu.ac.uk/

4 Key Topics and Main Metaphor Patterns in the Corpus

4.1 Introduction

Having described our 1.5-million-word corpus, the smaller sample corpus and the general research methodology in the previous chapter, we now turn in this chapter to an initial overview of our findings. This chapter has two major parts. Firstly, we will provide a general introduction to the differences in language usage across the three participant groups and the two genres that we have studied. This will take the form of a corpus analysis using a technique described in Chapter 3, that of keyness analysis, particularly as applied to semantic domains. This first part is not directly focused on metaphor analysis, but rather facilitates the beginnings of an understanding of the general shape and texture of the discourse in the corpus. In the second part of the chapter, we will focus on the main types of metaphor that we identified in the corpus using the computer-assisted techniques which we outlined in Chapter 3. The discussion will include quantitative and qualitative analyses of each type of metaphor across the various participant groups and genres in terms of topics and functions. From there, we will be able to draw some preliminary conclusions on variation in metaphor use in our corpus depending on genre and discourse community, and the role of different types of metaphors in talking and writing about cancer and the end of life. This preliminary analysis will then set the scene for the remainder of the book, by determining the types of metaphor that deserve more detailed consideration in the following chapters.

4.2 Vocabulary Differences in the Subcorpora

For a general introduction to and overview of our 1.5-million-word corpus, we begin here by applying exploratory corpus methods to expose the main topics and concepts mentioned in each of the subsets of the data from the three participant groups and two genres, and how these topics and concepts differ across subcorpora.

The keyness method we employ here has already been briefly introduced in Chapter 3. This method is very often used in corpus linguistics in an exploratory and comparative fashion to discover the 'aboutness' of a text or dataset, i.e. what is distinctive about it in terms of vocabulary (Scott and Tribble 2006). The method typically works at the word level. It involves taking a frequency list for a given text or corpus, that is, a list of distinct words (types) in the text along with how often they occur (tokens), and comparing the list to another word frequency list from a much larger reference corpus, or from another comparable corpus of similar size. For each word in the two lists, the frequencies in each corpus are compared by setting up a contingency table taking into account their expected relative sizes against the sizes of the two corpora. In general, some of the closed class ('grammatical' or 'function') words, such as 'the', 'of' and 'and', appear with similar relative frequencies in most corpora and therefore are usually not considered significant by the keywords procedure. However, if a word appears relatively more frequently in the text than might be expected compared to the reference corpus (including such function words), then it is considered 'key' (Scott 1997). Various filters can be applied to help thin out the list of words to be considered of interest for further analysis through methods such as concordances or collocations. For example, we may wish to remove low frequency items, of which there may not be enough examples to explain why the word is relevant. Alternatively, we could remove an item that is not well-dispersed (that is, spread evenly across different texts or sections in our corpus), since in such cases the higher relative frequency might be wholly due to just one writer or speaker who uses that word many more times than others, making the evidence of overuse across the whole corpus less convincing.

The same principle can be applied to any pair of comparable lists of quantifiable items. In this chapter, we apply this method to the comparison of the frequencies of semantic tags, which broadly correspond to topic areas in the data. We employ the Wmatrix software (introduced in Chapter 3), which runs each text through the semantic tagger and then prepares frequency lists for semantic tags. These lists are then compared so that we can see key semantic tags, also called key semantic domains (Rayson 2008), picked out by means of appropriate measures of statistical significance.

There are a number of different statistics that we can use in this comparison, from two main categories: significance and effect size. Significance tests can tell us how likely it is that we would observe a result if the difference between the two relative frequencies is due to random chance. In this book, we use the log-likelihood significance statistic for keyword calculation (Rayson and Garside 2000). Usually, if the statistics tell us that there is a 99% chance of non-randomness ($p < 0.01$; 1 d.f.; log-likelihood cut-off of 6.63), then we can say that the result is significant. In this chapter, we use the higher log-likelihood cut-off of 15.13 (99.99%, $p < 0.0001$, 1 d.f.). It should be noted that with larger frequencies and bigger corpora, there tends to be more evidence for any given comparison, and therefore usually higher significance values. This is why we use a more than usually stringent cut-off; it is also why we consider, as well as the significance test, certain effect size calculations.

Effect sizes emphasise the size of the difference between the two relative frequencies, rather than combining the size of the difference with the size of the corpora as significance statistics do. For our analyses we use the Log Ratio statistic (the binary log of the ratio of the relative frequencies) to calculate effect size. For example, a Log Ratio value of 1 indicates that the word is twice as common in our corpus as in the reference corpus, and higher Log Ratio values indicate much higher multiples. Using measures of significance and effect size in combination allows us both to see the amount of evidence for a frequency difference and to judge how important it might be. Further details of these statistics can be found in Rayson and Garside (2000) and Hardie (2014).

Having identified a set of key semantic tags in a particular section of our corpus, we can then use Wmatrix to see which words fit into each of the key categories, and to examine concordance lines by word or by semantic category to reconnect back with the underlying text. Thus, this approach combines corpus linguistics (keyness, concordance analysis) and natural language processing (tagging), as discussed in Chapter 2. As with all methods that involve one or more steps of automated analysis, we must always be aware of the potential for the computer to make mistakes. In this case, we have to bear in mind that the automated semantic tagger (UCREL Semantic Analysis System) is not perfect. It has a known, fairly small error rate (9%) in the semantic categories that it assigns to words or multiword expressions, and this has to be taken into account when drawing conclusions based on its results.

The following three subsections examine in turn the key semantic domains—or, in less technical terms, key topics—that emerge from a Wmatrix comparison of each participant group to the other two groups combined, highlighting where appropriate how these differ across our two genres (interviews and online fora). The complete lists of key semantic domains in each of the three subcorpora are provided in Appendix 2.

4.2.1 Key Topics: Patients

We began with the patients, comparing their interviews and online forum posts (600,993 words in total) with the combination of the carers' and professionals' data (924,931 words). There are 43 semantic tags that are statistically significantly overused by patients (with log-likelihood greater than or equal to 15.13), of which 5 items have a relative frequency at least twice as high as in the rest of the corpus (Log Ratio greater than or equal to 1) and another 15 items are around 50% more frequent in the patients' data (Log Ratio greater than 0.58).

Not surprisingly, patients talk about themselves a lot more than carers and professionals do. Wmatrix highlights the tag Z8 (Pronouns) as the most significant difference, and this is accounted for by words such as 'I', 'my' and 'me' being much more frequent in the patients' data. This trend is reflected in both the interviews and the online fora. We might also expect patients to focus in on certain elements of their medical treatment and to talk about their own bodies, and this is borne out with semantic tag B1 (Anatomy and physiology). This domain is very varied, covering 515 different word types. Moreover, there can be variation even in how a single word type is used; for example, patients talk about 'head' both literally and figuratively as in Examples 4.1 and 4.2 respectively (NB: in the examples presented in this section, we underline the words that were automatically tagged as belonging to the relevant semantic domain, whether or not they are used metaphorically; we also use the labels [I] and [O] to indicate whether an example is drawn, respectively, from the interviews or the online data; as in the rest of the book, original spellings are retained in extracts from the online forum data).

Example 4.1

My fiance kisses my head every morning and says hello peanuthead! [O]

Example 4.2

So sorry to hear its reared its ugly head and moving into other organs. [O]

References to other body parts ('hair', 'back', 'liver', 'breast', 'bowel' and 'brain') occur frequently in this semantic domain, along with words that refer to consequences, emotional or physical, of the treatment or condition (e.g. 'sleep', as in Example 4.3).

Example 4.3

Losing sleep seems to be one key side effect of a cancer diagnosis. [O]

One finding was perhaps surprising in data drawn from an online forum where patients and carers discuss life-threatening illness, medical treatment and other aspects of cancer: the key semantic tag E4.1+ (Happy). The most frequent words and phrases categorised in this group by the semantic tagger are 'lol' (i.e. laugh out loud), 'happy', 'fun', 'laugh(s/ing/ter)', 'funny', 'smile', 'sense of humour' and 'relief'. This reflects the fact that the forum contributors support one another, and suggests that this is often achieved by focusing on the positive, and by using humour to cheer each other up, as in Examples 4.4 and 4.5.

Example 4.4

Fight every inch of the way, but take the time to have fun, go to places you love, go to the woods and the sea to chill out.

[O]

Example 4.5

I think your encounter with the dye typifies the sense of humour we blooming well need to have to deal with what being's thrown at us!

[O]

Chapter 10 will explore such aspects of creativity and humour specifically in relation to metaphor on one particular thread of the online forum.

Negative emotions, on the other hand, are represented by the semantic tag E5− (Fear/shock), at about half the relative frequency of E4.1+ but still statistically significant. Patients tend to talk about being 'scared' of cancer or elements of the medical treatment; about their 'fear' of hospitals, of recurrence of the cancer, and of upsetting those around them; and about the 'shock' of the initial diagnosis. We will see later in this section, and in Chapter 9, how similar negative emotions are reflected and discussed by carers.

Two other key semantic domains serve to highlight potential differences between the use of language by patients and professionals in particular. F1 (Food), with terms such as 'eat', 'lunch', 'dinner' and 'meal', shows how much of the discussion centres around the social experiences and culture of eating with friends and family, as in Example 4.6. But we also see here words related to nutrition and nutritional advice given by health professionals, in references to different 'diets' such as 'high fibre' and 'low iodine'. The contexts of use of the word 'food' themselves bring out the difficulties of eating during or after cancer treatment, due to its effects on appetite, as shown in Example 4.7.

Example 4.6

but erm, and that's very nice, you go out and have a nice, nice meal and chat to people, and they bring you back

[O]

Example 4.7

Hi I know where you are coming from about no interest in food, I used to love my grub but after the operation I hated food

[O]

Similarly, the tag K5.1 (Sports) allows us to home in on terms which differentiate patients from the medical profession. It does include words and multiword expressions which refer to physiotherapy ('regular walks and exercise', 'exercise diary', 'post-op exercises'). But in addition, this category is a potentially good source of metaphors used by patients themselves such as 'waiting game' and cancer as a 'marathon' rather than a 'sprint'. We return to these metaphors in section 4.3.4.

Along with the focus on themselves, the patient section of the corpus also shows a large element of interpersonal discourse, which seems to serve a similar purpose to the supportive, humorous vocabulary described earlier. The key semantic tags A1.4 (Chance/luck) and A1.4+ (Lucky) alert us to the use of many expressions of support and solidarity, particularly in the online forum data, as in Examples 4.8 and 4.9.

Example 4.8

Good luck to those of you embarking on chemo or surgery soon.

[O]

Example 4.9

Fingers crossed this end as well for tomorrow and that she is feeling well.

[O]

The semantic tag Y2 (Information technology and computing) also allowed us to find many instances of the expression 'cyber hugs', which is used by some forum contributors as a closing formula at the end of their posts.

4.2.2 Key Topics: Professionals

Turning now to the professionals subcorpus (343,111 words), we compared this to the combined patients and carers subcorpora (1,182,813 words in total). In terms of statistical significance (a log-likelihood value greater than or equal to 15.13), there are 123 semantic tags that are worthy of further study. Of those, 72 show considerable size differences, that is, a Log Ratio value above 1, indicating at least a doubling in frequency in the professionals' language relative to patients and carers combined.

The fact that a greater number of significant differences arise from this comparison than from the other two comparisons among participant groups serves to illustrate the greater relative difference of the professionals' language to the other two subcorpora (partly related to the differences in data collection outlined in Chapter 3).

Two of the three most significant differences in frequency are the semantic tags L1– (Dead) and L1+ (Alive). These domains contain words and phrases such as 'death', 'dying', 'die(d)' and 'life threatening' (from L1–) and 'life', 'lives' and 'alive' (in L1+). To some extent, this is also a consequence of how we collected the data, and of the professionals' practice of discussing end-of-life care in terms of the whole process, both before and after death. But this result also suggests that carers in particular avoid explicit terms to do with death itself: we will return to this in the next subsection. In the professionals' data, these two semantic tags are also related to debates over ethically sensitive issues such as assisted suicide and to discussions about processes and experiences such as a 'good death' and a 'bad death'. We prompted the expression of views on the latter topic in the professionals' interviews by asking questions about the quality of alternative ways of dying. In Chapter 8, we will look in much more detail at how health professionals use metaphors to describe what they see as positive or negative experiences of death, and how these are differentiated according to the language and metaphors used in our corpus.

Many other key semantic tags in the profile of the professionals subcorpus serve to highlight discussion of professional practices, professional identity and the systems within which professionals operate. Both in the professionals' interviews and online fora, they are speaking and writing in a professional capacity, rather than a personal one. This leads to differences in style, which are reflected in the keyness of the semantic tag Z5 (grammatical bin) in particular. This domain is highly frequent in all English corpora, since it includes closed class words ('the', 'and', 'of', 'to'), but in this comparison it is significantly more frequent in the professionals' dataset than the rest of the corpus. The fourth most significant key domain, B3 (Medicines and medical treatment), points to topics such as healthcare settings ('hospice', 'hospital', 'ward'), healthcare professionals themselves ('doctor(s)', 'consultant(s)', 'nurse(s)' and 'GP(s)'), and, more generally, entities and processes in healthcare ('drugs', 'treatments', 'diagnosis'). Professionals do also talk about 'patient(s)', 'ill(ness)' and 'disease(s)' in domain B2– (Health and disease). Ethical issues and morality of medical decisions (G2.2+: Ethical), 'government' and 'state' (G1.1: Government) involvement in the National Health Service, the legalities around death and dying (G2:1: Law and order), and education and training (P1: Education) are all discussed more by professionals than by carers and patients.

As we previously noted, patients talk about themselves as individuals more, and we can observe the mirror image of this in the professionals subcorpus, which contains relatively more discussion about S5+ (Belonging to a group). Professionals refer to many different types of teams that they work in or liaise with: 'community team', 'physiotherapy and occupational therapist', 'chaplaincy and spiritual support team', 'hospice team' and 'palliative care team'. The same semantic tag also marks 'institutions' and 'organisation(s)' that they belong to. In particular, I3.1 (Work and employment) shows how much professionals talk about their working practices, working hours, roles and conditions, along with the importance of communication and of end-of-life care itself (in A11.1+, Important).

Professionals are bound by an ethical code of conduct, and as a result they do not disclose patient details from individual medical cases, whether in the interviews or on the online forum. They therefore use terms from semantic domains such as S2 (People) to create generalised, vague references when talking about their work in end-of-life care, as in Examples 4.10 and 4.11:

Example 4.10

That can be reassuring erm but so so actually giving people information again is very empowering erm for them.

[I]

Example 4.11

So lots of people will ask what is going to happen to me what will it be like.

[I]

Finally, in this subsection, professionals speak and write more than carers and patients do about religion and other terminology around faith. Semantic tags S9 (Religion and the Supernatural) and A7+++ (Likely) are key due to the higher relative frequency of terms such as 'Karma', 'religious', 'God', 'spiritual' and 'prayer'. Interestingly, many instances of these arise in contexts of reporting of beliefs and actions of patients and carers.

4.2.3 Key Topics: Carers

The final step in this initial overview of the corpus data is the comparison of the carers subcorpus (581,820 words) to the combination of the patients' and professionals' interviews and forum data (944,104 words). There are 45 significant semantic tags (with a log-likelihood of 15.13 and above). The effect sizes for the differences in relative frequency are typically lower than those we observed when looking at the healthcare professionals, with only 3 tags more than twice as frequent in the carers' data as elsewhere (Log Ratio of 1 or more). A further 9 semantic tags are between 50% and 100% more frequent here (Log Ratio above 0.58).

A large part of the carers' discourse in our subcorpus relates to other people in their lives. Semantic tag S4 (Kin) is the most significant key semantic tag here, with carers talking about close relations who are either patients themselves or people indirectly affected by another's illness: 'mum', 'dad', husband', 'son' and 'wife'. This is also reflected in the second key domain (Z1: Personal names), where they refer to the same types of people by name.

Time is a prominent domain for the carers. Semantic tag T1.1.2 (Time: present, simultaneous), which covers words and phrases such as 'now', 'today', 'at the moment' and 'tonight', highlights the focus in the carers' writing on the here and now. Just below the list of 12 main domains mentioned previously, but still significantly more frequent, are eight further time-related domains, including the future T1.1.3 ('will', 'tomorrow', 'soon'), the past T1.1.1 ('yesterday', 'last year', 'ago') and time periods T1.3 ('day', 'days', 'weeks', 'night'), for example. In the discourse around these terms related to time, carers talk about their uncertainty about the future and their sense of imminent loss and uncertainty; as well as the (possible or probable) death of the patient they care for, they also have to consider an additional time frame, namely that *following* the future death.

Bereavement itself emerges in discussions around the semantic tag X9.2– (Failure), in particular via words such as 'lost', 'losing' and 'lose'. Carers tend to use these terms instead of words such as 'death' itself, as we saw in the previous subsection, when talking about 'losing mum' for example. This domain also reflects, to a lesser degree, talk about 'losing' weight due to illness, but also the metaphorical expression of emotions ('feeling lost'). These also emerge in the domain O4.5 (Texture) via words such as 'hard' and 'wobbly', which carers use metaphorically to describe their own feelings and those of their loved one. Negative emotions ('upset', 'despair', 'regrets', 'suffering') are more specifically referred to by terms classed under the key semantic tag E4.1– (Sad), as illustrated in Examples 4.12 and 4.13. This domain is in direct contrast to the positive emotions expressed by patients that that we presented earlier. The metaphors used by carers to describe emotions following bereavement will be further and systematically considered in Chapter 9.

Example 4.12

His family say that I shouldn't <u>cry</u> in front of him what am I suppose to do

[O]

Example 4.13

I've been a bit sad this morning so I am going to rally and get out [O]

Just as in the patient subcorpus, we see key domains that reflect the supportive nature of the online fora in particular. The carers significantly overuse the tag S3.2 (Relationship), with the two most frequent words in this domain occurring very often together in sign-offs at the end of forum posts: 'love and hugs'. Similarly, the keyness of the semantic tag X2.6+ (Expected) is overwhelmingly a function of the high frequency of the single word 'hope', whose use reflects many instances of expression of support for fellow forum members, as in Example 4.14.

Example 4.14

there isn't really much I can say, I hope your dad doesn't get to poorly with the chemo [O]

The domain S1.2.5+ (Tough/strong) pulls together two of these topics, as the words within it are used to refer to the difficulties of getting through the days ahead ('tough times') but also emotional support to others ('I admire you and your inner strength'). Positive emotions and messages of support come through additionally in the domain E4.2+ (Content), representing words such as 'proud', 'pleased' and 'glad', used where carers write about their own achievements and those of others—including both the person that they are caring for and others in the forum.

4.2.4 Preliminary Summary

The three preceding analyses of key semantic domains amount to a comparative analysis of the contrasting topics observed in our data, focusing in turn on patients, professionals and carers and comparing each group to the other two. In our subcorpora, we have seen that patients tend to talk about themselves, elements of their treatments and their own bodies more than carers and professionals do. Patients' language also shows remarkable elements of humour in talking about their experiences of illness and end of life, but also negative emotions. The professionals subcorpus highlights discussions of professional issues and practices, healthcare settings and ethical decision-making, and the differences between 'good' and 'bad' deaths. Carers, as might be expected, talk about their close relations who are either ill or those who are directly affected, but also focus on many aspects of time (past, present and future), e.g. in terms of uncertainty about the future. Negative emotions also feature prominently, as do terms related to 'loss'.

As these preliminary results show, the corpus approach is a vital aid for getting to get to know the data better. The particular benefit of the keyness method for our purposes here is that the significant semantic categories lead us to read particular snippets of the corpus in concordances which we know merit attention because of their quantitative prominence.

4.3 Metaphor Patterns in the Corpus

We now move on from our overview of topics driven by the keyness method to a consideration of our central question—that is, the use of metaphor. Overall, the application of the method described in the previous chapter resulted in the identification of 6,686 instances of metaphor relevant to our topic in the corpus.

In Table 4.1, we show how these instances of metaphor are distributed across the different sections of our corpus. Given the differences in size between the different sections (see Chapter 3), in the table we provide both raw frequencies and normalised frequencies per 1,000 words.[1]

Overall, the metaphors we identified occur 4.4 times per 1,000 words in the whole corpus. Apart from the interviews with patients and family carers, the frequencies of metaphors in the different sections of the corpus are roughly similar to the overall frequency, ranging between 4.1 instances per 1,000 words (professional interviews) and 5.2 instances per 1,000 words (patients online). It is nonetheless noticeable that the highest relative frequency of metaphors in our corpus was found in the online patient data.

But Table 4.1 also shows that the interviews with patients and carers have much lower frequencies of metaphor than the mean for the corpus as a whole: 2.1 and 2.3 instances per 1,000 words respectively. This is likely to be primarily because the factual kinds of questions that were asked in these interviews were not conducive to emotional disclosure and evaluative comments, which are often conveyed through metaphor in other sections of the corpus. More generally, there is evidence from experimental studies that the use of metaphor is perceived to be more appropriate in interactions involving people who have more intimate rather than more distant relationships (see Katz 2017 for an overview). This may be relevant to our data. It is possible that patients and carers perceived their relationship with the interviewer as relatively more distant and formal than did the hospice managers we interviewed. Moreover, there is evidence in our data and from previous studies that relationships in peer-to-peer online patient fora are perceived and constructed as intimate even if contributors do not know one another's full identities and never meet offline (e.g. Allen et al. 2016). In fact, as mentioned in Chapter 3, it is this opportunity to maintain at least partial anonymity that fosters openness

Table 4.1 Raw Frequencies and Normalised Frequencies of Instances of Metaphor We Identified Through Our Main Method

Corpus Sections	*Interviews*		*Online Fora*		*Overall*	
	Raw Frequencies	*Per 1,000 Words*	*Raw Frequencies*	*Per 1,000 Words*	*Raw Frequencies*	*Per 1,000 Words*
Patients	209	2.1	2,613	5.2	2,822	4.7
Carers	187	2.3	2,228	4.5	2,415	4.2
Professionals	366	4.1	1,083	4.3	1,449	4.2
Overall	762	2.8	5,924	4.7	6,686	4.4

in communication and a perception of close personal relationships (Seale et al. 2010).

In Table 4.2, the raw frequencies of instances of metaphor are broken down according to the 10 main groups/types of metaphors we identified in the data, i.e. linguistic metaphors with literal meanings falling under one of the following broad semantic fields: Animals, Journey, Machines, Obstacles, Openness, Religion and the Supernatural, Restraint, Sports and Games, Violence, and Wholeness. This involved grouping the domains expressed by the semantic tagset under the broader headings we developed in the analysis of the sample corpus (see Appendix 3).

Overall, Violence and Journey metaphors are the two most frequent types, in the corpus as a whole and in all six sections. More specifically, what we call Violence metaphors[2] are the most frequent type of metaphor overall and in each section of the corpus except for professional interviews, where Journey metaphors are the most frequent and Violence metaphors the second most frequent type of metaphor. Both types of metaphors were introduced in the discussion of the example from the online carer data we considered in Chapter 1. Given their frequencies in the corpus, and the attention they have received in relation to cancer and end of life (see Chapters 1 and 2), we will devote a chapter each to Violence and Journey metaphors (Chapters 5 and 6 respectively).

In the rest of this chapter, we consider each of the other eight types of metaphor in turn, in decreasing order of frequency in the corpus as a whole. In each case, we provide a brief overview, present some illustrative examples and indicate where each type of metaphor is discussed further in Chapters 7 to 10 of this book.

4.3.1 Restraint Metaphors

Both patients and carers talk about the consequences of cancer in their lives in terms of being physically restrained in a particular location. This applies particularly to the inability to leave their homes as much as was

Table 4.2 Raw Frequencies of 10 Types of Metaphors in the Corpus and Frequencies per 1,000 Words

Metaphors	*Patients*			*Carers*			*Professionals*			*Totals*
	Interviews	*Online*	*Total*	*Interviews*	*Online*	*Total*	*Interviews*	*Online*	*Total*	
Violence	72 (0.71)	899 (1.79)	971 (1.61)	80 (0.98)	807 (1.61)	887 (1.52)	73 (0.81)	337 (1.33)	410 (1.19)	2268 (1.48)
Journey	56 (0.55)	730 (1.45)	786 (1.30)	28 (0.34)	384 (0.76)	412 (0.70)	98 (1.08)	217 (0.85)	315 (0.92)	1513 (0.99)
Restraint	29 (0.29)	257 (0.51)	286 (0.47)	34 (0.41)	176 (0.35)	210 (0.36)	57 (0.63)	169 (0.67)	226 (0.66)	722 (0.47)
Animals	18 (0.18)	120 (0.24)	138 (0.23)	9 (0.11)	397 (0.79)	406 (0.69)	2 (0.02)	48 (0.19)	50 (0.14)	594 (0.39)
Openness	13 (0.13)	186 (0.37)	199 (0.33)	17 (0.20)	146 (0.29)	163 (0.28)	53 (0.59)	148 (0.58)	201 (0.58)	563 (0.37)
Sports and Games	1 (0.01)	124 (0.25)	125 (0.21)	5 (0.06)	72 (0.14)	77 (0.15)	18 (0.20)	50 (0.98)	68 (0.19)	270 (0.18)
Religion and the Supernatural	1 (0.01)	139 (0.28)	140 (0.23)	0	92 (0.18)	92 (0.16)	2 (0.02)	24 (0.09)	26 (0.07)	258 (0.17)
Obstacles	5 (0.49)	71 (0.14)	76 (0.13)	7 (0.08)	56 (0.11)	63 (0.11)	24 (0.27)	62 (0.24)	86 (0.25)	225 (0.14)
Wholeness	4 (0.39)	58 (0.11)	62 (0.10)	3 (0.04)	62 (0.12)	65 (0.11)	16 (0.18)	16 (0.06)	32 (0.09)	159 (0.10)
Machines	10 (0.09)	29 (0.06)	39 (0.06)	4 (0.05)	36 (0.07)	40 (0.07)	23 (0.25)	12 (0.05)	35 (0.10)	114 (0.07)
Totals	209 (2.1)	2,613 (5.2)	**2,822 (4.7)**	187 (2.3)	2,228 (4.5)	**2,415 (4.2)**	366 (4.1)	1,083 (4.3)	**1,449 (4.2)**	**6,686 (4.4)**

previously possible, so that the house becomes a 'trap'. The following example is taken from the patient online section of the corpus (NB: from this point in the book onwards, we will underline in each example the relevant metaphorical expression(s), or a complete simile or other figurative comparison):

Example 4.15

I feel so trapped in the house, all I am doing is either going to the hospital or hospice. The days of my going out shopping etc are over.

[O]

The same scenario of physical restraint is evoked by the use of 'escape' or similar expressions in reference to the rare occasions when it is possible to do what one wants (Example 4.16) or, in the case of carers, to be temporarily relieved from looking after a sick family member (Example 4.17):

Example 4.16

At least not having to keep visiting the hospital gives me a little bit more money (no taxi fares, no extra prescriptions which I'd been told I wouldn't need, but did), and unchains me to go off to stay with friends and do things.

[O]

Example 4.17

Well i hope you get a few minutes to yourself and recharge your batteries. or have a hot soak in the tub that does wonders to me when I can escape for half an hour.

[O]

Restraint metaphors are used by patients and carers for a variety of other unwelcome consequences of one's own or a family member's cancer. For example, one carer writing online describes the experience of living with her son's illness as being 'trapped in a nightmare'. Likewise, in Example 4.18, a patient uses a simile involving imprisonment to express how she feels about not being allowed by healthcare professionals to eat what she wants, and particularly ice cream:

Example 4.18

Am I pathetic wanting that or what but I feel like a prisoner with all the rules about don't eat this don't do that.

[O]

Overall, Restraint metaphors convey the negative perceptions and emotions associated with not being able to live as one wants, including the inability to be the person that one would like to be (or formerly was). In cases such as Example 4.15, these metaphors show how being at home becomes associated with frustration when it is due to the illness rather than one's choice. For carers in particular, metaphors to do with 'escaping' from the house or caring duties also provide a way of conveying implicitly some degree of frustration with or even resentment at their situation, where voicing these feelings explicitly would make them seem insensitive towards the person who is ill. In fact, by focusing on the 'escape' rather than the restraint, carers are being especially indirect about this negative aspect of caring. Healthcare professionals use similar metaphors in relation to the experiences of carers, as when one of our interviewees comments that 'carers can become isolated and trapped in the home'.

Overall, Restraint metaphors occur in all sections of the corpus, with minor differences in relative frequencies across the various subsections. We will return to these metaphors in Chapter 7 when we discuss healthcare professionals' descriptions of the emotional aspects of their relationships with patients.

4.3.2 Animal Metaphors

As Table 4.2 shows, Animal metaphors in the corpus are primarily used by patients and carers writing online, but are rather infrequent in the online healthcare professional section and in all three interview sections of the corpus.

Both patients and carers describe cancer negatively as a 'beast', as in the following extracts from, respectively, the patient and carer online data:

> *Example 4.19*
>
> Dear Gabrielle, I am so sorry to hear that the beast is back after all of your positivity and bravery
>
> [O]

> *Example 4.20*
>
> After todays test when you get the results you will have the name of the beast you both will have to beat together
>
> [O]

The use of 'beast' emphasises the seriousness of the disease and the vulnerability of the person who is ill. In cases such as Example 4.20, 'beast' frames the cancer as an aggressive opponent within an antagonistic Violence scenario where the goal of the patient and their family is to 'beat' the illness. We will discuss these scenarios further in Chapter 5.

Animal metaphors are also used by both patients and carers to describe themselves in self-deprecatory terms, usually because of attitudes or behaviours that are part of the experience of illness. Several patients use 'chicken' metaphorically to suggest that they perceive themselves as the opposite of the conventional notion of the 'brave' cancer patient, as in the following extract:

> *Example 4.21*
>
> I am sooooo not brave . . . I'm the worlds biggest chicken . . . it use to take me all the time to go for a damn blood test
>
> [O]

In Example 4.22, a carer uses the simile 'like a bloody limpid [i.e. 'limpet']' to suggest that she is overly fearful about leaving her husband alone:

> *Example 4.22*
>
> I would hate for him to take a funny turn when he was alone so I am like a bloody limpid all day and night.
>
> [O]

Both patients and carers use similes involving scared animals in headlights to describe patients' vulnerability, anxiety and disempowerment at particular points in the experience of illness. In the following extract, a carer shares her worries about how much more anxious and fearful her husband appears to have become in relatively routine situations:

> *Example 4.23*
>
> We bought a new tv [. . .] my son in law st [set] it up and stuff [NAME OF HUSBAND] is terrified of it not in the ill way I'm used to this is extreme he looks like a scared animal in car headlights or something
>
> [O]

Some Animal metaphors, by contrast, are humorous self-descriptions, particularly when patients writing online try to put a positive spin on the changes in physical appearance caused by treatment:

> *Example 4.24*
>
> I'm doing fine and no one can tell I have been ill except for my slow growing hair—but some even think it's fashionable—I think I look like a poodle and you can see my photo on my home page
>
> [O]

The humorous use of Animal metaphors is also the reason for their higher frequency in the online carer data, in contrast with the online patient data, as well as with other sections of the corpus. Some carers on our online forum use animal terms as their handles (i.e. visible usernames). These terms then provide the inspiration for humorous and creative uses of further Animal metaphors in some interactions.[3] As well as providing some light relief in the discussion of difficult and sombre topics, these uses of Animal metaphors seem to strengthen the mutual relationships among forum contributors, and to reinforce the sense of a discourse community that shares a number of in-jokes within the context of sharing a difficult life predicament. In Chapter 10, we present in detail the use of humorous metaphors for self- and other-empowerment and social bonding in one particular thread on the cancer online forum. We return to Animal metaphors in Chapter 7, when discussing the metaphors used by patients and healthcare professionals to describe their mutual relationships.

4.3.3 Openness Metaphors

The members of all three participant groups use Openness metaphors to describe the ability and willingness to talk honestly and explicitly about one's emotions, a cancer diagnosis and/or the imminence of death. The following examples are taken from an interview with a patient (Example 4.25), a forum post by a carer (Example 4.26) and an interview with a hospice manager (Example 4.27):

Example 4.25

she came on and said 'Mum I don't know what to say.' I said 'We talk about it.' I was so busy putting her at ease, and from then on we were <u>open</u> we talked about it,

[I]

Example 4.26

Perhaps if you can tell your mum how you feel it will be upsetting but if things are out in the <u>open</u> it will be easier to move on to the next stage

[O]

Example 4.27

I would worry more about someone who wasn't <u>open</u> with their emotions

[I]

Conversely, inability or reluctance to communicate in a frank and explicit manner about illness and death are described metaphorically using expressions such as 'shutting others out/off' or 'locking oneself away'. The following extracts are taken from, respectively, our patient and carer data:

Example 4.28

I love my family so much but tend to shut them out because of the way I am trying to cope with the unknown.

[O]

Example 4.29

My mum chose the same route as yours choosing to lock herself away and wasting the little time she had left and i found it very frustrating as i was her carer 24/7

[O]

The metaphorical contrast between Open and Closed has evaluative implications that are very much in evidence in our data: by and large, behaviours that are described as 'open' are evaluated positively, and behaviours that are described in terms of expressions to do with being closed are evaluated negatively. On the one hand, the general encouragement of honesty and explicitness in our data can be seen as a welcome move towards the reduction of isolation and stigma in the experience of cancer and end of life. On the other hand, the metaphorical opposition between Open and Closed can lead to a judgemental attitude towards the legitimate choice not to reveal one's emotions or not to wish to talk about one's illness or impending death.

We return to these implications of Openness metaphors in Chapter 8, where we discuss the metaphors that healthcare professionals use to talk about 'good' and 'bad' deaths. In that chapter, we focus particularly on our interviews with hospice managers, where, as shown in Table 4.2, Openness metaphors are more frequent, in both absolute and relative terms, than in the interviews with patients and carers.

4.3.4 Sports and Games Metaphors

As shown in Table 4.2, Sports and Games metaphors are almost absent from the patient and carer interviews, but feature to roughly similar extents in the other sections of the corpus. More specifically, as we mentioned earlier, the semantic tag K5.1 (Sports) is overused in the patient data as compared with the rest of the corpus, and this is in part due to metaphorical uses of Sports vocabulary in the online patient data.

Both patients and healthcare professionals use the opposition between a 'sprint' and a 'marathon' metaphorically to suggest that, like a marathon, cancer requires sustained effort, determination and resilience over a long period of time. In the following extract, a doctor writing online explicitly suggests that the 'marathon versus sprint' metaphor is a good way to prepare someone to care for a person with a terminal illness:

Example 4.30

> An explanation that can work well in this circumstance is that caring for somebody with a terminal illness is more of a <u>marathon</u> rather than a <u>sprint</u>.
>
> [O]

Sports metaphors are also used by patients and carers to praise and encourage one another. For example, a young woman with breast cancer who lives alone with her three children is described by another forum contributor as 'a BC Gold medallist'. In the following extract, a patient on the online forum is similarly described as a winner in a contest against cancer:

Example 4.31

> KNOW in your mind you will <u>beat</u> this whatever it throws at you, however hard it is and however weak at times you may feel . . . only one <u>WINNER</u>—YOU!!
>
> [O]

These uses of Sport metaphors share with some Violence metaphors the idea of an antagonistic and competitive relationship with the disease, so that the illness experience is framed as leading to the patient's victory or defeat. As we show in more detail in Chapter 5, these metaphors can have negative implications, for example if they generate unrealistic expectations or if they are used in the terminal phase of the disease. However, they can also be used, as in the preceding examples, to present oneself or others as determined and empowered in the experience of illness. Both the 'gold medallist' and 'only one WINNER' examples also implicitly frame other forum participants as admiring fans of the person who is being addressed.

Finally, the online patient data contains 35 references to a cancer 'card' or 'cards', which can be 'played' or 'used' to receive special treatment or to excuse anti-social behaviours on account of having cancer. Two examples are given here:

Example 4.32

I just get fed up with all the phone calls and visitors sometimes!!!! Never mind I am smiling and will just play the ole cancer card and see what I can get this afternoon

[O]

Example 4.33

I said yes to an invite out but really don't want to go so I have just used the cancer card to get out of it.

[O]

As these extracts show, the 'cancer card' usually describes in humorous terms the strategies that can be used to turn one's cancer into a social advantage. Here the opponents in the metaphorical game are people who are not ill, rather than the cancer itself (see Semino and Demjén 2017 for a more detailed analysis of the 'cancer card' metaphor in a particular thread on our online forum). As we have mentioned before, we return to the topic of humorous metaphors in the patient online data in Chapter 10.

4.3.5 Religion and the Supernatural Metaphors

Metaphors drawing from the broad domains of religion and the supernatural are almost completely absent from the interview data, and are more frequent in online forum contributions by patients than by the two other participant groups.

Both patients and carers on the online forum describe distressing situations as being in 'hell', and situations of uncertainty and lack of activity (e.g. waiting for hospital appointments or test results) as being in 'limbo'. Perhaps less conventionally, both groups also refer to cancer as a 'demon' and a 'monster'. Similarly to what we noticed in relation to 'beast' earlier, these expressions emphasise the vulnerability of patients in the context of a life-threatening and unpredictable disease. The following extract is by a patient who, like several others on the online forum, finds it more difficult to cope with anxiety while not being treated with chemotherapy:

Example 4.34

when I was on treatment I felt in control of the disease, now I just feel like a sitting duck waiting for the green eyed monster to come up and swallow me whole.

[O]

Here the description of the cancer as a 'green-eyed monster'[4] is part of a lengthy simile in which the patient places herself in an extremely disempowered position—that of a 'sitting duck' waiting to be 'swallow[ed] [. . .] whole'. This situation is explicitly compared with the feeling of being 'in control of the disease' during the treatment. Indeed, at an earlier point the same patient recounts how she used the metaphor of tumours as 'dragons' to explain cancer to her young children in terms they could understand. When she started chemotherapy, she reassured them by extending the same metaphor in a way that placed her in the empowered position of 'dragon slayer':

Example 4.35

> When I started chemo I told them I had to have yucky medicine to try and kill my dragons (that's what we called my tumours) my children are very much into star wars, light sabers and slaying dragons, so mummy was the biggest dragon slayer in town!
>
> [O]

We return to some of these metaphors in Chapter 7, where we show how patients and healthcare professionals draw from the supernatural and magic to describe their mutual relationships.

4.3.6 *Obstacle Metaphors*

All three participant groups in our corpus talk—quite conventionally—about different kinds of difficulties as 'obstacles' and 'hurdles'. Patients in particular use these expressions metaphorically to talk about the illness, their treatment and the aspects of the healthcare system that they perceive as difficult to deal with. In the following extract, for example, a patient describes a dispensary pharmacist and her GP's receptionists as 'blockers', while venting her frustration about not being able to obtain the new medication prescribed by the GP:

Example 4.36

> So add the dispensery pharmacist to the GP's receptionists and you've got the two big blockers to me getting what I need.
>
> [O]

In Chapter 5, we show how Violence metaphors are similarly used by some patients (and healthcare professionals) to convey the difficulties they experience within the healthcare system, and therefore to express a negative evaluation of some healthcare professionals.

On the other hand, some healthcare professionals in our data use words such as 'barrier' metaphorically to talk about difficulties in communication with patients. In the following extract, one of the hospice managers we interviewed reflects on the consequences of patients in hospices being angry that they are going to die:

> *Example 4.37*
>
> I think that's one of the things that I found most difficult as a <u>barrier</u> to communication.
>
> [I]

These metaphors are similar to the Openness metaphors we discussed earlier, in that they evaluate negatively patients' reluctance to talk explicitly about their emotions and their own end-of-life situation. We will return to these metaphors and their potential implications for end-of-life care in Chapter 8.

4.3.7 Wholeness Metaphors

Metaphors to do with Wholeness, and particularly loss of Wholeness, are primarily used by patients and carers writing online to talk about the consequences of illness or bereavement for their own mental states, self-perceptions and sense of identity.

Some patients writing online use what Lakoff (1996) calls 'split-self' metaphors to describe differences in their own attitudes or behaviours at different points in time, as in the case of expressions such as 'my normal/jokey/chatty self' (see also Emmott 2002). In such cases, patients also tend to convey, more or less explicitly, contrasting evaluations of the different 'selves' that metaphorically make up the whole person. Patients' own current self-perceptions are sometimes contrasted unfavourably with a previous 'normal self' that the person wishes they could be once again. Similarly, patients sometimes apologise for being unusually quiet or pessimistic on the online forum, and promise to be 'back to' their more socially acceptable selves as soon as they can. One patient, for example, says that she had not posted on the forum for a while because she had been 'not so good mentally', and later adds, 'I will be back to my jokey self in no time'.

Carers who continue to contribute to the online forum after the death of the person they cared for often convey their emotions in terms of loss of physical wholeness (e.g. 'you realise you are only half a person'). We will discuss these metaphors in more detail in Chapter 9.

4.3.8 Machine Metaphors

Machine metaphors are the least frequent of the 10 main types of metaphor we identified in our data, with just over 100 instances in the whole corpus (see Table 4.2). These include a number of highly conventional metaphorical expressions for people's mental lives, such as 'coping mechanism' or 'switching off' from worries. Here we will focus on two particular machinery-related metaphors that are used to capture situations that patients find themselves in at various points in the experience of illness: 'roller coaster' and 'treadmill'.

'Roller coaster' is conventionally used in English generally to talk about experiences that involve extreme and uncontrollable alternations between positive and negative situations or emotions. On the online forum, patients tend to use this expression to acknowledge others' difficulties or to prepare them for future difficulties. However, in most cases the notion of upward movement is used metaphorically to express or instil hope that things will eventually improve, as in the following example:

Example 4.38

i know you are on <u>rollercoaster</u> and many <u>downward hills</u> but it can't keep <u>going down</u>—i am willing for there to be a very big <u>up</u> just round the corner.

[O]

In one particular online forum post by a patient, the notion of a metaphorical roller coaster is part of a creative and humorous simile to do with fairgrounds, which the writer uses to both convey the gruesome effects of chemotherapy and simultaneously make light of them:

my blog's updated if you need proof that this chemo is <u>like a visit to the fairground</u>—<u>dodgems</u>, <u>ghost train</u>, <u>waltzer</u>, <u>dive bomber</u> and <u>roller coaster</u> all combined in one <u>ride</u>—at least I have not been sick yet

[O]

The expression 'treadmill' is also used metaphorically to talk about the experience of treatment. Like 'roller coaster', it places the patient in a disempowered position, but it also emphasises repetitiveness and a perception of lack of individuality, as in the following example from the patient online forum:

Example 4.39

I'm not really happy about being back on the <u>treadmill</u> of treatment especially weekly but I've done it before so I suppose I can get through it again

[O]

In Chapter 7, we will discuss other similar uses of Machine metaphors for treatment and the healthcare systems, as used by both patients and healthcare professionals.

4.4 Conclusions

In this chapter, we began by using the semantic tagger software, and the facilities for keyness analysis and concordances afforded by the Wmatrix tool, to identify the semantic domains that are overused to a statistically significant extent by each of the three participant groups in our corpus as compared with the other two combined. This has revealed that patients use more pronouns than the other two groups, as well as more words that relate to the body, food, positive and negative emotions, and the creation and maintenance of supportive relationships on the online forum. Family carers, on the other hand, overuse words that relate to kinship, time and negative emotions, particularly in relation to grieving. And healthcare professionals overuse words to do with their professional concerns, including death and dying, medicine and healthcare, groups of people, and religion and spirituality. We have pointed out how this kind of analysis sheds light on the different perspectives and concerns of each group regarding illness, the end of life and healthcare, and led us to identify certain prominent topics which will be considered in more detail later in the book, i.e. how metaphors are used by healthcare professionals to talk about quality of death (Chapter 8) and by family carers to talk about bereavement and grieving (Chapter 9).

In the second half of the chapter, we began by presenting the frequencies and distributions of the 10 most frequent groups of metaphors identified in the corpus using our main method. While we devote the following two chapters to the two most frequent types (Violence and Journey metaphors), here we considered in turn the remaining eight types, through brief overviews and illustrative examples. On the basis of that discussion, we can now make several important observations, to which we will return in the rest of the book. A range of different types of metaphor are used in our data to frame the experience of cancer and the end of life in different ways. This is especially significant since media attention and policy decisions (as outlined in Chapters 1 and 2) have only focused on Violence and Journey metaphors. In our data, for example, the 'marathon' metaphor for having cancer emphasises the need for sustained effort and perseverance over a long period of time, while the 'roller coaster' metaphor emphasises lack of control and a constant alternation between emotional extremes. Some metaphors are used for specific aspects of the experience of illness, such as 'treadmill' for treatment and being 'trapped' for the inability to leave the house as much as one wishes. In contrast, some other metaphors can be used in different ways in different contexts, resulting in different framings, especially in terms of the (dis)empowerment of patients. We observed this many times throughout the analyses. For example, the metaphor of cancer as a 'dragon/monster' is used in two contrasting ways by the same patient—first to present herself as an empowered 'dragon slayer' for the benefit of her children, then to present herself as a helpless 'sitting duck' when not receiving treatment.

We also repeatedly pointed out how metaphors are used to evaluate situations, people and behaviours. This applies, for example, to Animal metaphors for describing oneself or others, and to metaphors of Openness or lack of it for people's approaches to communication during illness or at the end of life. As we mentioned in previous chapters, such evaluation is related to the framing effects of metaphors. We return to both of these in the following chapters. The analysis has also begun to show the variety of interpersonal functions that metaphors are used for, such as to explain, comfort, encourage or entertain others, and to form and strengthen social bonds, especially on the online forum.

Concerning the distribution of metaphors in our data, we have noted that metaphors are less frequent in the patient and carer interviews than in the other sections of the corpus, possibly because the questions and level of formality in these interviews were less conducive to eliciting discussion of the topics and functions that metaphors are used for in the other sections of the corpus. This reinforces previous research showing that metaphor use is dependent on genre (e.g. Deignan et al. 2013). Finally, we have pointed out patterns of metaphor use that are more or less typical of particular participant groups. For example, cancer is described as a 'beast', 'monster' or 'dragon' by patients and carers, but not by healthcare professionals. On the other hand, the metaphor of communication problems as 'barriers' is more characteristic of the discourse of healthcare professionals.

In the next two chapters, we turn to the two most frequent types of metaphors in our data—Violence and Journey metaphors.

Notes

1. We will not compare frequencies in our corpus with those found in other studies (e.g. Steen et al. 2010), as our approach focuses on particular topics and semantic domains, rather than attempting to identify all instances of metaphor in the corpus.
2. As we explain in more detail in Chapter 5, these include the different kinds of metaphors that have been variously referred to as Battle, Fight, War or Military metaphors.
3. We do not discuss these Animal metaphors in detail because that would involve mentioning the online handles of some contributors, which goes against the approach to preserving anonymity we have adopted.
4. The expression 'green-eyed monster' is used in Shakespeare's Othello to describe jealousy, but this potential allusion does not seem relevant here.

References

Allen, C., Vassilev, I., Kennedy, A., and Rogers, A. (2016). Long-term condition self-management support in online communities: A meta-synthesis of qualitative papers. *Journal of Medical Internet Research*, *18*(3), e61.

Deignan, A., Littlemore, J., and Semino, E. (2013). *Figurative language, genre and register*. Cambridge: Cambridge University Press.

Demjén, Z., and Semino, E. (2017). Using metaphor in healthcare: Physical health. In E. Semino and Z. Demjén (Eds.), *The Routledge handbook of metaphor and language* (pp. 385–399). London and New York: Routledge.

Emmott, C. (2002). 'Split selves' in fiction and in medical life stories: Cognitive linguistic theory and narrative practice. In E. Semino and J. Culpeper (Eds.), *Cognitive stylistics: Language and cognition in text analysis* (pp. 153–181). Amsterdam: John Benjamins.

Hardie, A. (2014). Log ratio—an informal introduction. *CASS Blog*. Retrieved June 16, 2016, from http://cass.lancs.ac.uk/?p=1133

Katz, A. (2017). Psycholinguistic approaches to metaphor acquisition and use. In E. Semino and Z. Demjén (eds) *The Routledge handbook of metaphor and language* (pp. 472–485). Abingdon: Routledge.

Lakoff, G. (1996). Sorry, I'm not myself today: The metaphor system for conceptualizing the self. In G. Fauconnier and E. Sweetser (Eds.), *Spaces, worlds and grammar* (pp. 91–123). Chicago: University of Chicago Press.

Rayson, P. (2008). From key words to key semantic domains. *International Journal of Corpus Linguistics*, *13*(4), 519–549.

Rayson, P., and Garside, R. (2000). Comparing corpora using frequency profiling. In *Proceedings of the workshop on Comparing Corpora, held in conjunction with the 38th annual meeting of the Association for Computational Linguistics (ACL 2000)*, October 1–8, Hong Kong, pp. 1–6.

Scott, M. (1997). PC analysis of key words—and key key words. *System* (ITALICS), *25*(2), 233–245.

Scott, M., and Tribble, C. (2006). *Textual patterns: Key words and corpus analysis in language education*. Amsterdam: John Benjamins.

Seale, C., Charteris-Black, J., MacFarlane, A., and McPherson, A. (2010). Interviews and internet forums: A comparison of two sources of qualitative data. *Qualitative Health Research*, *20*(5), 595–606.

Steen, G. J., Dorst, A. G., Herrmann, J. B., Kaal, A. A., Krennmayr, T., and Pasma, T. (2010). *A method for linguistic metaphor identification: From MIP to MIPVU*. Amsterdam: John Benjamins.

5 Violence Metaphors

5.1 Introduction

Controversies around the use of Battle, War or Military metaphors in the context of cancer regularly surface in the UK and US media. In April 2014, Kate Granger, a consultant geriatrician with advanced cancer,[1] began an opinion piece in the UK's *Guardian* newspaper with:

> 'She lost her brave fight.' If anyone mutters those words after my death, wherever I am, I will curse them. [. . .] I do not want to feel a failure about something beyond my control. I refuse to believe my death will be because I didn't battle hard enough.
>
> (Granger 2014)

A few months earlier, Bill Keller (2014), writing in the *New York Times*, implicitly critiqued the online behaviour of Lisa Bonchek Adams,[2] a writer and activist with metastatic breast cancer, as a 'very public cage fight with death'. As we outlined in Chapters 1 and 2, critiques of this kind date back at least to Susan Sontag's work in the 1970s and 1980s. On the other side of the debate, people like the Pulitzer Prize-winning journalist Amanda Bennett argue for the benefits of such 'heroic' narratives. Bennett (re-)claimed War metaphors in a 2013 TED Talk focusing on the experience of her husband's death from cancer.

The many critiques of Violence metaphors (e.g. also Miller 2010; Hurley 2014; McCartney 2014) cogently spell out why these metaphors can be harmful for patients: they position patient and illness as opponents, and suggest that not recovering is a personal defeat. On the other hand, it has also been suggested that these metaphors can be motivating for some (e.g. Reisfield and Wilson 2004, as well as Bennett 2013). There is, however, no systematic evidence to date of how often and in what ways these metaphors are actually used, and of the specific circumstances and uses that result in (dis)empowering framings (see Chapter 1 for our definition of (dis)empowerment). For example, debates such as those just described tend to assume that there is such a thing as a homogeneous

'War metaphor' when it comes to cancer, and that its implications tend to be consistent across contexts. It is also clear that, regardless which side of the debate one favours, the tendency to talk about cancer (and other difficult enterprises) in terms of these metaphors is highly conventional in English. Indeed, as we outlined in Chapter 4, Violence metaphors were the most frequently used type of metaphor in our corpus.

With this in mind, this chapter presents a quantitative and qualitative analysis of the ways in which Violence metaphors are used by the three participant groups in our corpus, and how these different uses can be variously interpreted as empowering or disempowering, particularly for patients. In the next section, we begin by introducing the specific aspects of our corpus linguistic method that are applied in this chapter. We then address our analysis in two phases: quantitative and qualitative. First, we give a quantitative overview—looking at the frequencies of Violence metaphors across the different participant groups and genres present in our corpus. Already in this quantitative section we show that Violence metaphors have multiple specific linguistic realisations, which are in turn used to different degrees by our three groups of participants. These quantitative findings inform the subsequent phase of qualitative analysis. By considering specific examples of Violence metaphor use in context, we demonstrate that members of all three groups use a much wider set of Violence metaphors than has been noted in previous studies, and each group uses them in a range of ways for different topics. We will organise our discussion of these uses based on topic and participant group, and comment on their likelihood to have empowering or disempowering effects for the participants concerned, discursively speaking. In this way, we address directly the debates and controversies surrounding the use of Violence metaphors in the context of cancer and the end of life.

In our conclusion to this chapter, we summarise our findings and briefly consider some issues regarding their implications for the practice of healthcare communication. However, a full treatment of these implications is reserved for the end of the next chapter, and we recommend that the present chapter be read together with Chapter 6 on Journey metaphors. Journey metaphors are, of course, also highly conventional in English, and are indeed the second most frequently used metaphor in our corpus (see Chapter 4). More importantly for the present discussion, the critique of Violence metaphors has tended to go hand in hand with a promotion of Journey metaphors as more positive and helpful alternatives, including in policy documents in the UK (see section 6.1 in the next chapter for more detail).

5.2 Methodology for the Retrieval of Potential Violence Metaphors

The details of method given in this section will be largely of interest to linguists; readers in other disciplines may wish to continue directly to section 5.3. In line with our methodology outlined in Chapter 3, we identified Violence metaphors in the manual analysis of a sample of our data. Following the manual analysis of our sample corpus, we regarded as Violence metaphors any metaphorical expressions or similes whose literal meanings suggest scenarios in which, prototypically, a human agent intentionally causes physical harm to another human, with or without weapons. Less prototypical scenarios involve non-human agents, the threat or consequences of violence, or non-physical harm. The linguistic metaphors (tokens) fitting this definition were then matched with the corresponding USAS (UCREL Semantic Analysis System) semantic tags in Wmatrix using the database/tool described in Chapter 3. We found that USAS used a number of different tags for the expressions in question:

- G3 (Warfare): e.g. 'fight' as a verb; 'battle';
- E3– (Violent/angry): e.g. 'hit'; 'attack';
- S8+ (Helping): e.g. 'defend'; 'protect';
- S8– (Hindering): e.g. 'fight' as a noun;
- X8+ (Trying hard): e.g. 'struggle';
- A1.1.1 (General actions, making): e.g. 'blast' and 'confront';
- A1.1.2 (Damaging and destroying): e.g. 'destroy'; 'shatter'.

As this list shows, the semantic categories in question overlapped in various ways, and the overlaps were increased when the broadsweep function of Wmatrix was enabled (see Chapter 3 for details on this). For instance, while 'struggle' has the first-place tag X8+, G3 is part of its extended list. Therefore, to avoid repetition, for this particular analysis we decided not to use the broadsweep function of Wmatrix; i.e. we used standard searches of the first-place tags only. We looked through each example in the USAS categories listed here to determine whether or not it was an instance of metaphor for some aspect of the experience of cancer and the end of life. In the remainder of this chapter, we present findings based on the metaphor patterns that we thus identified.

5.3 Violence Metaphors in the Corpus: Frequencies

As noted in Chapter 4, Violence metaphors were the single most frequent type of metaphor that we identified in our corpus data (2,268 instances). In the first part of this section, we will consider how these instances of metaphor, considered collectively, are distributed quantitatively across the different sections of the corpus. However, it cannot be assumed that any *specific* Violence metaphor (e.g. 'fighter' or 'battle') will show the same pattern of distribution as do Violence metaphors overall. Therefore, we will also look at the frequencies and distributions of different Violence metaphors, in section 5.3.2.

5.3.1 General Frequencies of Violence Metaphors

Of the 2,268 examples of Violence metaphors, 225 were found in the interview data and 2,043 in the online data, though the difference is smaller than it looks since the interview subcorpus is much smaller (see Chapter 3). Table 5.1 breaks down the frequency across all six sections of the corpus and includes both raw frequency and frequency normalised per 1,000 tokens of running text. In other words, normalised frequencies for the online forum data, for example, mean that one would expect to see on average 1.63 examples of words or multiword units expressing a Violence metaphor every 1,000 words. Figure 5.1 represents the normalised frequencies of the various genre/participant group combinations graphically.

As noted in section 5.2, the figures we give include *only* Violence metaphors that are used to talk about aspects of the experience of cancer and (care at) the end of life. Of course, there are more instances in the corpus of Violence metaphors being used to talk about *other* matters, as Violence metaphors are highly conventional in talk about a variety of common topics; but we do not include such instances in our analyses, as explained in Chapter 3.

The results in Table 5.1 show that members of all three participant groups use Violence metaphors to talk about cancer and the end of life in both genres. This, in itself, is an interesting finding, given the criticism that these metaphors have received in the context of cancer. But there are differences across participant groups and across genres, as the normalised frequencies per 1,000 tokens show.

- Online, patients use Violence metaphors more frequently than carers or professionals do, and this difference across groups is statistically significant (using a log-likelihood test for uniformity: $p < 0.05$, 2 d.f., log-likelihood = 23.22).

Table 5.1 Distribution of Violence Metaphors in the Corpus

	Patients		*Unpaid Family Carers*		*Healthcare Professionals*		*All Groups Combined*	
	RF	*NF*	*RF*	*NF*	*RF*	*NF*	*RF*	*NF*
Interviews	72	0.71	80	0.98	73	0.81	225	0.83
Online forum posts	899	1.80	807	1.61	337	1.33	2,043	1.63
Whole corpus	971	1.62	887	1.52	410	1.19	2,268	1.49

Note: RF = raw frequency and NF = frequency normalised per 1,000 tokens of running text.

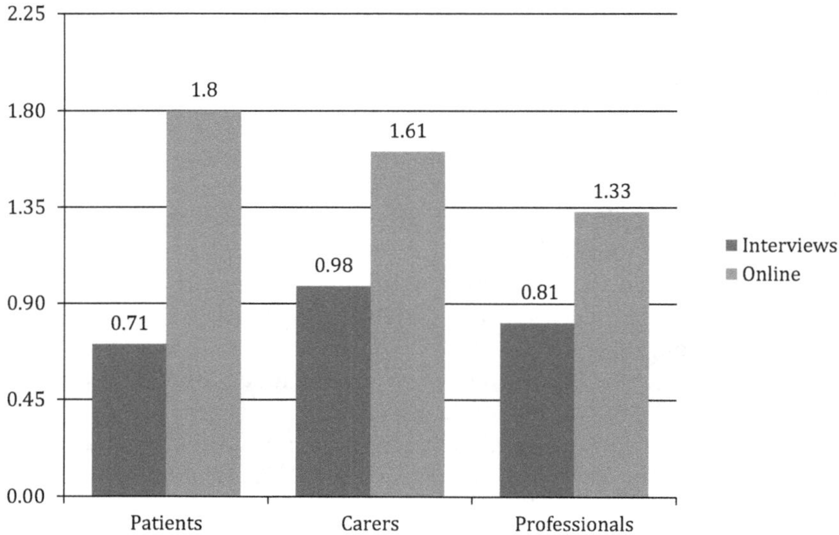

Figure 5.1 Frequencies of Violence Metaphors in the Corpus per 1,000 Words

- In interviews, members of all three participant groups use fewer Violence metaphors than does any group in the online data—less than 1.0 per 1,000 tokens. While the figures in the interview data are somewhat different for the three groups, this difference is not statistically significant (again using the log-likelihood test for uniformity: 2 d.f., log-likelihood = 3.86).

To begin to explain the reasons for these variations in frequency of use, we need to look closer at the forms and functions of Violence metaphors in our corpus. In the next section, we consider the variety of different types of Violence metaphors—different linguistic realisations—that are used by our three participant groups.

5.3.2 Frequencies of Different Violence Metaphors

To identify broad patterns in the use of Violence metaphors across different participant groups, we divided Violence metaphors into more specific lexical groups. The categories in Figures 5.2 and 5.3 still represent multiple tokens, but they only group together words that are related either grammatically, via inflection (e.g. 'fight', 'fighting', 'fought') or derivationally (i.e. they share a common root-word; e.g. 'fight', 'fighter'). We refer to these as *lexical groupings* and represent them using double

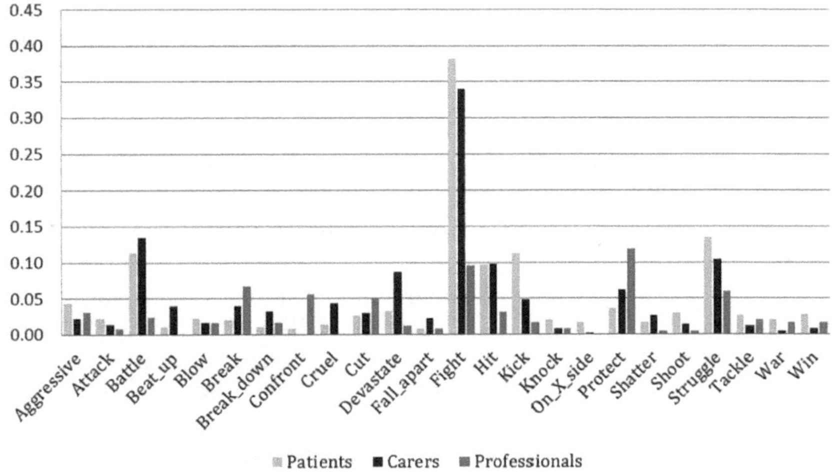

Figure 5.2 Frequencies per 1,000 Words of the Main Lexical Groupings of Violence Metaphors in the Online Data

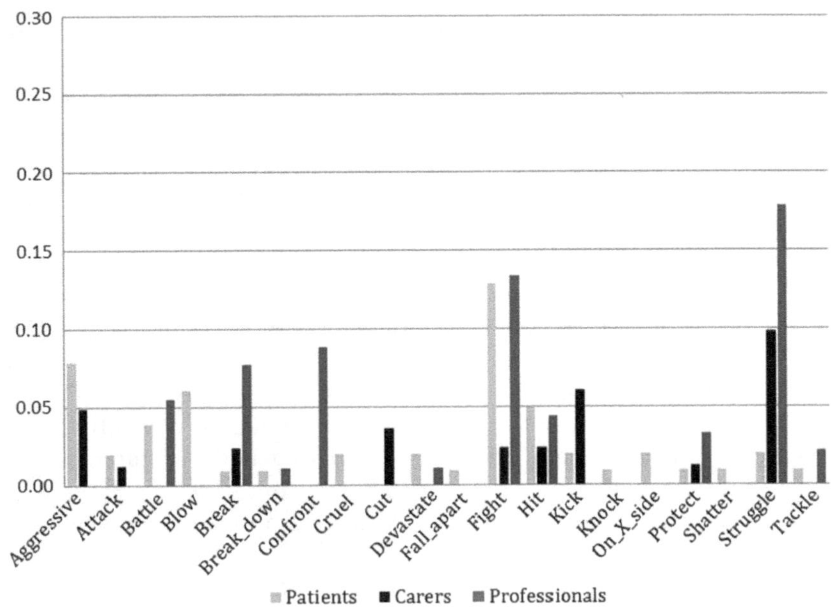

Figure 5.3 Frequencies per 1,000 Words of the Most Frequent Lexical Groupings of Violence Metaphors in the Interview Data

quotation marks. That is, "fight" refers to the lexical grouping of 'fight', 'fighting', 'fought', 'fighter' and so on. Lexical groupings are a useful basis for quantitative analysis at this stage because they make it possible to provide a broad comparative overview of the frequencies of Violence metaphors in the main sections of the corpus.

The full list of lexical groupings includes many infrequent items, so in Figures 5.2 and 5.3 we show only the lexical groupings which occur at least 10 times in at least one of the sections of the corpus. The frequencies are normalised per 1,000 words, as in the quantifications described above.

As Figure 5.2 shows, a fairly small number of lexical groupings stand out as especially frequent in the online data: "battle", "fight" (the most frequent of all), "hit", "kick", "protect" and "struggle". Interestingly, these lexical groupings all also show variation across the participant groups, and all but one show a similar pattern of contrast. "Battle", "fight", "hit", "kick" and "struggle" are all used more frequently by patients and carers than by healthcare professionals (the latter two are also used more frequently by patients than by carers), while "Protect" is relatively more frequent in the online writing produced by healthcare professionals. This might be related to the fact that "protect" is the only one of these lexical groupings that relates to the defensive rather than the offensive Violence scenario.[3] Two additional lexical groupings stand out for frequency of use by just one group: "devastate" is used by carers specifically (possibly referring to the consequences of the illness or death of a loved one), but not by patients or professionals; and "confront" is used by professionals but much less by patients and carers.

Similarly to the online data, in interviews "fight" is also prominent (Figure 5.3), but is the most frequent lexical grouping only for patients. For professionals "fight" takes second place, and for carers "fight" is not notably prominent at all. "Battle" shows a similar pattern to "fight", albeit at lower frequencies. For both carers and professionals, the most common grouping is "struggle"; the carers' prominent use of "struggle" was also a feature of the online data (and at about the same frequency of roughly 0.1 per 1,000 tokens). Meanwhile, "aggressive" stands out for its use by patients, and "break" and "confront" for professionals (the pattern bearing similarity to the online data, though at a slightly lower frequency). "Battle" and "devastate", used frequently by carers in the online data, are not used by them at all in the carer interview data.

It is likely that the differences in Violence metaphor patterns between the participant groups are a result of the differences in how these interviews were structured and collected (as detailed in Chapter 3). In addition, the raw frequency of any given lexical grouping in a particular participant group/genre combination is low in the interviews due to the relatively lower frequency of metaphor use in this genre, as outlined earlier in this chapter and in Chapter 4. As such, at this level of granularity, a detailed qualitative analysis of individual examples in context is a more appropriate means to arrive at valid interpretations of these patterns. It is to just such a qualitative analysis that we will now turn.

5.4 Violence Metaphors in the Corpus: Topics

In this section, we consider the topic areas that are talked about by means of the most common lexical groupings of Violence metaphors in our corpus: the relationship with cancer; the consequences or effects of the illness and its treatment, and death; and the relationship with the healthcare system (including healthcare professionals and higher authorities). We will focus our discussion of each topic on the usage of prominent lexical groupings, but here we will also comment on less common linguistic manifestations of Violence metaphors which are used for the same topic.

As we discussed in Chapters 1 and 2, we are focusing on metaphor in this book because of its potential to frame topics in particular ways. Metaphors frame topics and experiences by highlighting certain aspects of them while backgrounding others. They also often suggest implicit evaluations. The criticisms that Violence metaphors have received are based on their potential to frame the experience of illness, specifically cancer, in a way that puts patients and the illness in opposition, encourages the perception of the body as a battlefield and suggests that not getting better is a personal defeat. However, this disempowering framing is not the only one that Violence metaphors can evoke. As we show in the following, our data suggests that a particular framing is only partly a result of the broad type of metaphor used (e.g. Violence versus Journey) but also depends on specific linguistic realisations of the metaphor, who uses it and the purpose to which it is put (see also Semino et al. 2016).

More specifically, a detailed analysis of all Violence metaphors for the experience of illness in the patient data shows variation in three main respects:

a. Whether a Violence metaphorical expression occurs on its own or as part of an extended and partly creative metaphor;
b. The kind of Violence scenario that is evoked;
c. The kind of framing suggested by Violence metaphors.

Concerning (b), there is variation in terms of:

- What kind of metaphorical violence is involved;
- Who is the agent and who is the receiver of the metaphorical violence;
- To what extent the metaphorical violence is (likely to be) successful.

Concerning (c), we will show that different Violence metaphors frame the experience of illness and caregiving in different ways, including in terms of who is (dis)empowered and how, and of the associated evaluations and emotions.

5.4.1 Violence Metaphors for Relationships With the Disease

All three participant groups use Violence metaphors to talk about how they relate to cancer, both in the interviews and in the online data. There are, however, differences in the specific aspects of the relationship they focus on and in how different lexical groupings and specific metaphorical expressions tend to frame these aspects. In this section, we take each participant group in turn.

Patients' Use of Violence Metaphors for Relationships With the Disease

As we noted in section 5.3.2, the "fight" lexical group was the most commonly used by patients and carers in the online forum data. This lexical group often frames the experience in terms of combat, i.e. a prototypical Violence scenario. Often the combatant is the patient (sometimes with carers cast as co-combatants), and, on the other side, cancer is the enemy. These metaphors often express a desire and effort to get better, and present patients themselves as active and determined. The following examples illustrate this (note that here and throughout, [O] and [I] are appended to examples drawn from our online and interview data respectively; only the relevant metaphorical expressions or similes are underlined; and, as in previous chapters, original spellings are retained in quotes from the online forum data):

Example 5.1

Thus far in my fight against terminal cancer I have been very fortunate, fortunate that I am the person that I am [. . .]. I was also fortunate that my Consultants recognised that I was a born fighter and saw my determination

[O]

Example 5.2

I don't intend to give up; I don't intend to give in. No I want to fight it. I don't want it to beat me, I want to beat it.

[I]

Example 5.3

I have not hunkered down in my trench to just merely defend myself against the demon but have picked up my sword and taken the fight to the demon

[O]

Many examples, such as the first two here, make straightforward and conventional use of the "fight" grouping. In Example 5.2, however, the 'fight' metaphor occurs alongside another metaphor, 'beat', that characterises the relationship with the cancer in a similarly oppositional way. This is taken even further in Example 5.3, in which a highly vivid and specific extended warfare scenario is envisioned, with references to trench warfare, on the one hand, and heroic, sword-wielding, hand-to-hand combat, on the other. In these examples, the patient is in the subject position in the sentence, and is cast as an active agent in the metaphorical scenario. This is most clearly brought out in the speaker's reformulations in Example 5.2 (i.e. 'I don't want it to beat me, I want to beat it'). The use of 'fighter' in Example 5.2 is typical of the patient online data, where 'fighter' or 'fighters' always suggests a determined and optimistic attitude. These particular expressions tend therefore to be associated with a sense of pride, and function interpersonally as a way of expressing praise for oneself or others (e.g. 'You're such a fighter and so inspirational', 'I'm new to the forum and wanted to know if there are any other younger bowel cancer fighters amongst us').

Similar combat scenarios are also constructed by lexical groupings other than (or in addition to) "fight". For instance, in Example 5.4, the same scenario is expressed solely via the use of the noun 'enemy', while 'hit', 'kick' and 'beat' in Examples 5.5 to 5.8 are used by online contributors to express their efforts and determination to get better. In each case, the co-text makes clear that the same suggestion of active determination is in play.

Example 5.4

I BEGGED the prof who gave me my diagnosis to show me the scans, as I felt psychologically I would like to see the enemy's face, as it were

[O]

Example 5.5

I respect Cancer and never underestimate the power it has, but if you can face up to it and hit it back head on then I think you stand a good chance of beating it for just a bit longer.

[O]

Example 5.6

Your words though have given me a bit more of my fighting spirit back. I am ready to kick some cancer butt!

[O]

Example 5.7

Don't let the Demon get you down, spit it in it's eye and give it a swift kick up the wahoola.

[O]

In addition to their grammatical subject positioning, these lexical realisations of Violence metaphors also put the patient in the active role of the scenario, as the party who is able to exert physical violence against the disease. Comparable uses of the "kick" grouping are also used by patients for obviously self-motivational purposes, as in:

Example 5.8

So I woke up this morning and gave a very large kick to myself!

[O]

Example 5.9

What I needed was a very large kick up the backside.

[O]

The use of colloquial terms for body parts such as 'butt' (Example 5.6) and 'wahoola' (Example 5.7) typifies a frankness and strength of feeling that is often apparent in our online data. These informal expressions add humour and strengthen intimacy in the online forum discussions, where relationships between participants build up over many months. On several occasions, Violence metaphors are used as motivational greetings for the rest of forum contributors at the end of posts, as in: 'keep up the good fight' and 'soldier on everybody'. This contrasts with the interview situation, which inevitably involves a brief and more formal one-off relationship between interviewee and interviewer. We will explore the role of humour in depth in Chapter 10.

The expression 'fighting spirit' also appears to function as a means of self-motivation and self-comfort, or as a way of encouraging others, when patients tell each other to 'Keep up your fighting spirit'. The concept of 'fighting spirit' has been noted in other studies with regard to the feelings and emotions of patients with cancer. Salmon and Hall (2003: 1975) argue that the concept of the 'fighting spirit' of cancer patients has become culturally popular because it underlies an idea that fighting can improve the chances for survival. This echoes research by Stephen Greer and colleagues in the 1970/1980s that suggested that cancer survival was dependent on a positive attitude and a fighting spirit, while 'helplessness/hopelessness and denial' were regarded as negative approaches to cancer (e.g. Greer and Watson 1987). While there is no scientific consensus around these claims, the metaphorical scenarios here appear to function in ways which are arguably positive and empowering for patients: they suggest optimism and determination, and express a sense of agency and control. The disease is invariably evaluated negatively (e.g. 'Demon' in Example 5.7, but also referred to as 'Goliath' elsewhere), but its presence and power are also acknowledged and respected (e.g. in the capitalisation of both 'Cancer' and 'Demon'), which makes the successful fight against it a potential source of pride. This is expressed explicitly by a contributor to the patient online forum who comments: 'Cancer and the fighting of it is something to be very proud of'. These particular empowering framings of Violence metaphors are especially prominent in the patient online data.

Other lexical realisations of Violence metaphors, notably the "battle" grouping (and sometimes also "fight"), however, tend to be used to evoke, or highlight, extreme difficulties and unsuccessful outcomes. In the following examples, patients are still the grammatical subjects of the sentences and therefore agents, but are positioned as unsuccessful fighters.

Example 5.10

it must be dispiriting when you are <u>battling</u> as hard as you can, not to be given the <u>armour</u> to fight in,

[O]

In this example, the lack of success is attributed to an external source: the lack of adequate treatment provided by the healthcare professional. Here the treatment or medication would be an aid to the patient's fight, were they given access. In the next section, we discuss examples where medication and treatment are constructed rather differently.

In other cases, when the reality of someone's experience is that treatment fails, and the patient's 'fight' is unsuccessful, Violence metaphors construct the patient as similarly disempowered, characterising their end-of-life experience as a, potentially personal, defeat or failure, as in the following examples:

Example 5.11

we become ill to a point where we cannot <u>fight</u> any more, then we die.

[O]

Example 5.12

I feel such a failure that I am not winning this battle

[O]

Example 5.13

Do I wither or retreat from this weary battle?

[O]

Example 5.12 is particularly negative and disempowering, as the idea of 'not winning [the] battle' results in feelings of personal failure for something that is not the person's fault. In these examples, Violence metaphors tend to be used in combination with grammatical negation (Examples 5.10 to 5.12), expressions of negative emotion or metaphors from different metaphor groups with negative valence (e.g. 'wither' in Example 5.13).

A crucial aspect of these Violence metaphors that leads to such potentially disempowering effects is the fact that, in the terms used by Dancygier and Sweetser (2014), they can be subsumed under the general scenario of 'Competition' (alongside Argument, Business Competition and Sports metaphors). Dancygier and Sweetser (2014: 67) describe this scenario as involving 'at least two parties, consciously acting towards incompatible goals'; critically, then, 'only one of the parties can achieve her desired result'—one must win, and the other must therefore lose. This duality is reflected in the fact that the Violence scenario can be used in both empowering and disempowering ways. However, it is important to emphasise that detailed analysis at the discourse level, as already described, demonstrates that the specific linguistic realisation of the metaphor ("fight" versus "battle") and the co-text (presence or absence of negation, for example) contribute to the (dis)empowering framing; the nature of the framing cannot be established just on the basis of the broad type of metaphor. In addition, the positive and negative aspects of this duality can even intermingle, as in Example 5.14, where the empowering aspect of the 'fight' metaphor is seen as potentially causing future disempowerment in the context of how other people perceive the patient's loss of the metaphorical battle.

Example 5.14

I sometimes worry about being so positive or feel I am being cocky when I say I will fight this as I think oh my god what if I don't win people will think ah see I knew she couldn't do it!

[O]

For a patient to understand their possible lack of recovery as involving humiliation in the eyes of others demonstrates just how powerful and potentially negative the framing effects of Violence metaphors can be.

Carers' Use of Violence Metaphors for Relationships With the Disease

Online, carers use metaphors from the "fight" grouping nearly as much as patients, and similarly employ them in empowering scenarios to describe patients' attempts at getting better:

> *Example 5.15*
>
> HOPE YOUR DAD IS STILL FIGHTING THE FIGHT WITH ALL GUNS BLAZING
>
> [O]

Carers also repeatedly refer to those they care for as 'fighters', to positively evaluate their behaviour and signal their determination. These examples are very similar to the empowering patterns we noted in the patient data in the previous section. In some cases, carers position themselves as allies in the patient's fight, as in:

> *Example 5.16*
>
> he's vowed to fight, I've vowed to back him no matter what.
>
> [O]

> *Example 5.17*
>
> For me and especially for my wife it was about knowledge. If we could discover what we faced, we felt better able to tackle it. OK we didn't win but we made a jolly good fight of it.
>
> [O]

In these examples, it is not just the patient who is placed in an agentive role in the metaphorical scenario, but also the carers. This is signalled either by the parallel subject positioning of 'he' and 'I' involved in similarly active activities in Example 5.16, or by the use of 'we' in Example 5.17. In other cases, carers represent patients as fighting on their own, for example by means of the repeated use of the pronouns 'his' and 'he' in the following extract:

Example 5.18

It is his battle and I have to respect his wishes how he wants to fight it. [O]

Examples like Example 5.18 still suggest an active agentive role for the patient, but the reference to 'his battle' and 'his wishes' potentially suggests some degree of discord. Also significant is the choice of 'battle' as opposed to 'fight' at the beginning of Example 5.18. Similarly to the patient data, 'battle' tends to be used more in scenarios that evaluate the experience negatively, or that describe or anticipate a negative outcome. In the case of Example 5.18, the implication, supported by the obligation expressed in 'I have to', is that the carer does not necessarily agree with the patient's approach to their illness, but feels the need/pressure to support it nevertheless. The patient is empowered in this scenario, but the carer appears more bound by duty and therefore relatively disempowered.

This tendency for "battle" to be associated with negativity and potential disempowerment seems to hold true in the case of other examples of carer language too. In the case of terminal cancer, the 'battle' inevitably ends in 'loss', and many carers focus on this:

Example 5.19

My husband lost his battle after 10 ½ months.

[O]

Example 5.20

My son and I had battled on for nearly two weeks at home watching him struggle to try and do things

[O]

Example 5.21

he has had another fight but couldn't win this time and it had spread to his liver and chest

[O]

Example 5.22

sorry to hear about your husband its hard to believe there still not here with us. mine had stomach cancer diagnosed 2007 sadly he too lost the battle at just 47 in january this year.

[O]

In these cases, the lexical item from the "fight" or "battle" lexical grouping is often (though not always) realised via a noun rather than a verb, and combined with a verb from the "lose" or "struggle" lexical grouping or with grammatical negation (as in Example 5.21). These examples demonstrate once again that the specific linguistic realisation of the Violence metaphor (e.g. "fight" versus "battle") and what these combine with in the co-text contribute to the framing effects of the metaphor.

Professionals' Use of Violence Metaphors for Relationships With the Disease

This same general topic is also present in the healthcare professional data, and again draws on (among others) the "fight" and "battle" lexical groupings, particularly in online discussions. However, there are notable differences in the relationships among parties to the scenario. In the patient and carer data, the patients are usually the combatants, whether successful or not, with the carer as an ally or co-combatant in some cases. Professionals, on the other hand, tend to use Violence metaphors in ways that present themselves as leading or commanding their patients as a military commander, e.g. Example 5.23. The professional may even position themselves as the primary 'fighter'—entering combat on behalf of others in a vulnerable position, that is, the patients and carers, whose role is thereby backgrounded, as in Example 5.24.

Example 5.23

You are now the <u>general</u> and you see your <u>troops</u> killed in <u>battle</u>. [O]

Example 5.24

sometimes one is <u>fighting</u> for patient survival against the odds [O]

On the one hand, this 'fight on behalf of' framing casts professionals as the definitive agents in saving their patients in an almost heroic way, which can be seen as minimising or even ignoring the role and efforts of patients and carers. This could be interpreted as disempowering for patients. On the other hand, this framing also inevitably reflects the different approach that professionals have to the illness. Healthcare professionals, by definition, have chosen a particular relationship with illness, and it is part of their professional role to hold a position of relatively greater expertise and authority. In Chapter 7, however, we will show how this antagonistic approach to illness can frame patients' deaths as professional failure.

Overall, the fact that healthcare professionals do not tend to describe patients as agents within Violence scenarios can also be a reflection of their awareness of the critiques of such metaphors as outlined in the introduction of this chapter. This awareness is in fact made explicit by a healthcare professional in one of our interviews:

Example 5.25

> it's difficult to have advanced care planning discussions with somebody mainly or thoughts about how you'd like your end of life to be if they're still focused on do, don't like using the word but, fighting fighting the fight, fighting the illness fighting you know. So sometimes we get quite often I think we get in the middle of that one party still has with the fighting the battle scenario and maybe somebody's else in a completely different place.
>
> [I]

Although the patient is described as 'fighting' the illness here, our interviewee's discomfort with this phrasing is made clear in 'don't like using the word'. What is also notable in Example 5.25 is that, while reproducing the Violence scenario where the patient is 'fighting' the illness, the speaker here actually critiques that way of conceptualising the situation as counterproductive to advance discussion of end-of-life care (see Demjén et al. 2016 and Chapter 8 for further discussion). This may also explain why professionals in general make little use of metaphorical framings in which patients 'fight/battle' against cancer.

The discussions of Violence metaphors for relationships with the disease in this section show that different framings are suggested depending on what specific linguistic realisations of Violence metaphors are used, who uses them, what the specific topic is and what occurs in the text surrounding the metaphors. We can already begin to see that Violence metaphors can be disempowering in ways that justify the criticism they have received, but evidence from our data suggests a somewhat more complicated picture.

5.4.2 Violence Metaphors for the Effects of Disease, Treatment and Death

Another topic that all three groups describe via Violence metaphors is that of the effects or consequences that cancer, its treatment or death can have. Again, we take each participant group in turn.

Patients' Use of Violence Metaphors for the Effects of Disease, Treatment and Death

Violence metaphors other than the lexical groupings "fight" and "battle" tend to be used by patients to describe the consequences or effects of cancer and cancer treatment on themselves. One prominent lexical grouping that often serves this function is "hit". In the following examples, patients use the verb 'hit' to express the emotional consequences of being ill with cancer. In Example 5.26, the patient is arguably implicitly 'hit' by both the illness itself and its emotional effects (in the wider co-text, the reference of 'it' is left non-specific), but in the subsequent two examples, emotions are explicitly mentioned:

Example 5.26

it <u>hits</u> people in so many different ways.

[I]

Example 5.27

It's interesting what you say about emotional things can take a long time to <u>hit</u> home.

[O]

Example 5.28

so many people seem to manage to be so positive about it all and I just am not. The emotional side of it has <u>hit</u> me far harder than I ever imagined

[O]

In these examples, the emotions cancer causes are placed in the role of aggressor or initiator of the violence, and the patients are on the receiving end with little control over the situation. As such, these types of examples convey a sense of disempowerment, but they allow patients to express a key aspect of their experience nevertheless. These types of metaphors are in line with more general metaphors for emotions, which often present them as uncontrollable irrespective of whether they are positive or negative (more on this in Chapter 9).

Violence metaphors in the lexical grouping "hit" are also used in the online data to convey the patients' perception of the effects of cancer treatment:

Example 5.29

Deep breath, before the big wave <u>hits</u> you! [chemotherapy]

[O]

Example 5.30

They <u>hit</u> me with radiation for 10 days.

[O]

As Examples 5.29 and 5.30 demonstrate, patients seem to perceive cancer treatment as another attacker, alongside the illness itself. Similar Violence scenarios are also constructed via less frequent lexical realisations such 'a battering from chemo', 'a "hammering" from medication' (scare quotes in the original) and the particularly poignant Example 5.31, which involves the personification of the person's 'normal cells' and a 'sledgehammer':

Example 5.31

what did i think all my normal little cells were doing after being hit by a sledgehammer of both toxic chemicals and radiation

[O]

Here the treatment is positioned as an attacker in a similar way to the illness, rather than being presented as the patient's ally, as might have been anticipated.

Overall, in all of these examples, the patient is on the receiving end of metaphorical violence that they either are not able to resist (in the case of emotions) or should not resist (in the case of treatment). Cumulatively, this reflects a deeply disempowered perception of the patient's position in the experience of illness and treatment.

Carers' Use of Violence Metaphors for the Effects of Disease, Treatment and Death

Carers, like patients, use 'hit' metaphors to describe the effects of cancer on their loved ones or themselves. Once again, these effects can be both physical and emotional.

Example 5.32

It hits indiscriminately and without remorse.

[O]

Example 5.33

This disease is awful and often hits the ones that deserve it the least.

[O]

Example 5.34

it does get easier. Not better, but definitely easier. But it still hits like a sledgehammer sometimes.

[O]

Example 5.35

Now grief is <u>hitting</u> me every day.

[O]

However, as the last two examples show, in contrast with patients, carers use the "hit" grouping not just for the effects of cancer, but also for the effects of death. As we discuss in detail in Chapter 9, some of the carers in our online data continue to contribute to the forum after the person they cared for has died. As a consequence, their Violence metaphors often relate to the experience of bereavement. They express these experiences not just via the prototypical Violence metaphors in the "hit" grouping, but also via metaphors that reference the effects of violence, particularly 'devastate'. This particular linguistic realisation is indeed rather more frequent in the carers' data than the patients' or professionals':

Example 5.36

I know the <u>devastation</u> and sadness you feel.

[O]

Interestingly, 'devastate' metaphors used by carers are often oriented towards other carers (as in Example 5.36), rather than self-oriented. They seem to be used to provide comfort, empathy and solidarity among people who have had similarly unhappy experiences. This means that, although these metaphors position carers as disempowered (in the sense that they cannot control the emotional consequences of illness and death), the interpersonal function of those metaphors can be seen as empowering, in that they are used to support others.

It is worth noting that 'devastate' metaphors are not used at all by carers in interviews. This is most likely because all the carer interviewees were still caring for someone with cancer at the time of interviews, whereas some of the online carers were bereaved, and discussing their feelings of grief (although 'devastate' was sometimes used in the context of the diagnosis of cancer as well). In addition, the interview setting is relatively more formal in contrast to the perceived informality and intimacy of the online forum environment, where carers perhaps feel able to express their emotions more freely.

Professionals' Use of Violence Metaphors for the Effects of Disease, Treatment and Death

Metaphorical violence involving the emotional effects of cancer and death is also evident in the professionals' data, but in a somewhat different form. The primary lexical group involved is the highly conventional "struggle", which, as we noted in our quantitative analysis, is the single most frequent violence-related lexical group in the interview data for professionals. Healthcare professionals use 'struggle' metaphors to express the problems they face in the process of caring for and communicating with people who are dying, e.g. Examples 5.37 and 5.38; to describe conflicted feelings they observe in dying patients, as in Example 5.39; and to describe the difficulties families face in end-of-life situations, as in Example 5.40:

Example 5.37

we're all human and we're all struggling and trying our best.

[I]

Example 5.38

as healthcare professional we really struggled with that because we would always be honest with patients.

[I]

Example 5.39

I think these patients really struggle deeply because they are ready to die, they've given up and they want to die and they find it very difficult to live in those last few days or weeks.

[I]

Example 5.40

the family are struggling with them being at home.

[I]

In all cases, 'struggle' metaphors suggest that the people involved cannot fully overcome the difficulties they are dealing with.

Another Violence metaphor often used by professionals in reference to the (emotional) consequences of illness and death is "confront". In the following examples, metaphors from the "confront" lexical group are used in relation to the uncomfortable feelings and truths surrounding death (e.g. 'grief', 'helplessness').

Example 5.41

What do you think about being confronted to repetitive situations of death, feeling the grief of the patient relatives, ruminating all this, getting a deep feeling of helplessness even if it is known and admitted that in such situations the patient's death is expected, and the logic says that the doctor can't do more than his current efforts

[O]

Example 5.42

I think there is a fascination about erm . . . confronting yourself with the most frightening thing in life maybe, there's like a knife-edge thing you know so if there's something that's really that's personally challenging, there's a perverse bit of me that wants to confront myself with it fully.

[I]

In Example 5.43, the metaphorical scenario is extended by the subsequent use of 'conflict':

Example 5.43

What I do not think I ever realized at the time was that "serving" in the PM Room also helped me to confront the essential fallibility inherent in my profession and started me off on my lifelong conflict with the inescapable uncertainty and error

[O]

In the same way as 'struggle', 'confront' metaphors help to communicate a negative evaluation. The examples show that patients' deaths are negative experiences for healthcare professionals that they need to actively deal with. Sleeman (2013) argues that part of the difficulty stems from the problematic view that patient death potentially represents failure on the part of the professional, as we have mentioned earlier (see also Chapter 7). Interestingly, this view is comparable to the kind of problematic responsibility that patients can feel if their cancer experience is framed in terms of the Violence metaphor and they do not get better. However, in these examples (especially Examples 5.42 and 5.43), professionals demonstrate agency by actively challenging or addressing these negative feelings.

The discussions of Violence metaphors for the consequences of cancer and death in this section provide further evidence that different linguistic realisations of Violence metaphors in context frame experiences in different ways. Violence metaphors in the "hit" grouping, for example, seem to mostly suggest disempowerment for both carers and patients. We also have further evidence that it matters who uses these metaphors. While patients generally only use Violence metaphors with reference to themselves, professionals and carers use them both with reference to patients and with reference to themselves. This is beginning to suggest that patients not only use Violence metaphors more frequently than others, but also potentially use them with a more homogeneous referent. In addition, the examples in this section show that the interpersonal functions of Violence metaphors also matter. For example, while 'devastate' metaphors suggest a disempowering scenario, the way carers mostly use them to support each other can also be seen as empowering. Once again, the framing implications of Violence metaphors are influenced by multiple factors.

5.4.3 Violence Metaphors for Relationships With the Healthcare System

Violence metaphors are also used to describe the relationship patients and carers have with their healthcare professionals and/or the healthcare system. The latter—the relationship with the healthcare system—is something that healthcare professionals also describe using Violence metaphors. It is to these usages that we turn in this section.

Patients' Use of Violence Metaphors for Relationships With the Healthcare System

Some of the prominent linguistic realisations of the Violence metaphor we have already discussed are also used by patients to describe their relationships and interactions with healthcare professionals, especially when it comes to access to medication:

> *Example 5.44*
>
> that first lady that was well publicised about <u>fighting</u> and getting the Herceptin;
>
> [I]

> *Example 5.45*
>
> I will <u>fight</u> for Avastin.
>
> [O]

Here patients describe as a 'fight' their own or others' efforts to get the treatment they need. Because they are active and agentive in these scenarios, one could argue that, discursively, patients are empowered. However, the fact that medication needs to be fought for in this way, and the negative evaluation that the Violence metaphor communicates, suggests unnecessary and in principle avoidable problems with the healthcare system and with patients' relationships with healthcare professionals. These can be seen as in marked contrast with the way some healthcare professionals construct their role as fighters for the patients in section 5.4.1.

Carers' Use of Violence Metaphors for Relationships With the Healthcare System

Carers, like patients, also use "fight" and 'battle' metaphors for their interactions with the healthcare system, e.g.:

Example 5.46

It seems to me that while my husband <u>fights</u> cancer, I am <u>fighting</u> the system.

[O]

Example 5.47

wondering why everything is a <u>battle</u> with the NHS.

[O]

In these examples again, carers are ostensibly empowered, as they are expressing their own agency. They are also allied with the patient, as in Example 5.46. However, arguably, this particular fight is only necessary because the healthcare system itself is perceived not to function for the benefit of patients and their families. As with the patients' examples, the metaphorical combat also involves a marked imbalance of power and control in favour of the healthcare system and those who make decisions within it.

Professionals' Use of Violence Metaphors for Relationships With the Healthcare System

Perhaps surprisingly, a very similar framing also occurs in the professionals' data. However, whereas patients and carers both construct scenarios in which they are fighting against the healthcare professionals, the professionals present themselves as fighting with a higher authority, i.e. the government administrative body which provides the funding for treatment of patients, for example:

Example 5.48

<u>fighting</u> with health authorities and PCTs for a reasonable level of funding.

[I]

Example 5.49

it's a constant <u>battle</u> to get the funding.

[I]

What unifies the use of this framing across patients, carers and professionals is that in all cases we see the construction of a metaphorical scenario where they must engage in metaphorical violence against the 'next level up' of healthcare authority in order to obtain access to resources: medication, services and funding. The examples in this section are interesting because in the case of all three groups, the person speaking is presented as having agency: patients, carers and healthcare professionals are equally active in these scenarios. However, this is arguably a type of agency that should not be needed, and that is therefore likely to feel unwelcome (cf. the notion of agency as being 'desired' by the relevant person/people in our definition of (dis)empowerment in Chapter 1). More generally, relationships that should be collaborative are presented by these metaphors as antagonistic.

5.5 Conclusions

This chapter has given the first detailed exposition of findings around a single class of metaphor—Violence metaphors—arrived at via our combination of corpus-based quantitative and qualitative methods. We began our detailed analysis with a focus on Violence metaphors for two reasons: they were the most frequent type of metaphor in our data; and they have repeatedly been the subject of heated debate in the context of cancer.

Our combination of semi-automated quantitative and detailed qualitative analysis permits us to arrive at a more comprehensive account of Violence metaphors than would have been possible otherwise. We started, for example, by showing that, when it comes to cancer, there is not just one kind of Battle/War/Military metaphor (e.g. as suggested by Miller 2010), but rather that multiple specific lexical groupings can be subsumed under the general label of Violence metaphors, with different frequencies, uses and functions. We also showed that, although Violence metaphors are the most frequent type of metaphor in our corpus, the frequency varies across both the two genres and the three participant groups in our corpus. Broadly speaking, they are used more frequently when writing online than in interviews, and health professionals use them less frequently than the other two participant groups represented in our corpus.

We suggested that the difference between genres can be understood in terms of the contrast in formality and anonymity between interviews and online fora. The online forum setting fosters a sense of being able to express views and emotions more freely, including by means of Violence metaphors, than is the case in one-to-one face-to-face interactions with a relative stranger. As shown in Chapter 4, this applies to metaphors generally in the patient and carer sections of the corpus. We also argued that healthcare professionals might use Violence metaphors less frequently than patients and carers because they are aware of their potential detrimental effects for patients.

We also identified quantitative variation in terms of how Violence metaphors are realised linguistically: different lexical groupings are quantitatively most prominent in different sections of our corpus. For example, in online data "fight" is very commonly employed by patients and carers but not professionals, whereas interviews with healthcare professionals exhibit frequent examples of "struggle". However, explaining these differences required an understanding of how the metaphors were actually being used. This is where our qualitative analysis highlighted the different topics participants tend to focus on, the mental states they express and the different roles and perspectives they take in relation to each other, the illness and care.

Throughout our analysis, we considered how different uses appeared to frame participants' experience, and we showed repeatedly that the framing does not just depend on the overarching metaphor used. The discussions of Violence metaphors for relationships with the disease, for example, showed that the specific linguistic realisations of Violence metaphors mattered. 'Fighter(s)' tends to be used by patients to describe themselves or others positively. 'Battle' metaphors tend to suggest scenarios where patients are disempowered, while "fight" and "kick" metaphors often evoke more empowering scenarios. This, however, only holds true if the co-text does not include grammatical negation or negative evaluative expressions. Our discussion of Violence metaphors for the consequences of cancer and death reinforced this point, showing that the "hit" lexical grouping mostly suggests disempowerment for both carers and patients. However, it also matters who uses these metaphors and for what aspects of the experience of illness and caregiving. When patients use these metaphors for progressive cancer or the terminal phase of the disease, the framings can be particularly negative and disempowering. Professionals, on the other hand, cast themselves as senior military officers, and the patients as their troops, or alternatively as fighting on behalf of the patients (and carers), not only against the disease, but perhaps more prominently against unpleasant or uncomfortable feelings and truths that may arise in the end-of-life situation. The precise way in which Violence metaphors are used also matters: while 'devastate' metaphors suggested a disempowering scenario, the way carers mostly use them to support each other is in fact empowering from an interpersonal perspective. And we observed a similar trend in relation to Violence metaphors for the relationship with the healthcare system. While the metaphors themselves constructed a scenario where patients, carers and healthcare professionals were agentive, exerting control over their higher-ups, relationships that should have been collaborative were being presented as unnecessarily antagonistic. This suggests a very real disempowerment experienced regularly by some participants, and points out areas where practices and systems may be in need of attention and improvement.

These observations suggest that, while there is certainly evidence for the disempowering effects of Violence metaphors that justifies the criticism they have received, the reality is somewhat more complicated. Regardless of the complexity of the different metaphorical scenarios that the different participant groups make use of, we have seen across the board that Violence metaphors are not necessarily negative. The overarching metaphor cannot be evaluated separately from the details of the context and manner of use of specific instances and patterns. This means that broad generalisations concerning the implications of metaphor patterns need to be made with caution when making decisions about practice in healthcare. While we can confirm that it would be unwise for healthcare professionals to actively introduce Violence metaphors in interactions with patients, it would probably also be misguided to attempt to censor them, given that some Violence metaphors appear to be used to express personal determination and encouragement. They are also used, by all participants, to express criticism of the healthcare system, which is important to take note of and address in the provision of healthcare generally, and cancer care and end-of-life care in particular. The priority in healthcare communication should therefore be to encourage and enable people, and particularly patients, to use the metaphors that represent their experiences as faithfully and helpfully as possible.

Of course, no discussion of any single pattern of metaphorical language can provide a wholly comprehensive account of how patients, carers and professionals discuss cancer and the end of life. As we noted, the second most frequent type of metaphor we found was the Journey metaphor—which is precisely the metaphor advocated as a replacement for Violence metaphors by many of those who have cast doubt on the appropriateness of the latter. We therefore return to these arguments after a discussion of Journey metaphors at the end of Chapter 6.

Notes

1. Kate Granger died on 23 July 2016.
2. Lisa Bonchek Adams died on 6 March 2015.
3. The quantitative prominence of "protect" in the professional online subcorpus is mainly due to the fact that it is used as a common rhetorical move in discussions of euthanasia (opponents of euthanasia characterise their stance as 'protecting' patients). This debate is present at several points in our data, but is not sufficiently relevant to this chapter to be discussed in detail.

References

Bennett, A. (2013). We need a heroic narrative for death. *TED Talk*. Retrieved March 2017, from www.ted.com/talks/amanda_bennett_a_heroic_narrative_for_letting_go

Dancygier, B., and Sweetser, E. (2014). *Figurative language*. Cambridge: Cambridge University Press.

Demjén, Z., Semino, E., and Koller, V. (2016). Metaphors for 'good' and 'bad' deaths: A health professional view. *Metaphor and the Social World*, *6*(1), 1–19.

Granger, K. (2014). Having cancer is not a fight or a battle. *The Guardian*. Retrieved March 2017, from www.theguardian.com/society/2014/apr/25/having-cancer-not-fight-or-battle

Greer, S., and Watson, M. (1987). Mental Adjustment to cancer: Its measurement and prognostic significance. *Cancer Surveys*, *6*, 439–453.

Hurley, K. E. (2014). To fight, or not to fight: A cancer psychotherapist with cancer confronts the battle metaphor. *Women & Therapy*, *37*(3–4), 311–318.

Keller, B. (2014). Heroic measures. *New York Times*. Retrieved March 2017, from www.nytimes.com/2014/01/13/opinion/keller-heroic-measures.html?_r=1

McCartney, M. (2014). The fight is on: Military metaphors for cancer may harm patients. *The BMJ*, *349*, g5155.

Miller, R. S. (2010). Speak up: 8 words & phrases to ban in oncology! *Oncology Times*, *32*(12), 20.

Reisfield, G. M., and Wilson, G. R. (2004). Use of metaphor in the discourse on cancer. *Journal of Clinical Oncology*, 22(19), 4024–4027.

Salmon, P., and Hall, G. M. (2003). Patient empowerment and control: A psychological discourse in the service of medicine. *Social Science & Medicine*, *57*, 1969–1980.

Semino, E., Demjén, Z., and Demmen, J. (2016 advance access). An integrated approach to metaphor and framing in cognition, discourse and practice, with an application to metaphors for cancer. *Applied Linguistics*.

Sleeman, K. E. (2013). End-of-life communication: Let's talk about death. *Journal of the Royal College of Physicians Edinburgh*, *43*, 197–199.

6 Journey Metaphors

6.1 Introduction

In January 2005, journalist Melanie McFadyean wrote a piece on her experience of breast cancer for the UK *Guardian* newspaper, and had this to say about different metaphors for being ill with cancer:

> I read obituaries and always look at the dates of birth. Those of my vintage have often died 'after a long battle with cancer'. People with cancer have enough to deal with without feeling that every day of their lives must be a battle with the disease. [. . .]
>
> [W]hy should people with cancer be expected to take up arms? It is better to see cancer as a journey. Everyone says that being positive helps you to come through, and being positive during a journey seems easier to me than being positive during a war in which the enemy is all around you.
>
> (McFadyean 2005)

In line with some of our discussion in Chapter 5, McFadyean's criticism of 'battle' and 'war' metaphors is particularly to do with the framing of the disease as an 'enemy [. . .] all around you', and the negative emotional consequences this can have for the daily lives of people with cancer. In contrast, the alternative idea of cancer as a 'journey' makes it easier, in her view, to adopt the kind of positive attitude that is believed to be helpful for patients.

McFadyean is not alone in her preference for 'journey' as a metaphor for the experience of cancer. The same metaphor is adopted, for example, in self-help books such as *The Cancer Journey: Positive Steps to Heal Yourself* (Evans et al. 2011), and in recent official documents and guidelines in several different countries. Both the 2007 National Health Service *Cancer Reform Strategy* and the 2015–20 *Cancer Strategy for England* avoid references to 'battles' or 'wars', and adopt instead the notion of the patient's 'cancer journey', with different treatment and care plans referred to as 'pathways' (Department of Health 2007, 2015). The same pattern is apparent in, for example, the 2008 End of Life Care Strategy for England and Wales (Department of Health 2008), the *Journey of Change* initiative of the Irish Hospice Foundation, the *Cancer Journey* section of the website of Cancer Care Ontario in Canada and the 2017 *Writing About Cancer Guidelines* of the Cancer Institute of New South Wales. For our purposes, this raises the question of to what extent and how Journey metaphors are used in our corpus, and whether any evidence can be found that they are indeed more helpful and appropriate than Violence metaphors.

We dealt with the Violence metaphor half of this question in Chapter 5, and in this chapter, we discuss the use of 'cancer journey' and other Journey metaphors in our corpus (e.g. 'slow road to death' and 'palliative pathway'). The structure of this chapter is similar to the previous one. We begin by introducing the specific aspects of our corpus linguistic method that are applied in this chapter. We then compare the frequencies of Journey metaphors in the different sections of our corpus, focusing particularly on differences between different participant groups. To make sense of these differences, we then present a detailed qualitative analysis of the use of Journey metaphors to talk about two specific topics: the experience of illness (including the end of life) and treatment options. We show how Journey metaphors can be used in a variety of empowering and disempowering ways, and particularly to express both positive and negative views and emotions. This is similar to what we observed for Violence metaphors in Chapter 5. The final section of the analysis therefore reconsiders the opposition between Journey and Violence metaphors by focusing on the individuals in our online data who use both types of metaphors, whether in combination or separately.

6.2 Methodology for the Retrieval of Potential Journey Metaphors

In the manual analysis of the sample corpus (see Chapter 3), we classified movement-related metaphors under four semantic groupings:

- Movement: e.g. 'I'm scared of what is to <u>come</u>';
- Location: e.g. 'there's often been times where where I'd had someone so stuck in a bad <u>place</u> that we couldn't help at all';
- Direction: e.g. 'you are very young to be <u>going through</u> such a tough time';
- Journey: e.g. 'I am humbled by courage and dignity of my patients on their final <u>journey</u>'.

The tokens for all four groupings in the sample corpus were matched with the corresponding USAS (UCREL Semantic Analysis System) semantic domain tags in Wmatrix using the database/tool described in Chapter 3. The majority of tokens were found to fall under the following USAS tags:

- M1 (Moving, coming and going);
- M3 (Vehicles and transport on land);
- M6 (Location and direction);
- M7 (Places).

In contrast with the Violence metaphors analysed in Chapter 5, however, pilot semantic concordances revealed that the majority of tokens under each USAS tag in the whole corpus were used literally. Whereas there is little talk of actual physical violence in our data, there are, not surprisingly, many non-metaphorical references to movement and places (e.g. 'So I decided I must go to the doctor'). For this reason, concordancing the semantic tags just listed was an inefficient way to identify Journey metaphors in our corpus.

We therefore selected a group of expressions from each of these semantic tags that, on the basis of the analysis of the sample corpus, were likely to be used metaphorically in our data to discuss topics relevant to our study. These were: 'journey*', 'path*', 'road*', 'step*', 'route*', 'way* through', 'go*/com* through', 'forward*', 'backward*', 'run*', 'move*', 'travel*', 'turn*', 'direction*' and 'place*' (NB: here the asterisk functions as a wildcard; i.e. it stands for any sequence of zero or more characters. In other words, for each expression, we searched for all inflectional forms: e.g. 'journey' and 'journeys', and 'come through' and 'coming through'.). This approach privileges efficiency over exhaustiveness: we were able to identify metaphorical expressions faster than by using semantic concordances, but our findings were limited to the expressions we actually searched for (cf. L'Hote 2014 for a similar approach to Journey metaphors using the tools in Wmatrix). Moreover, this set of search words identified a fairly broad set of movement-related metaphors, which some analysts might prefer to label as Movement rather than Journey metaphors specifically. However, we will stick with Journey as our umbrella label for all these metaphors, given how prominent the term 'journey' itself is in current discourse around cancer and the end of life.

6.3 Journey Metaphors in the Corpus: Frequencies

As we mentioned in Chapter 4, Journey metaphors are the second most frequent type of metaphor we identified in the corpus, after Violence metaphors (1,513 and 2,268 instances respectively). This is not surprising, given the prominence of Journey metaphors in English generally, and particularly of the metaphor LIFE IS A JOURNEY (e.g. Lakoff 1993). However, the Journey metaphors we have identified in our data relate to the very specific topics of cancer and end of life, and display some degree of variation in terms of distribution within the corpus. In this section, we begin by presenting the overall frequencies of Journey metaphors in the different sections of the corpus. We then consider the frequencies of specific Journey metaphors across genres and groups.

6.3.1 General Frequencies of Journey Metaphors

Of the 1,513 instances of Journey metaphors we identified in the whole corpus, 182 were found in the interview data and 1,331 in the online data. The frequency of use among each group and in each genre is shown in Table 6.1, including raw frequencies and frequencies normalised per 1,000 tokens. Because online forum data makes up a large proportion of the corpus, it will strongly influence results where the two genres are combined. Therefore, in Table 6.1 we also break the data down to consider interviews and online forum discussions as separate genres.

The figures in Table 6.1 show that members of all three groups use Journey metaphors to talk about cancer and the end of life in both genres. There are differences in frequency, however, both across genres and across participant groups.

Overall, the normalised frequencies per 1,000 tokens in Figure 6.1 show that patients use Journey metaphors more frequently than the other two groups (using a log-likelihood test for uniformity: $p < 0.0001$, 2 d.f., log-likelihood = 109.27), and that Journey metaphors are more frequent in the online data than in the interviews ($p < 0.0001$, 2 d.f., log-likelihood = 38.53). However, these overall trends need to be qualified by taking into account the intersections between groups and genres:

- Online, carers and healthcare professionals use Journey metaphors with similar frequencies, while patients use them considerably more often than the other two groups;

Table 6.1 Distribution of Journey Metaphors in the Corpus

	Patients		*Unpaid Family Carers*		*Healthcare Professionals*		*All Groups Combined*	
	RF	*NF*	*RF*	*NF*	*RF*	*NF*	*RF*	*NF*
Interviews	56	0.56	28	0.34	98	1.09	182	0.67
Online forum posts	730	1.46	384	0.77	217	0.86	1,331	1.06
Whole corpus	786	1.31	412	0.71	315	0.92	1,513	0.99

Note: RF = raw frequencies and NF = frequencies normalised per 1,000 tokens.

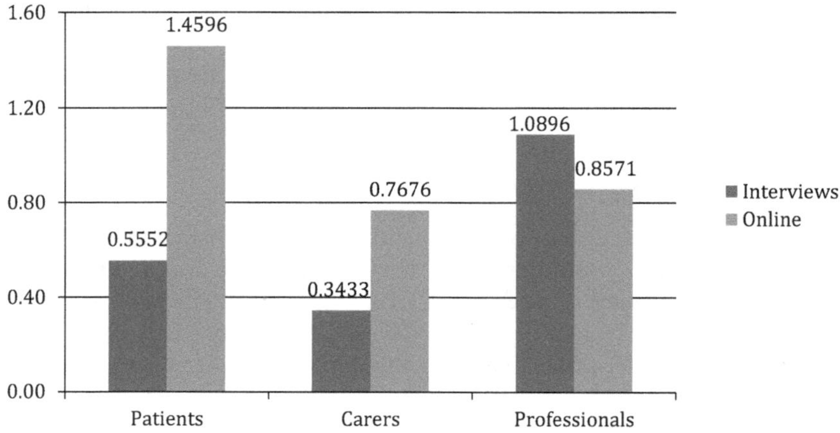

Figure 6.1 Frequencies of Journey Metaphors in the Corpus per 1,000 Words

- In the interviews, carers and patients use Journey metaphors with similar frequencies, while healthcare professionals use them considerably more often;
- Healthcare professionals are the only group who use Journey metaphors more frequently in interviews than in online forum posts in our corpus.

To begin to explain these variations in frequency of use, we now consider the frequencies across genres and participant groups of different *kinds* of Journey metaphors.

6.3.2 Frequencies of Different Journey Metaphors

To identify broad patterns in the use of Journey metaphors in the corpus, in Figures 6.2 and 6.3 we have grouped together inflectionally and derivationally related expressions (e.g. 'journey' and 'journeys'; 'path' and 'pathway'), as in the previous chapter. For the sake of exposition, we have also combined pairs of metaphorical opposites ('come' and 'go'; and 'forward' and 'backward'). As in the previous chapter, we refer to these lexical groupings by means of double quotation marks, such as "journey" and "path".

In the online data (Figure 6.2), patients use "journey" metaphors, 'go/come through' metaphors and 'forward/backward' metaphors more often than the other two groups. Healthcare professionals use 'path' metaphors more often than the other two groups.

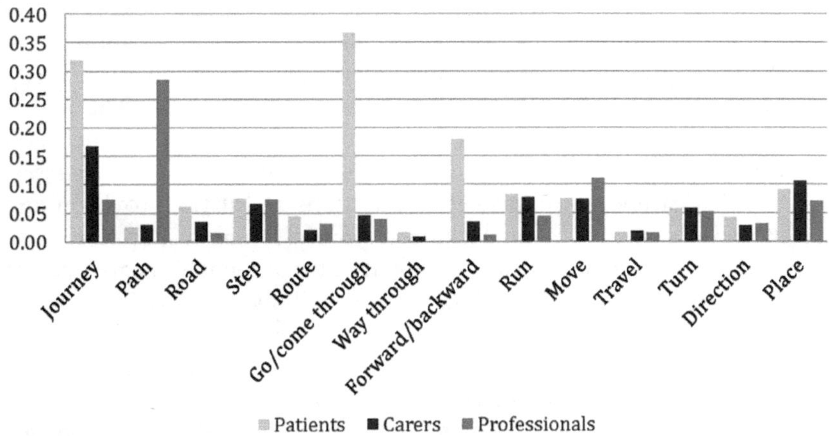

Figure 6.2 Frequencies per 1,000 Words of the Main Lexical Groups of Journey Metaphors in the Online Forum Data

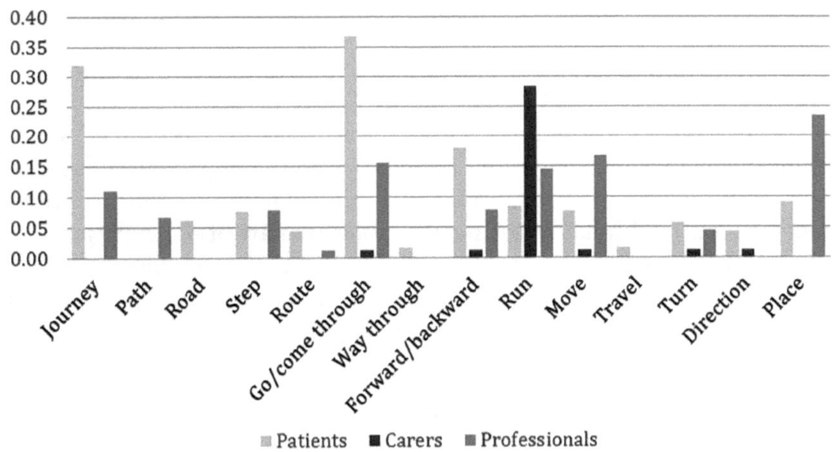

Figure 6.3 Frequencies per 1,000 Words of the Main Lexical Groups of Journey Metaphors in the Interview Data

In the interviews (Figure 6.3), the patients' higher frequency of "journey" and 'go/come through' metaphors is more marked. In addition, carers use "run" metaphors more often than the other two groups, and healthcare professionals use 'place' metaphors more often.

As we show in the following, all three groups use "journey" metaphors to refer to the experience of illness ('cancer journey') and the end of life ('final journey'). However, patients use these expressions more frequently, as they relate to their own experience, and that experience is central to both the interviews and the online forum (see section 6.4.1). For the same reason, patients more often talk about that experience as something they 'go through'. Similarly, they talk more often about positive change or success in terms of 'coming through' or moving 'forward', and about negative change in terms of moving 'backward'. The higher frequency of "run" metaphors in carer interviews is due to our inclusion of expressions such as 'She was there too to run part of the first session', which carers use in answer to questions about the provision and use of services in their area. Healthcare professionals use 'pathway(s)' more than the other two groups to talk about treatment and care options within the UK National Health Service, especially when writing online (see section 6.4.2). They also use 'place' metaphors in the interviews in answer to questions about their work with patients and families, and about different ways of dying (see Chapter 8).

Overall, these broad patterns also show the variety of topics expressed via Journey metaphors in our data. In the next section, we discuss the main topics that are discussed in terms of Journey metaphors by members of the three participant groups. This will enable us to provide more nuanced explanations for the frequency differences we have reported so far.

6.4 Journey Metaphors in the Corpus: Topics

In this section, we consider two main topic areas that are talked about by means of Journey metaphors in our corpus: the experience of illness, including (care at) the end of life (section 6.4.1) and treatment options (section 6.4.2). Although treatment options are part of the experience of illness, we deal with them as a separate topic as they involve a specific subset of metaphorical expressions in our data, and a notable contrast between healthcare professionals and the other two groups.

6.4.1 Journey Metaphors for the Experience of Illness

All three participant groups use Journey metaphors to talk about the experience of illness, and specifically cancer, both in the interviews and in the online data (e.g. 'going through the cancer journey changes you forever', from the patient online data). Carers and healthcare professionals also use Journey metaphors to talk about the final phase of life and the process of dying ('my husband's slow road to death', from the carer online data).

As with Violence metaphors in the previous chapter, a detailed analysis of all Journey metaphors for the experience of illness shows variation in three main respects:

a. Whether a Journey metaphorical expression occurs on its own or as part of an extended and partly creative metaphor;

b. The kind of Journey scenario that is evoked;
c. The kind of framing provided by Journey metaphors.

Concerning (b), there is variation in terms of:

- Whether someone is in control of the journey, and who that is;
- Whether there is a single road/route or many;
- Whether there are travelling companions and, if so, who/what they are;
- The terrain or location of travel and/or the condition of the road;
- The destination or end point of the journey.

Concerning (c), Journey metaphors in our data are used to frame the experience of illness in a range of different ways, particularly in terms of the degree of agency and general (dis)empowerment of the patient him/herself, and the emotions that are expressed or evoked, which may be both positive and negative. The examples we discuss in the following demonstrate this variation, and also show the resulting variety of interpersonal functions that different Journey metaphors help to perform (e.g. expressing emotions, providing encouragement and strengthening group cohesion).

Patients' Use of Journey Metaphors for the Experience of Illness

The patient data contains 162 metaphorical uses of the word 'journey', mostly in the online data (160 instances in the online data versus 2 in the interviews). As shown in Figures 6.2 and 6.3, this corresponds to higher relative frequencies in both genres than for the other two groups (but the raw frequencies in the interviews are too low to be meaningful). In 145 out of 162 cases, the metaphorical journey is the experience of being ill with cancer, including 13 instances of the phrase 'cancer journey'. The nouns 'road' and 'path' are also repeatedly used metaphorically for the experience of illness (in 21 and 10 cases respectively).

Some metaphorical uses of '(cancer) journey' in particular occur in isolation from other related metaphorical expressions and are rather neutral. For example, an online forum contributor mentions 'the time line of a thyroid cancer journey' while suggesting a way of organising future posts that would be maximally useful for people with new diagnoses. In many other cases, however, several Journey-related metaphorical expressions are used together to put forward a particular view of the illness experience, including a positive or negative evaluation.

The notion of cancer as a 'journey' is sometimes used quite explicitly to put forward a view of being ill that facilitates acceptance (NB: in quotations from our data, we underline the journey-related metaphorical expressions that are relevant to the topics of cancer and end of life, even if they were not among the search terms mentioned in section 6.2; as in previous chapters, original spellings are retained in quotations from the online data):

Example 6.1

> if you can think of this chapter in your life as a reluctant journey and each procedure a place along that journey that must be completed before you move onto the next it may help you better deal with it.
>
> [O]

This can also apply in the difficult situation where the disease has become progressive, and where the use of a Violence metaphor would result in a framing in which the person has 'lost the battle/fight':

Example 6.2

> There are certain points in the cancer journey where the plan has to change. You could say diagnosis is the first of them. The end of useful chemotherapy is another. At each of these change points, a new care plan must be discussed and put into place effectively. It is imperative that you do not get the impression that the doctors are giving up.
>
> [O]

In both cases, extended Journey metaphors are used to provide encouragement and empathetic advice to people who are finding it difficult to cope with a new or worsened diagnosis. The idea of a journey emphasises continuity and purposefulness over lengthy periods of time, even in situations that are unwelcome ('reluctant journey') or where there is no hope of curative treatment ('end of useful chemotherapy'). In Example 6.1, the use of the signalling expression 'if you can think of' explicitly suggests the intention to help the addressee reconceptualise their situation in a less negative way. In the same example, 'chapter' is also used metaphorically to present the illness as part of a sequence of entities that make up the person's life.

Journey metaphors are also used in our online data to highlight some positive aspects of the mostly negative experience of being ill with cancer, and particularly a new appreciation of different aspects of one's life:

Example 6.3

> My journey may not be smooth but it certainly makes me look up and take notice of the scenary!
>
> [O]

Here the Journey framing makes it possible to combine the idea of difficult travelling conditions with the appreciation of new places. Likewise, in Example 6.4, the notion of 'enjoy[ing] the good scenery' is used in a lengthy simile aiming to encourage another patient to focus more on the positive than the negative aspects of the experience of cancer:

Example 6.4

> Cancer is just like a long and winding country road enjoy the good scenery and get past the rough areas as quickly and as safely as you can.
>
> [O]

In these examples, the person with cancer is also placed in a position where they have at least some degree of choice and agency in the journey and how they approach it ('makes me look up and take notice', 'enjoy [. . .] and get past'), even if the journey itself cannot be avoided.

In other cases, Journey metaphors are used in ways that more explicitly place the patient in an active, empowered position:

Example 6.5

> But most of all I passionately believe we all need to choose our own road through this and be our own health advocate, not to be a passive patient but to feel an empowered collaborator in our road back to full health
>
> [O]

Here the idea of a choice of 'road' seems to allude to different treatment options (see section 6.5.2): the readers of the post are being encouraged to take charge of what happens to them. Moreover, the destination of the journey is described as 'back to full health'. In other words, the destination is positive, and the health condition that the patient aims for is the same as prior to the cancer diagnosis. This example shows both the positive, motivating ways in which Journey metaphors can frame the experience of cancer, and a possibly unrealistic view of the outcome of treatment, i.e. fully restoring the person to a pre-cancer state of health. This notion of full health as the destination in Journey metaphors for the illness experience recurs in a number of other posts.

A final positive framing of the illness experience that is provided by some Journey metaphors in our corpus is the notion of other people with cancer as fellow travellers:

Example 6.6

> The rocks in our paths are easier to handle when we're all in it together. My biggest learning point from the whole cancer experience is that the best people to help you are the ones who've been there before or are heading there with you.
>
> [O]

Here the reference to 'rocks in our paths' suggests difficulty, but the writers and other people on the forum are presented as benefiting from being companions on the same path, and from the help that can be provided by people with more experience.

In addition, in 42 cases, Journey metaphors are used as parting formulae to sign off at the end of a post, as we have also observed for some Violence metaphors in Chapter 5 (e.g. 'keep up the good fight'). These formulae display some degree of variation, but all involve wishing others well in coping with their illness, as in: 'best of luck on your journey', 'all the best on your journey', 'safe journey', 'stay strong on your journeys', 'peace be the journey' and so on.

Conversely, however, Journey metaphors are also used by patients in our data to express negative emotions, and to suggest extreme difficulty and helplessness—or what can be summarised broadly as disempowerment. Often, this specific framing is evoked via the co-text of the metaphor at hand (similarly to what we noted with Violence metaphors in Chapter 5). The adjectives that modify 'journey' and related metaphorical expressions include: 'fearsome', 'difficult', 'long and arduous', 'infernal', 'unenviable', 'hardest' and 'very tough'. Our data also includes phrases such as 'nightmare of a journey' and 'hell of a journey' in relation to the experience of cancer.

In Example 6.7, the writer negatively evaluates her progress on the 'cancer journey', but for reasons outside her control:

Example 6.7

> Well, I have not done so well with my own "cancer journey" through the wilderness of my own local hospitals
>
> [O]

Here what is metaphorised as a journey is not the illness experience generally but the specific experience of being a patient in the writer's local hospitals, which are themselves metaphorically described as inhospitable environments ('wilderness').

An even greater sense of lack of control on the cancer 'journey' or 'road' is conveyed by the following examples:

Example 6.8

How the hell am I supposed to know how to navigate this road I do not even want to be on when I've never done it before

[O]

Example 6.9

As much as I have found this thread painful (and scarey) because I am [. . .] a brain tumour patient myself. I have often said that I only pop by every now and again because it saddens my heart to read of the passengers nearing the end of their journey and those recently having finished their journey.

[O]

The author of Example 6.8 expresses lack of acceptance and frustration via the notion of being an unwilling traveller on an unfamiliar road. This example also suggests that even Journey metaphors can potentially put some responsibility for success or failure on patients; they need to know how to navigate the road. Example 6.9 is part of a long series of posts in which the writer describes the contributors to the online forum as travelling on the same train. This particular Journey metaphor places the patients in the disempowered position of 'passengers' with no control on the journey, and spells out the end point of the journey as death rather than recovery.

A negative framing is also suggested by Journey metaphors in which the person is travelling alone, as when someone comments that 'every person's cancer journey is different'. In the following extract, the difficulties experienced by both patients and family carers are described as lonely journeys:

Example 6.10

as much as we have support from family and friends, we go through the cancer journey on our own, as much as you, as a carer, go through your journey on your own

[O]

The expression 'go through', which is repeated twice in Example 6.10, is used metaphorically by patients in our data more often than by the other two participant groups (see Figures 6.2 and 6.3), and tends to suggest slowness and difficulty on the journey. Therefore, similarly to what we noted regarding the linguistic realisations of the Violence metaphor (e.g. 'battle' versus 'fighter') in Chapter 5, the specific lexicalisation of the metaphor also matters with Journey metaphors. In a few cases, the illness itself is presented as the patient's travelling companion, as in:

Example 6.11

On my journey so far with cancer I have learnt to expect the worst. [O]

Overall, Journey metaphors in our patient data involve a variety of different scenarios, which can be used to express different degrees of agency and (dis)empowerment, different attitudes and a range of positive or negative emotions. As we have shown, the patients contributing to the online forum use Journey metaphors for a variety of interpersonal purposes, including not just expressing their own views and emotions, but also supporting others via advice, encouragement and a sense of companionship and solidarity.

Carers' Use of Journey Metaphors for the Experience of Illness

The family carers in our corpus also use Journey metaphors for the experience of cancer when writing online, although less frequently than patients. In the carer data, 66 out of 84 metaphorical uses of 'journey' refer to the illness experience of the person they care for, including eight instances of 'cancer journey'. Seven out of 17 metaphorical instances of 'road' are also used metaphorically in a similar way.

As in the patient data, a variety of pre-modifying expressions are used to indicate the difficulty of the overall experience. Metaphorical instances of 'journey' are pre-modified by expressions such as 'awful', 'hard', 'arduous', 'dreadful', 'horrific', 'tough' and 'old', as well as 'crap' and 'nightmare of a'. Similarly, the carer's experience of illness is described as a 'road' that can be 'rocky', 'hard' and 'long'. On the other hand, as with the patients, the notion of a journey allows for the possibility of positive moments:

Example 6.12

The journey is tough but my husband and I made some wonderful memories and had many wonderful moments

[O]

In other words, carers' Journey metaphors for the experience of illness display similar kinds of variation as we have noticed for patients, but from a different perspective. Different kinds of Journey scenarios are used to express a sense of isolation, on the one hand, and, on the other, feelings of companionship with the person who is ill or with other carers on the online forum. This depends on whether the journey is undertaken alone or shared with fellow travellers, and to what extent it is presented as feasible.

In the Journey scenario evoked by Example 6.13 (which we also quoted in Chapter 1), a recently bereaved husband provides emotional support and advice to a distraught contributor who has been writing about her husband's reaction to her cancer. This is one of several examples where a carer and a loved one are presented as travelling together, but on a path that is unique to them:

Example 6.13

Cancer is a journey, some people have similar experiences to others on that journey, but by and large the journey has many twists and turns that means no two people go the exact same route. I think it is like trying to drive a coach and horses uphill with no back wheels on the coach. You do need to stop occasionally and rest the horses, review the situation with your husband.

[O]

Here the idea of cancer as a journey is first extended to specify a difficult and lonely journey ('many twists and turns', 'no two people go the exact same route'), and then creatively elaborated via a lengthy simile. The simile outlines a scenario involving a difficult path ('uphill') and a specific but damaged vehicle ('coach and horses [. . .] with no back wheels on the coach'). This scenario is used to encourage and validate times of reflection within a couple experiencing cancer together ('stop occasionally and rest the horses').

In contrast, in several other cases the sick person's uniquely difficult situation is conveyed by suggesting that they are travelling alone. This applies particularly when a carer is writing after their loved one has died, so that the journey's end point is death, whether or not it is explicitly mentioned:

Example 6.14

may he rest peacefully noiw after his long and arduous journey

[O]

Example 6.15

The truth is that I think that my friend and I started our hell at almost the same time, she with her husband's sudden death and me with my husband's slow road to death.

[O]

Example 6.14 emphasises the sick person's difficulties by describing his journey as 'long and arduous', which justifies the use of the conventional euphemistic metaphor 'rest' for death. Example 6.15, in contrast, emphasises the emotional toll that incurable cancer takes on family carers. The expression 'hell' is used to capture both the friend's experience of her husband dying suddenly and the writer's experience of protracted illness with no hope of recovery. Here the description of the road as 'slow' involves a transfer of the notion of speed from the metaphorical travel to the travelling surface itself (similar Speed metaphors are used to describe 'bad deaths' by healthcare professionals, as we discuss in Chapter 8).

The most comforting and mutually encouraging uses of Journey metaphors for the experience of illness in the carer data are those where the journey is shared with other carers contributing to the forum, even if the circumstances are difficult:

Example 6.16

HI, we are on the same <u>journey</u> as you, My husband was also diagnosed in May

[O]

Example 6.17

Its a <u>rocky road</u> we are <u>travelling on</u> you and I, take care.

[O]

In a similar way to patients, a few carers use Journey metaphors to wish others well at the end of posts:

Example 6.18

Look after yourself and stay strong for the <u>road ahead</u> looks like a <u>rocky</u> one for you. I'm here if you need to chat. the biggest hug to you and your girls xxxhugsxxx

[O]

Professionals' Use of Journey Metaphors for the Experience of Illness

The health professionals' section of our corpus contains relatively few instances of Journey metaphors for the experience of illness, compared with patients and carers. The word 'journey' is used metaphorically in relation to the experience of illness 15 times (out of 29 metaphorical occurrences), and 'road' only once (out of two metaphorical occurrences). Where Journey metaphors are used for this topic, the focus is often on the end-of-life period in particular. This is due to the way in which we collected our data, and often involves euphemistic references to dying or proximity to death, as in 'last journey' or 'final journey'. Where Journey metaphors are extended beyond individual expressions, the professional perspective is very much in evidence:

Example 6.19

as health professionals we must shore up (our patients) dignity and bloster their self-confidence; facilitating acceptance of their illness and accompanying them on their uncertain journey.

[O]

Example 6.20

So erm hospice care has grown up out of erm somebody actually saying we should be alongside somebody when they're actually in extremis towards the end of their life erm and being alongside people you're actually trying to erm to to walk with them on their journey.

[I]

In Example 6.19, the metaphorical journey is illness generally, while in Example 6.20, from an interview with a hospice manager, it relates to the final stages of the person's life. In Example 6.19, 'shore up' and 'bolster' are also used metaphorically to refer to the doctor's role in ensuring patients' dignity and self-confidence. More importantly, in both examples, the healthcare professional is presented as a travelling companion 'accompanying' and 'walking with' or 'alongside' the patient. This role on the metaphorical journey reflects the professional aspirations and identities of the writer and interviewee respectively, but, in our corpus, is typical only of the Journey metaphors used by healthcare professionals. Although our patient and carer data includes many expressions of praise and gratitude towards healthcare professionals, we have not found comparable instances of patients' or carers' Journey metaphors where doctors or nurses accompany the patient and their families on the metaphorical journey of illness or end of life. As we have shown, where patients or carers mention companions on their metaphorical journey, they refer to their family members, or to other patients or carers.

We will return to healthcare professionals' use of Journey metaphors for the end of life in Chapter 8, where we discuss specifically the metaphors they use to describe 'good' and 'bad' deaths.

6.4.2 Journey Metaphors for Treatment/Care Options

In this section, we turn to the Journey metaphors that are used in our corpus to refer to options for treatment and care. This involves a specific subset of Journey metaphors, including particularly the "path" lexical grouping.

As shown in Figures 6.2 and 6.3, 'path' metaphors in our corpus are used significantly more frequently by healthcare professionals than by members of the other two groups, especially in the online data. The "path" grouping includes both the nouns 'path' and 'pathway', and it is the latter that is responsible for the differences among the participant groups. In the professional data, 74 out of 78 instances of 'path' metaphors involve the noun 'pathway'. In contrast, 'path' metaphors for patients and carer mostly involve 'path' rather than 'pathway' (12 out of 13 instances for patients and 9 out of 15 instances for carers).

Professionals' Journey Metaphors for Treatment/Care Options

In the UK National Health Service, the term 'pathway' is generally used to refer to a structured treatment plan or strategy. This use of the term dates from the early 2000s, when 'integrated care pathways' were introduced to reduce clinical variability and improve outcomes. In our data, 'pathway' relates primarily to palliative and end-of-life care: the top 10 collocates of 'pathway' in the professional sections of our corpus include 'dying', 'end' and 'life'.[1]

In the following example, one of our interviewees positively evaluates the 'pathways' that apply to people with cancer in need of palliative care, in contrast with patients with other conditions:

> *Example 6.21*
>
> if they [patients with gynaecological cancers] needed referring to palliative care I'd do the referral for palliative care and I felt those patients were quite well supported, my <u>pathways</u> were clear, I knew who I was referring to, I knew what services I could tap into for those patients erm for other disease groups like your you know stroke patients that type of thing who haven't got a traditional hospice diagnosis, <u>pathways</u> were much much less clear.
>
> [I]

As is often the case for metaphorical technical terms, 'pathway' in examples such as this has a context-specific meaning that, for healthcare professionals, has all but lost its connection with the physical source-domain meaning (see Deignan et al. 2013). This can be seen, among other things, from the fact that, in the professional data, 'pathway' does not tend to occur as part of extended and/or creative Journey metaphors, in contrast to, for example, the use of 'journey' for the experience of illness (see section 6.4.1). In Example 6.21, the other metaphorical expressions are highly conventional and do not form a single metaphorical scenario of which 'pathways' is a part ('clear', 'tap into'). Moreover, the use of the first-person singular pronoun in 'my pathways were clear' also emphasises the professional's rather than the patient's perspective.

In addition, in 43 out of 74 metaphorical instances of 'pathway' in the healthcare professional data, the term occurs as part of the phrase 'Liverpool Care Pathway'. To these need to be added 110 instances of the acronym 'LPC' for this particular pathway in our online data. Indeed, the top three collocates of 'pathway' in our healthcare professional data are 'Liverpool', 'LPC' and 'care'. The Liverpool Care Pathway for the Dying Patient was a particular approach to the care of the dying that was initially introduced in the late 1990s to ensure the comfort and dignity of dying patients. It involved, among other things, the cessation of non-essential medication and treatment for patients who were deemed to be close enough to death not to benefit from further intervention. In 2012, the LCP became publicly controversial after numerous media reports that it was not always correctly implemented. In 2013, an independent review recommended that it should be phased out. Our healthcare professional data, which spans the period 2008–13, reflects this controversy. Some uses are supportive, usually by emphasising the original goals of the pathway:

Example 6.22

The Liverpool Care pathway (LCP) was introduced to do just that—make dying as comfortable and as dignified a process as possible.

[O]

Other references are more critical, or minimally recognise the negative perceptions that came to be increasingly associated with the pathway, in spite of its stated intentions:

Example 6.23

The liverpool care pathway is in widespread use across all health care.

I am now asked by terrified patients not to admit them in case they are put on the dreaded Liverpool Care Pathway, given a lethal injection and even whether it represents some kind of punishment for bad behaviour in hospital.

[O]

In contrast with this technical use of 'pathway', the healthcare professionals in our data seldom use other expressions for treatment options. 'Route' is used metaphorically on two occasions to refer to treatment options available to physicians (e.g. a 'conservative route' to deal with chronic kidney disease), while 'path' is used on four occasions to refer to the choices that patients can make:

Example 6.24

> It is somehow counter-intuitive that a 13 year old should choose a <u>path</u> that will inevitably result in her death, when treatment is available.
>
> [O]

In contrast, these and other less formal terms are preferred by patients and carers.

Patients' Journey Metaphors for Treatment/Care Options

Our patient data contains only one metaphorical instance of 'pathway', as follows:

Example 6.25

> I wish you and your mum all the best and a speedy <u>pathway</u> to getting the best advice and treatment for her.
>
> [O]

Although this use of 'pathway' is broadly related to treatment or care options, it refers specifically to the process that the patient has to go through to receive 'the best advice and treatment'. It is therefore different from the technical use we have described in relation to healthcare professionals. Moreover, the use of the adjective 'speedy' as a pre-modifier of 'pathway' may suggest more active metaphoricity than in the technical use of 'pathway' in the healthcare professional data: the idea of the speed of metaphorical travel towards 'getting the best advice and treatment' is applied to the travelling surface ('pathway'), which is therefore implicitly presented as capable of movement.

The patient data contains a number of other expressions that are used metaphorically to refer to different options for treatment and care. In the following example, 'path' is used metaphorically in the context of encouraging another patient to take charge of making decisions about treatment:

Example 6.26

> Its your disease, your life and your <u>path</u> to choose. Good luck with whichever <u>way</u> it <u>takes</u> you.
>
> [O]

Eight out of 33 metaphorical instances of 'road' are used in a similar way, including by positioning the patient in an empowered decision-making position:

Example 6.27

You aren't anywhere near the end of your personal treatment road yet and there are plenty of people living with and managing the disease

[O]

Example 6.28

Wishing you a safe journey, whichever road you choose.

[O]

In the patient data, 17 out of 24 metaphorical instances of 'route' are also to do with care/treatment options, although they vary in terms of whether they present the patient in an empowered (Example 6.29) or disempowered role (Example 6.30):

Example 6.29

In the end, you can only take one route through treatment, and you can only achieve one outcome. Having achieved that outcome, you can never know whether a different treatment would have made a difference. We all have to come to terms with that uncertainty.

[O]

Example 6.30

Don't get me wrong, being a patient is hard, but we follow whatever route the doctors decide is best for us, and we know we have very little control on what is happening or going to happen to us.

[O]

In all these cases, the main metaphorical expression is not a technical term in the institutional healthcare context, and several metaphorical expressions are used in close proximity to one another to outline a Journey scenario, e.g. 'your path [. . .] whichever way it takes you' (Example 6.26); 'aren't anywhere near the end of your personal treatment road' (Example 6.27); 'safe journey, whichever road' (Example 6.28); and 'follow whatever route' (Example 6.30). Although all the underlined expressions involve conventionalised metaphorical meanings, they cumulatively suggest a greater degree of active metaphoricity than in the professionals' technical use of 'pathway'.

Carers' Journey Metaphors for Treatment/Care Options

When 'pathway' is used metaphorically in the carer sections of our corpus, it is mostly to do with the experience of caring for someone with cancer in general terms, as in: 'you are not alone. I have walked the same pathway as you for the last three years' (see section 6.4.1). In fact, our carer data only includes one instance of 'pathway' in reference to a structured care plan:

Example 6.31

On Friday the Macmillan nurse did his Care Pathway and got all the drugs together for the anticipated syringe driver.

[O]

The use of capital letters and the reference to the Macmillan nurse suggests that the writer has picked up 'Care Pathway' as a technical term in interaction with the healthcare professionals caring for her husband. It is noteworthy that this is the only such use in the whole of our patient and carer data.

Carers also use other non-technical Journey metaphors for care/treatment options, although less frequently than patients. In the following example, the expression 'chemo route' is used in a context where the patient is given agency in deciding whether or not to have a further course of chemotherapy for an incurable lymphoma:

Example 6.32

The consultant wants an answer TODAY because if he wants to take the chemo route, then they have to start it as soon as possible.

[O]

Overall, therefore, the members of all three groups use Journey metaphors to refer to different care or treatment options. However, in the healthcare professionals' data, this overwhelmingly involves the frequent use of 'pathway' as a technical term, including in reference to the Liverpool Care Pathway. As is generally the case for originally metaphorical technical terms, 'pathway' is therefore unlikely to retain any potential metaphoricity for the members of the professional discourse community. This is evident, among other things, from the fact that it is not used by healthcare professionals as part of extended metaphors evoking rich Journey scenarios. In contrast, patients and carers in our data almost never use 'pathway' in this technical sense. Instead, both groups, and especially patients, use other, more informal metaphorical expressions such as 'road' and 'route', usually in combination with other Journey metaphors. This suggests that, as argued in previous studies of metaphorical technical terms, 'pathway' may retain its metaphoricity for patients and carers, even when it is used in a specialised technical sense by healthcare professionals (see Deignan et al. 2013). This can be a source of misunderstanding if the term is used in interactions with patients and their families, or in informational materials, without awareness that non-experts may have difficulties understanding it, or may understand it differently from healthcare professionals. For example, literal, physical pathways often cross one another, so that a traveller has the option of moving from one to another, but this does not apply to clinical pathways in the National Health Service, where patients cannot normally choose to change pathways even if they wish to.

6.5 Journey and Violence Metaphors in Combination

In this and the previous chapters, we have shown how Journey and Violence metaphors for cancer and the end of life broadly contrast in terms of the framings they provide, but are not as opposed in terms of their evaluative, emotional and potentially (dis)empowering implications as is often suggested in the scholarly literature, media opinion pieces and policy decisions. In this section, we consider in more detail the relationship between these two broad types of metaphors in our corpus.

6.5.1 Journey and Violence Metaphors Used Together

Violence and Journey metaphors are sometimes used alongside each other in our data. For example, one contributor to the patient online forum signs off at the end of a sombre post by presenting 'battle' and 'journey' as alternative but equally acceptable descriptions of having a brain tumour ('BT'):

> *Example 6.33*
>
> Love and Strength to all those involved in a BT battle or journey
>
> [O]

Another patient writing online uses a Violence metaphor and a novel Journey metaphor as alternative descriptions of another patient's 'journey':

> *Example 6.34*
>
> Did you find your journey a battle or a steady work(wo)manlike trudge?
>
> [O]

First, the fact that 'battle' is used as a possible gloss for the person's 'journey' suggests that the writer does not perceive the two framings as incompatible, possibly because they are both rather general and conventional. Second, the more precise description of the metaphorical 'trudge' as 'steady' and 'work(wo)manlike' gives some indication of how that is perceived to contrast with a 'battle': it involves long-term effort and persistence as opposed to the short-term intense burst of energetic and aggressive activity associated with battles.

In several posts, Violence and Journey metaphors are combined in complementary ways rather than contrasted. In the following two examples, a patient and a carer respectively present the destination of the cancer 'journey' as the site of a battle with the disease:

Example 6.35

Continued strength to everyone on this journey, whatever your situation, we are united in our journeys to slay the BC Beast :)

[O]

Example 6.36

I am totally convinced that as you will help and guide him through this part of his journey, he will come out the other end in a much better place to fight this disease.

[O]

In Example 6.35, the use of 'slay' and 'Beast' may be seen as allusions to mythical battles, such as that between St George and the Dragon. The fact that this description is applied to people with breast cancer suggests that Violence metaphors are not perceived by at least some of the patients in our data as unsuitable for a type of cancer that overwhelmingly affects women. In Example 6.36, a carer writing online describes the addressee's role metaphorically as that of a guide on a journey, and the preposition 'through' is used, as is often the case in our data, to emphasise difficulty (as opposed to 'on this part of his journey', which would be more neutral). This help and guidance will result in the patient being able to get better, conveyed metaphorically as being in a most suitable place to 'fight' the cancer. Both descriptions involve the kind of metaphorical creativity that has been described as 'combining' different conventional metaphors into a single coherent whole (Lakoff and Turner 1989; see also Leech 1969). This combination also has a narrative element, as the metaphorical journey is presented as prior to the metaphorical fight or battle.

In other cases, the use of Violence and Journey metaphors in close proximity does not, strictly speaking, outline fully coherent scenarios, but the result seems rhetorically effective nonetheless. Example 6.37 is part of a post in which a woman with incurable metastatic cancer talks about training for the London Marathon for the first time as a way of continuing to live life to the full. In the extract, she talks about the metaphorical cancer 'journey' itself as an aggressor that 'tears [her] apart':[2]

Example 6.37

My journey so far with cancer has torn me apart but I am insistent that something positive has to come out of it.

[O]

In Example 6.38, another patient talks about the difficulties in 'fighting' the (cancer) 'Demon' in terms appropriate for difficulties on a journey ('twists and turns'):

Example 6.38

I would just like to wish you all the best with your operation in March, I am so glad your fortunes have changed for the better, so many twists and turns when it comes to fighting this Demon.

[O]

Examples such as these are traditionally described as 'mixed metaphors', and negatively evaluated for being incoherent and confusing. More recently, research on metaphor has shown that the 'mixing' of metaphors is a frequent phenomenon that does not, for the most part, impede comprehension or necessarily reflect a poor command of one's language (e.g. Kimmel 2010; Gibbs 2016; Semino 2016).

Finally, there are also cases where a writer rapidly shifts from one type of metaphor to another. In the following extract (already quoted as two separate examples), a healthcare professional talks about his patients' 'final journey' just before they die:

Example 6.39

I am humbled by the courage and dignity of my patients on their final journey. You are now the general and you see your troops killed in battle.

[O]

Here the euphemistic reference to the patients' 'final journey' helps to express the doctor's admiration for the way in which they accept their imminent death, while the following 'battle' metaphor emphasises the patients' vulnerability (as 'troops' being 'killed') and the doctor's sense of responsibility (as the 'general').

6.5.2 Journey and Violence Metaphors Used Separately by the Same Individuals

Many of the individuals represented in our online data use Journey and Violence metaphors at different points in the same post, or in different posts.

Our opening example in Chapter 1 is taken from a lengthy online forum post that a recently widowed carer, whom we referred to as Peter, addresses to a woman who is finding it difficult to understand her husband's reaction to her cancer diagnosis. Peter tries to help by recounting in some detail his own experience of and reactions to his late wife's cancer. He talks about alternating between conflicting thoughts and emotions, and uses the extended and creative Journey metaphor in Example 6.13 to express the loneliness and difficulties caused by cancer and the need to take the time to reflect quietly about the situation with one's partner ('no two people go the exact same route', 'like trying to drive a coach and horses uphill with no back wheels on the coach', 'stop occasionally and rest the horses'). He then remembers how, soon after her diagnosis, his wife of 40 years wanted him to leave her to spare him from suffering, and uses a Violence metaphor to express his response to this:

Example 6.40

> Naturally, being kind of stubborn, I refused to go, I worked on the basis that this was an enemy attacking my loved one and it had picked a fight with me as well. I wish I could say that we won all the battles, and that she is alive and well and cancer free. We did however win a significant number of the skirmishes to make me proud to have been worthy to be by my darling's side.
>
> [O]

Here Peter creatively exploits the notion of a 'fight' with cancer to express how he felt involved, motivated and strong in trying to help his wife survive her illness. The cancer is explicitly personified as an 'enemy' 'attacking' his wife but also 'pick[ing] a fight' with him, and the small successes that preceded his wife's death are presented as 'win[ning]' some 'skirmishes', in contrast to 'all the battles' that he wishes they could have won. This sense of being a determined (if defeated) combatant alongside his wife leads to the pride that Peter explicitly mentions at the end of the extract.

Something similar can be observed in the writings of a patient who is one of the most prolific contributors to the online forum we analysed. For the purposes of this discussion, we will call him Dave. We cannot do full justice to the creativity and variety of metaphors that Dave uses to talk about his own and others' experiences of cancer. Among other types of metaphors, Dave repeatedly uses both Journey and Violence metaphors at different points, as in the following two examples (already quoted above and in Chapter 5):

Example 6.41

> if you can think of this chapter in your life as a reluctant <u>journey</u> and each procedure a <u>place</u> along that <u>journey</u> that must be completed before you <u>move onto</u> the next it may help you better deal with it.
>
> [O]

Example 6.42

> if other people see me as brave then ok, after all I have not <u>hunkered down</u> in my <u>trench</u> to just merely <u>defend</u> myself against the <u>demon</u> but have <u>picked up</u> my <u>sword</u> and taken the <u>fight</u> to the <u>demon</u>
>
> [O]

In Example 6.41, an extended Journey metaphor is used to encourage another person to accept a recent cancer diagnosis and to develop an attitude that will help them cope with their treatment. The person's attitude is transferred to the journey itself via the adjective 'reluctant', but overall the idea of a journey with interim destinations is used to suggest that it is possible to cope with being ill by focusing on one 'procedure' at a time, even when, as in the case of the particular addressee, there is little or no hope of being cured. This also helps to normalise cancer as part of life's longer 'journey'—something also suggested by the metaphorical use of 'chapter'.

In Example 6.42, Dave uses a creative Violence metaphor to express how he has come to accept being described as 'brave' by other people. He uses two different Violence scenarios to contrast two possible approaches to being ill: passive acceptance as 'defending' oneself by 'hunker[ing] down' in one's 'trench', versus active determination to get better as having engaged in a 'fight' with 'the demon' (as he repeatedly describes cancer; see also our discussion of Supernatural metaphors in Chapter 4). The latter approach is positively evaluated and corresponds to his view of bravery as a person with cancer.

These extracts from Peter's and Dave's posts, and the other examples in this section, provide yet more evidence that it is overly simplistic to contrast Violence and Journey metaphors as respectively bad and good for cancer patients: both can provide empowering or disempowering framings, and reflect and reinforce both positive and negative attitudes and emotions. Moreover, our analysis shows that the two types of metaphors are best suited for different functions. The notion of cancer as a metaphorical journey is particularly suited to emphasise the lengthy duration of the illness, the presence of a succession of phases, the need for long-term perseverance, and a focus on the future. The notion of violent confrontation with the disease is particularly suited to expressing lack of fear, dogged determination, intense effort to get better and a focus on the moment. Some versions of Violence metaphors also include a competitive element, which can be negative when the illness is incurable, but positive in the context of coping with difficult side effects of potentially curative treatment.

This explains why the same individuals sometimes use both types of metaphors, separately or in combination, depending on what they are trying to express. Rather than mutually exclusive alternatives, these two broad types of metaphors are therefore best seen as different resources that people dealing with cancer and the end of life may exploit for different purposes. This is not in contradiction with the possibility that some people may prefer one type of metaphor or the other (or neither), and that Violence metaphors can be particularly harmful when *imposed* on people with cancer, or applied when the disease is incurable.

Because of the size of our corpus, we cannot provide definite figures for how many people in our data use *both* Violence and Journey metaphors. We do, however, have evidence that a sizeable proportion of patients and carers do. We separated the online writings of each of the individuals included in our patient and carer subcorpora and identified those who use both the singular noun 'journey' and words belonging to the semantic tag S8– (Hindering): 'journey' is mostly used metaphorically in our data, and so are the tokens under S8–, which include 'fight' and 'fighting'. Out of 56 carers in our online data, 20 use 'journey' at least once, 35 use items included under S8–, and 15 use both (i.e. just over a quarter). And out of 56 patients, 33 use 'journey' at least once, 44 use items included under S8–, and 27 use both (i.e. just under half). Given that these figures are based only on the use of one word and one semantic domain, they are likely to underestimate the proportion of people in the two subcorpora who use both Journey and Violence metaphors.

6.6 Conclusions

Journey metaphors are the second most frequent type of metaphor in our corpus (after Violence metaphors), in spite of the fact that our methodological constraints (see section 6.2) only enabled us to identify a subset (albeit substantial) of all such metaphors. This high relative frequency can be seen as partly a reflection of the conventionality and versatility of Journey metaphors in English generally, and partly as a consequence of the specific topics that these metaphors help to express and the functions they perform in our data specifically. We have shown how all three participant groups in our corpus use Journey metaphors to talk about the experience of illness and treatment options, and to perform a range of functions, both personal (expressing views and emotions) and interpersonal (advising, encouraging, empathising).

The different topics and functions of Journey metaphors also help explain the quantitative differences we have observed in the different sections of the corpus. Patients use Journey metaphors more than the other two groups to talk about different aspects of the experience of illness. This explains a higher relative frequency of Journey metaphors in the patient online data in particular, and a more frequent use by patients of expressions such as 'journey' and 'go/come through'. In interviews, healthcare professionals use Journey metaphors more frequently than the other two groups and than in the online professional data, primarily because these metaphors are used to answer questions about end-of-life care and good/bad deaths (see Chapter 8).

Some of the quantitative and qualitative differences we have observed among the participant groups have potential implications for communication in healthcare. Healthcare professionals regularly use 'pathway' as a metaphorical technical term for a structured care plan, while patients and carers in our data do so extremely rarely. Instead, patients and carers use more informal Journey metaphors for treatment/care options, such as 'path' and 'road'. This, we have suggested, can lead to ambiguity or misunderstanding if 'pathway' is used in written or spoken communication with patients and their families, for whom it may retain a degree of active metaphoricity that it no longer has for healthcare professionals.

From a qualitative point of view, only healthcare professionals describe themselves as companions on patients' illness journeys, while patients and family carers never describe doctors and nurses as such in our data. This suggests a potential contrast between professionals' identities and aspirations, on the one hand, and the perceptions of the people they serve, on the other.

Taking Chapter 5 and the present chapter together, our analyses have shown that patients and carers use Violence and Journey metaphors more frequently when writing online than in interviews. This is partly because our interviews with patients and carers were conducted as part of previous studies concerned with people's experiences of healthcare services. This was less conducive to the expression of emotions, evaluations and personal views than our own interviews with healthcare professionals. Having said that, the frequency and variety of Violence and Journey metaphors in our online data for patients and carers in particular confirms the important role that peer-to-peer online communication can have for people living with their own or a loved one's cancer, or illness generally.

As we have shown, both types of metaphors are used to express moments of optimism, give vent to negative emotions and provide advice, support, encouragement and solidarity to others. They also help in the construction and negotiation of new identities for people whose lives and sense of self have been upset by an illness such as cancer, whether as fighters, travellers on a new journey or both. In this sense, metaphors help to perform some of the central positive functions associated with peer-to-peer online communities, including for people with cancer (e.g. Zhang et al. 2017).

Does our analysis support the view that Violence metaphors are harmful for people with cancer, and Journey metaphors a better alternative? As we have suggested throughout, the answer is no, or at least not straightforwardly. On the one hand, Journey metaphors for the experience of cancer do seem to have some of the advantages mentioned by McFadyean at the beginning of this chapter, and implicitly suggested by the preference for Journey metaphors in policy documents and initiatives. Journey metaphors can frame the experience in ways that emphasise continuity, companionship, agency, purpose and potentially positive aspects and emotions. The absence of an opponent against which one could win or lose also means that they do not have the same potential to cause the feelings of anxiety or guilt that we have noted for Violence metaphors, especially when the illness is incurable. On the other hand, Journey metaphors can also be used to reflect and reinforce a sense of powerlessness and loneliness, and to express negative emotions such as frustration, dejection and lack of acceptance. In Chapter 5, we showed that the same kind of variation applies to Violence metaphors, which can also be used to express positive or negative emotions, and to suggest both empowerment and disempowerment, especially as far as patients are concerned.

What seems to make a difference is not the type of metaphor per se, but the kind of Journey or Violence scenario that is evoked, and the emotions and degree of (dis)empowerment associated with the role of the patient (or carer/healthcare professional) in that scenario. This is in fact consistent both with earlier small-case studies of individual variation in relation to metaphors for cancer (e.g. Reisfield and Wilson 2004; Appleton and Flynn 2014), and with studies suggesting that, in areas such as education, it is important to provide learners with a variety of metaphors for a particular topic, as different metaphors provide different perspectives (e.g. Cameron 2003). In addition, we have shown that a crucial consideration in determining the nature of the framing suggested by a metaphor is the specific lexical realisations (e.g. 'fighter' versus 'battle', or 'journey' versus 'go through') and other lexical items, whether figurative or not, found in the co-text (e.g. the presence of negation or negative evaluative adjectives). The importance of specific metaphorical scenarios and linguistic realisations for the framing effects of different metaphors also has implications for metaphor theory, and particularly for the validity of generalisations made in terms of broad conceptual metaphors such as BEING ILL WITH

CANCER IS A VIOLENT CONFRONTATION WITH THE DISEASE and BEING ILL WITH CANCER IS A JOURNEY (see Semino et al. 2016 and Chapter 11).

Concerning the relationship between Violence and Journey metaphors, our analyses have shown that they are best suited to express different aspects of people's experiences and emotions, rather than being straightforwardly opposite ways of expressing the same things. Violence metaphors are best at expressing defiance, intense activity or concentration, and determination to succeed against the odds. Journey metaphors are best at expressing continuity, quiet perseverance over lengthy periods of time, and a new appreciation of life in the context of adversity. These different functions are particularly obvious when Journey and Violence metaphors are used together, or by the same people on different occasions.

Our findings therefore confirm the need for extreme caution in the use of Violence metaphors by healthcare professionals, charities and the media, but also emphasise the importance of accepting and encouraging individual variation in metaphor use, and valuing the different contributions that Violence and Journey metaphors can make to people's ability to express and cope with their experiences. Censoring Violence metaphors and promoting Journey metaphors uncritically across the board can deprive patients in particular of the advantages of the former, and ignore the inevitable limitations of the latter.

Notes

1. Collocates were computed within a window of five words to the left and five words to the right of 'pathway', and ordered by the Dice coefficient measure of collocation strength. The threshold for inclusion was set at five instances.
2. In Example 6.37, 'come out of' is also used as a very conventional metaphorical expression that constructs the journey/illness as a container from which the person can take out different kinds of entities/experiences.

References

Appleton, L., and Flynn, M. (2014). Searching for the new normal: Exploring the role of language and metaphors in becoming a cancer survivor. *European Journal of Oncology Nursing*, *18*(4), 378–384.

Cameron, L. (2003). *Metaphor in educational discourse*. London: Continuum.

Cancer Institute of New South Wales. (2017). Writing about cancer guidelines. Available online: https://www.cancerinstitute.org.au/about-us/Media/Writing-about-cancer-guidelines [Accessed 29/09/2017].

Deignan, A., Littlemore, J., and Semino, E. (2013). *Figurative language, genre and register*. Cambridge: Cambridge University Press.

Department of Health. (2007). *Cancer reform strategy*. Retrieved April 2017, from www.nhs.uk/NHSEngland/NSF/Documents/Cancer%20Reform%20Strategy.pdf

Department of Health. (2008). *End of life care strategy*. Retrieved April 2017, from www.gov.uk/government/publications/end-of-life-care-strategy-promoting-high-quality-care-for-adults-at-the-end-of-their-life

Department of Health. (2015). *Achieving world class cancer outcomes: A strategy for England*. Report of the Independent Cancer Task Force Retrieved April 2017, from www.cancerresearchuk.org/sites/default/files/achieving_world-class_cancer_outcomes_-_a_strategy_for_england_2015-2020.pdf

Evans, P., Noble, P., and Hull-Malham, N. (2011). *The cancer journey: Positive steps to help yourself heal*. London: Antony Rowe Publishing Services.

Gibbs, R. W. Jr (Ed.). (2016). *Mixing metaphor*. Amsterdam: John Benjamins.

Kimmel, M. (2010). Why we mix metaphors (and mix them well): Discourse coherence, conceptual metaphor, and beyond. *Journal of Pragmatics*, 42, 97–115.

Lakoff, G. (1993). The contemporary theory of metaphor. In A. Ortony (Ed.), *Metaphor and thought* (pp. 202–251). Cambridge and New York: Cambridge University Press.

Lakoff, G., and Turner, M. (1989). *More than cool reason: A field guide to poetic metaphor*. Chicago: University of Chicago Press.

Leech, G. N. (1969). *A linguistic guide to English poetry*. London: Longman.

L'Hôte, E. (2014). *Identity, narrative and metaphor: A corpus-based cognitive analysis of new labour discourse*. Basingstoke: Palgrave Macmillan.

McFadyean, M. (2005, January 22). Who knew? *The Guardian*. Available: https://www.theguardian.com/society/2005/jan/22/cancercare.weekendmagazine [Accessed 29/09/2017].

Reisfield, G. M., and Wilson, G. R. (2004). Use of metaphor in the discourse on cancer. *Journal of Clinical Oncology*, 22(19), 4024–4027.

Semino, E. (2016). A corpus-based study of 'mixed metaphor' as a metalinguistic comment. In R. W. Gibbs, Jr. (Ed.), *Mixing metaphor* (pp. 203–220). Amsterdam: John Benjamins.

Semino, E., Demjén, Z., and Demmen, J. (2016 advance access). An integrated approach to metaphor and framing in cognition, discourse and practice, with an application to metaphors for cancer. *Applied Linguistics*.

Zhang, S., O'Carroll, E. B., Owen, J., Bakken, S., and Elhadad, N. (2017). Online cancer communities as informatics intervention for social support: Conceptualization, characterization, and impact. *Journal of the American Informatics Association*, 24(2), 451–459.

Websites

Irish Hospice Foundation—journey of change. Retrieved April 2017, from http://hospicefoundation.ie/healthcare-programmes/residential-care/journey-change/

Cancer Care Ontario—cancer journey. Retrieved April 2017, from www.cancercare.on.ca/pcs/careoverview/cancercontrol/

Cancer Research Institute of New South Wales—writing about cancer guidelines. Retrieved April 2017, from www.cancerinstitute.org.au/about-us/Media/Writing-about-cancer-guidelines

7 Metaphors for the Relationship Between Patients and Healthcare Professionals

7.1 Introduction

The relationship between patients and healthcare professionals is a crucial aspect of healthcare. The quality of that relationship can make a big difference to the patient's experience, the success of a healthcare interaction and the professional lives of people who work in healthcare. A large literature exists on communication in healthcare settings from a linguistic perspective, and particularly on doctor-patient and nurse-patient interaction, focusing on communicative challenges and the negotiation of face needs, power and knowledge (for an overview, see Harvey and Koteyko 2013: 5–70). From a healthcare perspective, the therapeutic relationship is primarily considered in the context of training (e.g. the 'Sage and Thyme' approach developed at the University Hospital of South Manchester: www.sageandthymetraining.org.uk), but little evidence-based research has been carried out (e.g. Stevenson 2007).

Our data and methods enable us to take a different but complementary approach: in this chapter, we discuss the metaphors that are used by patients on the one hand and healthcare professionals on the other to describe their mutual relationships. For the purposes of our analysis, we take a broad view of what counts as a metaphor for this relationship. We include both metaphorical descriptions of members of the other group (e.g. patients describing healthcare professionals as 'vampires') and various metaphorical ways of referring to what each group does for or in interaction with the other (e.g. a healthcare professional patient talking about doctors 'fighting for patient survival' in Intensive Care Units). We consider the implications of the main metaphor patterns we identified for a better understanding of both patients' and professionals' experiences, attitudes and perspectives, and for fostering better relationships.

After some methodological details in section 7.2, we consider three broad topic areas where metaphors play a role in both datasets, but where differences between the two groups are important:

1. Descriptions of members of the other group (section 7.3);
2. Descriptions of what healthcare professionals do for patients (section 7.4);

3. Descriptions of particularly sensitive aspects of the relationship, i.e. interactions with healthcare professionals in the patient data and emotional involvement with patients in the healthcare professional data (section 7.5).

Section 7.6 provides some conclusions.

7.2 Methodology for the Retrieval of Relevant Metaphors

We employed a two-stage approach to the identification of metaphors that patients and healthcare professionals use in our corpus to talk about their mutual relationships. First, we collected relevant instances from the 1,449 linguistic metaphors we identified in the healthcare professional data and the 2,822 we identified in the patient data via the methodology described in Chapter 3 (see also Table 4.1). Second, we extracted concordances of the most relevant literal references to the members of the two groups from the patient and professional sections of our corpus, and checked the co-text in each case for metaphorical descriptions of the mutual relationships between them (cf. Stefanowitsch 2006 on concordancing lexical items from the target domain to study conventional metaphors).

For the healthcare professional data, we extracted and analysed concordances of the noun 'patient(s)' (in both singular and plural forms), which occurred 2,447 times. Other candidate expressions were considered ('cases' and 'people with'), but these did not generate useful data for our purposes, as they occurred infrequently and in close proximity to 'patients'. From the patient data, we extracted and analysed concordances for the main labels that the patients use to refer to the different types of healthcare professionals that they interact with. More specifically, we identified the 10 most frequent lexical items that were annotated by the USAS (UCREL Semantic Analysis System) tagger in Wmatrix with *both* the semantic tag B3 (Medicines and medical treatment) *and* S2 (People). The 10 lexical items were: 'nurse', 'doctor', 'GP', 'consultant', 'surgeon', 'sister', 'nurses', 'oncologist', 'doctors' and 'specialist'. We excluded 'sister(s)' from the analysis as this noun was in fact overwhelmingly used as a kinship term, but extracted concordances for all instances of the other nouns, in both singular and plural form in all cases,[1] i.e.:

- 'consultant(s)': 201 instances;
- 'doctor(s)': 323 instances;
- 'GP(s)': 216 instances;
- 'nurse(s)': 464 instances;
- 'oncologist(s)': 155 instances;

- 'specialist(s)': 143 instances;
- 'surgeon(s)': 179 instances.

This generated a total of 1,681 concordance lines for analysis.

7.3 Metaphorical Descriptions of Members of the Other Group

Both the patients and the healthcare professionals in our data use a range of metaphors to describe or refer to the members of the other group. However, both groups only use metaphors for this purpose when writing online, and not in interviews. This may be because, as we show, these metaphors often involve some form of evaluation, and focus on problematic and/or controversial issues. In addition, some of the patients' metaphors are light-hearted or humorous. It is likely that the interview setting discouraged this kind of description, in contrast with the anonymity and greater informality of online writing (cf. Seale et al. 2010). In this section, we begin with healthcare professionals and then discuss the metaphors used by patients.

7.3.1 Healthcare Professionals' Metaphorical Descriptions of Patients

In our online data, healthcare professionals do not often refer to or describe their patients metaphorically. When they do, the metaphors tend to be relatively novel and to occur as part of a broader argument or reflection about professional practices and challenges. For example, in the following extract, the writer describes patients as doctors' 'best teachers', and patients who have died as 'ghosts' (as in previous chapters, original spellings are retained in quotations from the online data):

Example 7.1

> Our patients are our best <u>teachers</u>. It is nice when they can stay alive and share their family stories. It is not so nice when despite your best efforts nature wins and death carries them to some other place. The <u>ghosts</u> of these patients remain with the physician, not in the sense of a <u>shadowy specter</u>, but, as a reiteration of thought. What was the ultimate cause of demise, could an intervention have been done differently, should the procedure be performed or deferred? These <u>ghosts</u> help us to make better decisions in the future. These <u>ghosts</u> point to new directions in research, new therapies, rejuvenation of old therapies turning a defeat into a victory. [. . .]
>
> As you accumulate <u>ghosts</u>—use them well.
>
> [O]

The use of 'best teachers' reverses the stereotypical view within which it is patients who benefit from the greater expertise of healthcare professionals, and emphasises instead the benefits that doctors can gain in interacting with and caring for patients. Similarly, 'ghosts' is used positively to indicate memories of deceased patients that can help doctors improve their future practices and decision-making, in contrast with the negative associations of the alternative metaphor 'shadowy specter'. This positive metaphorical role for patients is included within a broader and more conventional metaphor for the professionals' goal to keep patients alive (see 'nature wins' and 'defeat' versus 'victory'; see section 7.4.1). In response to Example 7.1, however, another forum contributor uses the expression 'a couple of ghosts who haunt me' more conventionally to refer to sad memories about two specific deceased patients with whose stories they became particularly involved.

Another writer, whom we will call Ulysses, criticises what he describes as 'Western Medicine' because, in his view, it has:

Example 7.2

> reduced the human being into pathological fragments which are dismembered and even psychiatry tends to do the same
>
> [O]

The metaphorical description of patients as 'fragments' emphasises the dehumanisation of patients that Ulysses aims to criticise. While 'dismembered' could be interpreted as partly literal when applied to patients who may need surgery, the reference to psychiatry requires a metaphorical interpretation: it can be taken as referring to an approach to care that only takes some aspects of patients into account, and ignores the individuality of the whole person. In a different post, Ulysses' critique involves a lengthy and sarcastic metaphorical comparison between some ward rounds from the beginning of his career and the court processions of the French king Louis the 14th. Within that metaphor, Ulysses casts the consultant as the king ('le Roi Soleil') and patients as 'royal subjects'. This highlights and negatively evaluates the way in which some consultants interpret their own role, resulting in patients having no control at all and seemingly relying on consultants' favours and whims.

Finally, a debate among online forum contributors involves the appropriateness of patients being described as 'work':

Example 7.3

> Patients are not Work! Rather they are Living, Breathing, Humans, Part of our great race called Humanity!
>
> [O]

Example 7.4

> By definition, work is carrying out a task in return for payment; i.e. employment. We would not be 'working' with patients if we were not paid. Therefore, patients ARE work. This does not however mean that work and compassion/empathy are mutually exclusive.
>
> [O]

This debate seems to involve different interpretations of 'work' as a description of patients. In Example 7.3, where capitalisation is repeatedly used for emphasis, 'work' seems to be intended as a (negated) metaphorical description that dehumanises patients. In Example 7.4, in contrast, 'work' seems to be intended as a metonymy: patients are associated with paid employment, so that referring to them as 'work' is simply a factual statement that does not deprive them of healthcare professionals' compassion and empathy. At a deeper level, however, the contrast between these two extracts seems to lie in whether healthcare is seen as a profession like any other or as something special and different, which is not primarily undertaken for the sake of remuneration. As we mentioned earlier, metaphorical descriptions of patients in the healthcare professional data tend to be evaluative, and the uses of 'work' in these two extracts have contrasting evaluative implications for the view of patients that this expression is used to capture.

7.3.2 Patients' Metaphorical Descriptions of Healthcare Professionals

Our patient online data contains a number of different metaphorical references to healthcare professionals. As this section shows, these are quite varied and tend to express some form of positive or negative evaluation. As we mentioned earlier, some also include an element of humour.

Praise for healthcare professionals is sometimes expressed by describing them in terms of conventional metaphorical expressions to do with celestial bodies or supernatural entities, such as 'star' and 'saint'. In our data, this applies particularly to descriptions of specialist cancer nurses, as in 'my mac nurse was my mega star' and 'I can honestly say I would put my mac nurse in the "saint" category'.

A more specific description in terms of a supernatural entity is the metaphorical use of 'vampire' for healthcare professionals who take blood samples. This is a case of a 'topic-triggered' metaphor (Koller 2004; Semino 2008: 222–225; Kövecses 2015), as drawing blood (which is associated with vampires) applies literally to the situation that the metaphor describes:

Example 7.5

I honestly don't think this vampire was drunk, just useless!

[O]

Example 7.6

Off for a bloodtest later, so gotta make myself purrrrrrty for the vampire

[O]

Example 7.7

it's funny but I call them the vampire doctors, there was only one guy on the ward who had fingers like divining rods so I was always pleased when he was on.

[O]

These descriptions suggest that the negative perception of the particular procedure of blood-taking is reflected onto the person who carries it out. However, this potential negative evaluation is partly mitigated by the humour that results from the contrast between predatory blood-sucking fictional creatures, on the one hand, and, on the other hand, healthcare professionals taking blood as part of their job for the patients' ultimate benefit. In Example 7.6, a humorous tone is also suggested by the use of 'purrrrrrty' as a spelling variant of 'pretty', and by the notion itself of wanting to look good for the healthcare professional taking the blood sample. The writer in Example 7.7 explicitly describes as 'funny' his metaphorical use of 'vampire' to refer to doctors who find it difficult to locate his veins. He then uses a simile involving a different supernatural scenario ('fingers like divining rods') to refer to the only nurse/doctor who could easily identify the right point for taking a blood sample.

Other patients in our data humorously refer to healthcare professionals by attributing supernatural powers to them:

Example 7.8

so you are trying to plan your future with starting work etc but not actually knowing whether you have a future yet until the great fortune teller aka GC tells you, so it there any point in spending time planning it when it might not happen and you could just sit and drink gin and admire the view instead,

[O]

Example 7.9

> No sleep not good last night—think i got myself worked into a pickle again—no magic nurse tonight but hopefully tomorrow.
>
> [O]

Example 7.10

> Off to see The Wizard of Onc today—to fetch my 4th cycle of Temodal
>
> [O]

In Example 7.8, 'fortune teller' is used metaphorically to refer to the consultant's role in making predictions about the person's outlook. In the other two examples, references to magic are used to praise particular healthcare professionals, in a light-hearted, humorous way, because of what they do for the patient (respectively, providing effective sleeping pills and the appropriate chemotherapy treatment). Example 7.10 is also an instance of a creative naming strategy: by shortening 'oncology' to 'onc', the writer makes a humorous intertextual reference to the eponymous character from *The Wizard of Oz*, who did not in fact possess the magical powers that are attributed to him.[2]

Our data contains a few other instances of metaphorical references to healthcare professionals that are both creative and humorous, such as the following:

Example 7.11

> paid a spontaneous visit to the Head Booby Hunter today to find his final opinion
>
> [O]

Here the use of 'Head Booby Hunter' for a breast surgeon metaphorically describes the identification and removal of tumours as hunting, and also creates a pun between the informal 'booby' (as a reference to breasts) and 'booty', which collocates with 'hunter' in different contexts.

Overall, mutual metaphorical descriptions of patients and healthcare professionals tend to be evaluative, and often highlight an imbalance in knowledge, power and control. However, in our data healthcare professionals describe (themselves and) patients metaphorically in serious reflections and discussions about professional challenges and practices, usually to support a particular argument (e.g. the failings of Western medicine). Patients, on the other hand, refer to healthcare professionals metaphorically in a more light-hearted fashion, seemingly to amuse themselves and others and to defuse accounts of stressful situations (e.g. blood tests and consultations about one's outlook). This is likely to be due, at least in part, to the fact that patients can write fairly freely on openly accessible online fora, while healthcare professionals are constrained by their role even when using pseudonyms. In some cases at least, the humour potentially mitigates negative evaluations of healthcare professionals, their activities and the greater degree of power and control they can exercise in relation to patients (see also Chapter 10).

7.4 Metaphors for What Healthcare Professionals Do for Patients

A variety of metaphors are used in our data to refer to or discuss what healthcare professionals do for patients. As in the previous section, we consider healthcare professionals first.

7.4.1 Healthcare Professionals' Metaphors for What Healthcare Professionals Do for Patients

The healthcare professionals in our data use many different metaphors to describe what they do for patients. Some are very frequent and conventional, such as the use of 'support' (which has a physical basic meaning) in 'so they're all senior nurses and they support patients at home', from one of our interviews with hospice managers. However, they also use the kinds of Violence and Journey metaphors we discussed in Chapters 5 and 6. As we have shown, these metaphors can be used to frame the role of healthcare professionals in relation to patients in very different ways.

In the following extract, several Violence metaphors are used to describe the care that doctors provide for patients in Intensive Therapy Units (ITUs):

> *Example 7.12*
>
> It can be particularly difficult for some of the more caring ITU doctors as sometimes one is fighting for patient survival against the odds without knowing just what the patient wants—or be under pressure to fight longer than seems reasonable. Despite expectations, the likelihood of losing the struggle are quite high.
>
> [O]

Here the attempt to prolong the patient's life is presented as a 'fight' or a 'struggle' that the doctor is likely to 'lose'. Although the writer explicitly recognises the challenges that result from not knowing the patient's wishes, and from unreasonable pressures to keep the patient alive, the use of Violence metaphors presents the prospect of the patient's death as something to be avoided at all costs, and the actual death of a patient as a professional failure.

The Violence metaphor in Example 6.39 in Chapter 6 ('You are now the general and you see your troops killed in battle) similarly positions doctors in an antagonist relationship with patients' deaths (see also 'nature wins' and 'defeat' versus 'victory' in Example 7.1). This can be seen as the health professionals' counterpart of patients describing themselves as 'losing' the 'battle' against cancer, and can be equally detrimental for morale and self-esteem.

In contrast, several online writers in our data explicitly question this metaphorical framing of their own role by saying that death is 'not the enemy', but rather should sometimes be seen as the 'best outcome' for the patient, as it can provide 'peace' and 'release' (see also our discussion of metaphors for 'good' versus 'bad' deaths in Chapter 8, particularly in our interviews with hospice managers). In a discussion of empathy with patients, a forum contributor uses a Sports metaphor to put forward a similar critique of an approach where:

Example 7.13

the tussle to cure or keep alive becomes an aim in itself which one has to try to win, irrespective of what the patient feels about this.

[O]

This writer goes on to compare this attitude to watching a football match, where wanting one's team to win 'may not reflect an empathy with the players on the pitch'.

Other metaphors for what healthcare professionals do for patients do not focus on the antagonistic relationship with the prospect of death, but rather on helping patients come to terms with their illness and prognosis. Example 7.14 is part of a discussion of how doctors find it difficult to tell patients that they are dying. Here Physical Support and Journey metaphors are used to describe the patients' experience and the healthcare professionals' role (see also Chapter 6):

Example 7.14

as health professionals we must shore up (our patients) dignity and bloster their self-confidence; facilitating acceptance of their illness and accompanying them on their uncertain journey.

[O]

The use of a Journey metaphor for the patient's experience casts the healthcare professional in the role of travelling companion. The notion of 'accompanying' the patient is consistent with the Physical

Support metaphors that the writer uses to describe the emotional and psychological care provided by healthcare professionals ('shore up . . . dignity' and 'bolster . . . self-confidence'). Both types of metaphors present healthcare as something that focuses on improving the patient's life rather than simply avoiding their death. This difference is of course due, in part, to the fact that here the topic is not intensive care in particular, as in Example 7.12. Nonetheless, the metaphors used in Example 7.14 provide a contrasting conceptualisation of healthcare professionals' goals in caring for patients, and have very different implications for what constitutes the most appropriate kind of professional behaviour and for the professional view of a patient's death.

The instances of metaphor we have discussed so far also contrast in terms of how they present the different roles of healthcare professionals and patients with respect to agency. In the Violence metaphors in Example 7.12, only the doctor is cast in an active, empowered role, which reflects the particular condition of patients in intensive care. In Example 7.14, the contrast is less marked, and the relationship is presented as a much more egalitarian one: on the one hand, the patients are in need of the professional help that is described in terms of physical support and companionship on a journey; on the other hand, it is the patients who are travelling, and the healthcare professional's role on the journey is that of fellow traveller rather than leader.

The power differential between consultants in particular and patients is the topic of several posts by the online writer we have called Ulysses, whom we have already quoted in section 7.3.1. In a particular post, Ulysses criticises a view of ward rounds which, in his view, metaphorically 'puts the doctor in the centre', rather than the patient. He then uses several different metaphors to evaluate negatively what he sees as the way doctors approach patients in 'Western Medicine':

Example 7.15

The doctor then thinks with the mentality of a <u>bomber pilot checking</u> his <u>instruments</u> and <u>flying</u> a <u>mission</u>. [. . .]

Alas, few of us "see" our patients. We see only a duodenal ulcer, or hypertension, or major depression. We <u>skate</u> along the <u>surface like water boatmen</u> and our ward rounds are like this too. A <u>spot weld</u> here, a bit of <u>panel beating</u> there, perhaps a new <u>muffler</u> or a <u>grease</u> and <u>oil change</u>.

Example 7.15 contains three different extended metaphors for the same topic, i.e. the inadequate ways in which, according to Ulysses, many doctors approach the care of their patients (cf. Goatly's 1997 notion of 'diversification' in metaphor use):

- A Violence metaphor ('the mentality of a bomber pilot. . . ');
- A Surface metaphor ('We skate along the surface. . . '), which also involves an Animal simile ('like water boatmen') and a Movement metaphor ('skate');
- A Machine metaphor ('A spot weld here. . .).

All three metaphors suggest a total lack of empathy and compassion on the part of doctors, and a tendency not to approach patients as whole human beings. The Violence metaphor ('bomber pilot. . . ') highlights the doctor's own activities as individual heroic enterprises that are ends in themselves, and backgrounds the interpersonal element of professional activities. In the Surface metaphor, the reference to 'skat[ing] along the surface' implicitly contrasts with the metaphorical 'depth' that would be required for ward rounds to be focused on patients' real needs (see Lakoff and Johnson 1980: 100–101; Kövecses 2000: 90–92). In the Machine metaphor, patients are dehumanised and fragmented as mechanical objects consisting of multiple parts. The expressions 'new muffler' and 'grease and oil change' suggest motor vehicles in particular, and therefore creatively extend the conventional metaphor THE BODY IS A MACHINE (e.g. Kövecses 2000: 103). This notion of fragmentation is consistent with Ulysses' claim that doctors only 'see'[3] conditions such as 'a duodenal ulcer', rather than a whole person to relate to. As has been noted elsewhere, in institutional healthcare settings patients are often referred to metonymically in terms of their illness (e.g. Dirven 1999: 276). While this can be seen as a useful communicative shorthand (e.g. Littlemore 2015), it has the potential consequence of discouraging an approach to care that takes the whole person into account.

In all three metaphors, the decision to adopt that particular approach to care is blamed on the healthcare professionals themselves: agency is first attributed generically to 'the doctor', then to a personified 'Western Medicine' and then to all the members of the profession via the first-person plural pronoun 'we', in which Ulysses also includes himself. In the rest of the post, Ulysses goes on to talk about the advantages of going below the 'tip of the ice-berg', which is a variant on the Surface metaphor in Example 7.15: in both cases, what is visible on the surface is assumed to be less important and worthwhile than what is hidden below the surface. This alternative approach, Ulysses claims, enables doctors to 'connect' with patients and 'takes [them] to a new land which is more satisfying and with better outcomes'.

While the length and complexity of Ulysses' metaphors are rather striking, there are several other cases in our data of doctors talking about having to treat patients as mechanical parts on a 'conveyor belt' or 'production line', so that their role is reduced to 'tightening screws and welding on the new bits on compliant production model people'. This is usually blamed on the way in which the UK healthcare system increasingly emphasises numerical targets and financial constraints at the expense of the human side of caring for patients.

Overall, different metaphors in our healthcare professional data frame the relationship with patients in a range of different ways, especially with respect to the professionals' roles, practices, approach and goals. As we have shown, this leads to different views of what counts as success or failure (particularly in relation to patients' deaths) and of what are perceived as dominant practices in healthcare.

7.4.2 Patients' Metaphors for What Healthcare Professionals Do for Patients

Several different metaphors are used by patients in our data to talk about what healthcare professionals do for them, whether as individuals, groups or parts of the healthcare system more generally. These metaphors tend to present the healthcare professionals as active/in control and patients as passive/disempowered, but vary in terms of the attitudes and emotions associated with this situation.

As we pointed out in Chapter 5, Violence metaphors can be used to express frustration when healthcare professionals do not prescribe the treatment that patients think would be best for them:

> *Example 7.16*
>
> it must be dispiriting when you are battling as hard as you can, not to be given the armour to fight in, but maybe [. . .] the side-effects would have been so unpleasant.
>
> [O]

Although the writer recognises the possibility of extreme side effects, here the metaphor of lack of provision of armoury to a fighter emphasises the imbalance of power between the patient and healthcare professionals, and the potentially negative consequences, from the patient's perspective, of that imbalance. In contrast with some of the metaphors used by healthcare professionals (e.g. Example 7.12), here the healthcare professional is not 'fighting' for the patient but rather withholding the equipment that would enable the patient to 'battle'.

A particularly strong sense of disempowerment and lack of control is expressed by the writer of the following extract, who recounts her experience of multiple tests for a lump in her thyroid:

Example 7.17

> MRI on the Monday—I lay back as they stuck the canula in my arm for the contrast injection and thought "How many times will I have to go through stuff like this?" I felt like my body was no longer mine and all the doctors were going to get access to it.
>
> [O]

The simile 'like my body was no longer mine' and the metaphor of 'access' to her body on the part of doctors suggest that actions taken for the ultimate benefit of patients are perceived as a threat to the integrity of body boundaries and to the person's sense of self and privacy.

Machine metaphors are used by some patients to refer to the processes and systems within which healthcare professionals operate. These metaphors also tend to have a strong evaluative dimension:

Example 7.18

> And I changed doctors and their fail-safe mechanism kicked in and they sent me with this surgery for a mammogram
>
> [O]

Example 7.19

> I think the worst thing was waiting for treatment to happen—once you get into it you get on the conveyor belt.
>
> [O]

Example 7.20

> They [medical staff] look on us all as just another appointment, and into the sausage machine we go.
>
> [O]

In all three examples, the use of Machine metaphors suggests a perception of healthcare as impersonal, and therefore insensitive to the individuality of patients. In the first two examples, however, the emphasis is on the contrast between lack of action on the part of healthcare professionals and the relative sense of safety and reassurance in receiving tests or treatment at all. Here 'fail-safe mechanism' and 'conveyor belt' suggest a perception of reliability and continuity in care processes, which are appreciated even if the patient is depersonalised and disempowered within them. This contrasts with the attitude expressed in Example 7.17, where medical tests are described in terms of loss of privacy and identity.

In Example 7.20, however, 'sausage machine' suggests a negative evaluation of the current approach to care in the National Health Service, and is part of a broader criticism, on the part of this particular forum contributor, of healthcare professionals' attitude to patients. Within this metaphor, patients are equated to sausages produced in such a way that they are all identical. This is consistent with the metonymic use of 'appointment' to suggest a depersonalised view of patients on the part of healthcare professionals, even though, in grammatical terms, patients are in fact positioned as agents (e.g. 'into . . . we go'). The rough mincing of meat that is involved in producing sausages also potentially contributes to the negative view of patients suggested by this metaphor.

A different patient makes a more creative use of metaphors involving mechanical objects to contrast different phases in treatment, and their consequences for her own emotional states. First she describes herself as having been 'Go-Go Action Barbie' ever since her surgeon decided to remove her tumour. Then she adds:

Example 7.21

and now I feel like I've been put in a holding pattern like a 747 circling Heathrow.

[O]

Both the 'Barbie' metaphor and the '747' simile describe the patient in terms of entities whose movement is under the control of others. The doll moves when someone presses the relevant buttons. The plane can only land when air traffic controllers allow the pilot to do so. The phrase 'Go-Go Action Barbie' suggests frenetic activity (during a period of surgery and treatment) that may not have been under the patient's control but that was clearly aimed at treating the illness and prolonging life. In contrast, being 'put in a holding pattern like a 747 circling Heathrow' suggests a sense of frustration and powerlessness in a subsequent phase in which nothing is happening in terms of tests and treatment. Here the patient is the subject of a passive grammatical structure ('I've been put'), and the 747 scenario is a creative variant on the more conventional metaphor of 'going round in circles', which suggests aimless/pointless activity. The 747 scenario is also of course an example of a very specific Journey metaphor, in which the patient is on a Journey controlled by healthcare professionals (e.g. Example 6.30 in Chapter 6: 'we follow whatever route the doctors decide is best for us'). Within Journey metaphors generally and the conventional LIFE IS A JOURNEY metaphor in particular, movement forward is presented as positive, as it corresponds to the ability to achieve one's goals, whereas lack of forward movement (as in 'circling') is constructed as negative.

A more positive type of metaphor for the care provided by healthcare professionals involves the notion of magic (cf. Supernatural metaphors in the previous section, and Religion and the Supernatural metaphors in Chapter 4). Example 7.22 is to do with cancer treatment itself, while the following two examples are to do with symptoms or the more general consequences of the illness (pain and sleeplessness respectively):

Example 7.22

Just waiting to see the oncologist to see if he thinks he can <u>work</u> the necessary <u>magic</u> to shrink the things.

[O]

Example 7.23

The Doc will <u>wave</u> his <u>magic wand</u> and make the pain go away!!

[O]

Example 7.24

No <u>magic potion</u> tonight fraid—think they waiting for thursday night now

[O]

As with several of the patterns we have already described, these Supernatural metaphors present healthcare professionals as entirely in control of what happens to patients, and patients as not being in a position to understand what happens to them. There is, however, a humorous and possibly even affectionate tone in how the various references to magic present the doctors/nurses as all-powerful and their interventions as mysterious. This contrasts with the frustration associated with other metaphors in which the patient is also presented as powerless, such as some of the Machine metaphors we have just discussed. The difference seems to lie in the fact that Supernatural metaphors do not involve the dehumanisation of patients, and also present healthcare interventions as quick and effective. Some patients also use the conventional metaphorical expression 'magic bullet' to refer to a possible future treatment that doctors may eventually be able to use to cure cancer completely.

In contrast to the patterns we have discussed so far, our patient data contains a few metaphors in which the role of healthcare professionals in relation to patients is described metaphorically in a way that places the patient firmly in charge. It is noticeable, however, that such cases tend to involve nurses rather than other types of healthcare professionals. One writer advises another patient to '<u>use</u> the Mac nurse to vent on'. Another person uses several metaphors for her relationship with nurses:

Example 7.25

> My number one source of support has been from my mac nurse—she has been the most valuable tool in my tool box not just for me but friends and family as well.
>
> [O]

Here the care and advice provided by the Macmillan nurse are described via the very conventional physical metaphor 'support'. Following that, however, the emphasis is on the importance of the patient being in control in the relationship with the nurse. This is expressed via the mechanical metaphorical description of the 'mac nurse' as 'the most valuable tool' in the person's 'tool box'. In contrast with the examples we have discussed so far, the Tool metaphor presents the healthcare professional, rather than the patient, as an object to be used in mechanical processes. This reverses the conventional power relationship between patients and healthcare professionals, and places the patient in charge, while also positively evaluating the nurse. This kind of description of the actual patient-professional relationships only occurs on a small number of occasions in our data, however, and, as we have mentioned, is mostly limited to the relationship with nurses.

Finally, light-hearted and potentially humorous metaphors are occasionally used by the patients in our data to describe what healthcare professionals do for them. The following extract is part of a list of experiences that were explicitly reported as 'good' by a patient, after a series of more negative ones:

Example 7.26

> Another GOOD—The registrar—all of 12 years old, but jumped in, all guns blazing, when I had a crisis.
>
> [O]

Here the registrar's intervention at a time of crisis is metaphorically described in terms reminiscent of action film heroes ('jumped in, all guns blazing'). The potential humour of this description is increased by the contrast with the writer's perception of the registrar's age ('all of 12 years old'). Nonetheless, the intervention is explicitly perceived as welcome.

With a few exceptions, however, the different metaphors that patients use to describe what healthcare professionals do for them tend to emphasise a perception of an imbalance of expertise, power and control, although this imbalance is evaluated differently within different metaphors. This shows a plurality of views: some patients seem to be happy to leave control to the healthcare professionals and see their activities as magic, while others seem to prefer a situation where they can be in charge of what happens to them. We have also shown how here too some metaphors are light-hearted and potentially humorous, which can help the writer accept or redress the perception of asymmetries in the relationship between patients and healthcare professionals.

7.5 Metaphors for Further Sensitive Aspects of the Relationship Between Patients and Healthcare Professionals

In this final section of the discussion of our findings, we do not discuss matching topics for metaphors in the patient and healthcare professional data, as in the previous two sections. Rather, we consider the metaphors used for two different but related aspects of the relationship that emerged as important for the respective participant group in our analyses of the data: communication with healthcare professionals in the patient data, and emotional involvement with patients in the healthcare professional data. Both aspects are highly sensitive for the relevant group, and both involve potentially negative emotions, as we will show.

7.5.1 Patients' Metaphors for Communication With Healthcare Professionals

In Chapter 5, we showed how the patients in our data use a variety of Violence metaphors to describe their interactions with healthcare professionals, as in the case of expressions such as: 'I will fight for Avastin'. These metaphors suggest an antagonistic perception of communication with healthcare professionals and, in some cases, the idea that considerable persistence and determination are needed for good care.

Other metaphors for the communicative behaviour of healthcare professionals also suggest an approach that is not satisfactory from a patient's point of view. For example, in the following extract the metaphorical use of the verb 'waft' indicates a dismissive attitude towards a suggestion that the patient had made concerning the possible environmental origin of their cancer:

Example 7.27

I put this to my endocrine consultant and of course he wafted such suggestions away.

[O]

A stronger sense of frustration and disempowerment can be conveyed by the use of a variety of other metaphors to describe interactions in which patients feel they are not given sufficient opportunities to consider and discuss their options:

Example 7.28

> Sometimes surgeons and doctors push you to do what is easier for them and you find yourself agreeing but afterwards it doesn't always turn out to be best for you or what you wanted.
>
> [O]

Here 'push' refers metaphorically to communicative behaviour that allows patients little or no chance to disagree. The use of 'find' in 'find yourself agreeing' also suggests that, as a consequence, patients have no control in the interaction and may verbally accept the recommendations of 'surgeons and doctors' without having had time to consider them properly.

Several patients in our data use similes to express how they are sometimes made to feel in unsatisfactory interactions with healthcare professionals. In Example 7.29, an online forum contributor uses the conventional expression 'like a bunny in the headlights' to acknowledge the disorientation, fear and helplessness that the addressee might feel when talking with some doctors:

Example 7.29

> Doctors [. . .] do seem to be pretty scary people. They use a lot of long words and you probably sit there like a bunny in the headlights and you just don't know what to ask them.
>
> [O]

In the rest of the post, the writer encourages another forum contributor to ask questions and play a more active part in future consultations.

More frequently, patients use similes to do with teacher-pupil or parent-child relationships to express the attitudes that they attribute to some surgeons or consultants:

Example 7.30

> so I generally see somebody off her [the surgeon's] team, and the last lady I saw I wasn't impressed with her she talked to me as if I was a child at school
>
> [I]

Example 7.31

> I am so sorry to hear about all the mets and recurrences. I really don't think you are at all to blame—but I know that feeling of the consultant looming over you like a naughty schoolgirl!
>
> [O]

Example 7.32

The most useful thing I saw on a thread of people ranting about HCC cells not picking up RAI was a post from a lady who said that it doesn't matter- the surgeons cut out the HCC and the RAI kills the remaining Thyroid cells. My doc smiled at me <u>like a proud parent</u> when I parotted that back at him.

[O]

In Example 7.30, the comparison with 'a child at school' is used by one of our interviewees to suggest a patronising attitude on the part of a member of her surgeon's team. In Example 7.31, the 'naughty schoolgirl' simile is used to express how some patients feel when their cancer re-occurs and the consultant seems to be disappointed in them. In Example 7.32, a forum contributor uses the 'proud parent' simile to convey the pride she saw in her doctor when she accurately repeated some medical information she had read online. Although this is reported as a positive experience, this simile also places the patient in the position of a child who is dependent on the approval of the doctor/parent. The use of the verb 'parrot' to refer to how the patient conveyed the information also suggests that what was perceived as positive was an uncritical report of information that the doctor regarded as accurate. These metaphors do not challenge the imbalance of expertise and power in the relationship with healthcare professionals. What is criticised, more or less implicitly, is the exploitation of such imbalance to belittle or patronise patients, or to ignore their wishes and opinions. This has implications for how a more person-centred approach to (communication in) healthcare might be operationalised.

Supernatural metaphors to do with magic are also used by patients in our data to talk about a particular aspect of their experience of communicating with healthcare professionals. The expression 'magic word(s)' is applied to words that are particularly salient to patients in conversations about diagnosis or prognosis. These 'magic words' can involve both good and bad news:

Example 7.33

The <u>magic words</u> from my surgeon after the op were 'no vascular spread'.

[O]

Example 7.34

When I convinced myself I would die (i.e. just after I heard the <u>magic word</u> cancer and just before I heard the word curable)

[O]

In Example 7.33 'magic words' refers to the good news from the surgeon that the cancer had not spread, while in Example 7.34 'magic word' refers to the word 'cancer' itself on first diagnosis. In contrast with the magic-related metaphors we discussed in the previous sections, here 'magic' does not apply to the abilities of healthcare professionals, but rather to the effect that some of their words have on patients during consultations in which important news is communicated about their condition. Example 7.34 in particular shows the immediate impact of the use of the word 'cancer' on the patient, who reports convincing herself that she would die in the short space between hearing the words 'cancer' and 'curable' in a particular consultation.

Overall, the metaphors used by patients for their interactions with healthcare professionals convey the tension and vulnerability they tend to feel, as well as a heightened perception of the imbalance of power and expertise, which can result in subsequent frustration and regret.

7.5.2 Healthcare Professionals' Metaphors for Emotional Involvement With Patients

In our healthcare professional data, a variety of metaphors are used to talk about the dilemmas, risks and opportunities involved in the emotional side of the relationship with patients, both during treatment and when patients die. This is not surprising. On the one hand, a central professional challenge in healthcare is finding a balance between being compassionate and preserving professionalism and one's mental health (e.g. Kearney et al. 2009). On the other hand, it is well-known that emotions and emotional relationships are among the subjective and sensitive aspects of human experiences that tend to be expressed through metaphor (e.g. Kövecses 2000; Stefanowitsch 2006).

Our online data includes one particular thread that is entitled 'Do you get emotional about patients?' The thread starts with a request for advice from a medical student:

Example 7.35

I find myself getting hugely <u>attached</u> to patients that I meet. I get <u>caught up</u> in their "story" who they were, what happened so that they became admitted and then I share their joy when they are discharged home and I feel great sadness when they pass away or they don't improve as we had hoped.

So, what I want to ask is how do you <u>detach</u> yourselves? As medical professionals, of course we should remain <u>detached</u> and objective, but do you go home, at the end of your shift and allow your emotions to <u>show through</u>?

[O]

The student's questions exploit a highly conventional metaphor in which empathy is a physical tie, and lack of empathy is absence of physical ties ('attached' versus 'detached'; cf. Restraint metaphors in Chapter 4). The use of 'show through' also suggests that the body is a metaphorical container for the emotions, and that emotions are only accessible to others when the container is transparent enough for its contents to be visible from the outside (cf. Kövecses 2000; and metaphors for the expression of emotions in Chapters 8 and 9).

This opening post is followed by 21 further contributions by 17 different contributors, in addition to the medical student. Most of the contributions are by more experienced doctors who give advice on the basis of their experiences. Contrasting views are expressed via different metaphors.

Several contributions express the dangers of emotional involvement in terms of metaphors that involve loss of control, and the solutions in terms of regaining control:

Example 7.36

You do need to <u>compartmentalise</u> your emotions a bit in order to cope. Don't allow yourself to feel <u>overwhelemed</u> by emotion.

[O]

Here the strategy needed to avoid becoming 'overwhelmed' is expressed in terms of a spatial metaphor for the person/mind, in which difficult emotions are objects that can be confined to a separate compartment.

Several contributors make a distinction between the need to control one's emotions while in the professional context and the freedom to experience them fully in private.

Example 7.37

If you can <u>suspend</u> the <u>rush</u> of emotions at the bedside and allow yourself to be <u>washed over</u> by them at a later, safer time, I think you will be ok.

[O]

As in Example 7.36, the writer in Example 7.37 talks about emotions as an external force that is hard to control ('rush', 'washed over') (cf. Kövecses 2000), but suggests that it is acceptable to lose that control outside the professional environment.

In contrast, the advice in Example 7.38 is to avoid experiencing any emotions about patients' deaths even after leaving the hospital, to safeguard one's private life:

Example 7.38

Personally, as I left the hospital on an evening everything was sealed up in a mental box in my head and filed under 'forget'. Since I had never previously known the patients and had no reason to know them after they left the hospital there was no reason to get emotional about them if they were not there the next day.

Allowing oneself to become too close to patients can be dangerous and affect your normal life outside work.

[O]

Here emotional involvement with patients is described via the conventional spatial metaphor of closeness (Grady 1997; Lakoff and Johnson 1999: 50), and is presented as 'dangerous'. Similarly to Example 7.36, the solution is proposed via a metaphor in which the healthcare professional's mind is a physical space with different sections, so that emotions are objects that can be permanently kept in a place where they have no influence. Another contributor similarly advises the medical student to 'learn to package negative emotions so they can be sealed up and thrown away'. In all these cases, negative emotions are presented as dangerous entities that can only be dealt with via some form of containment or removal. Within these descriptions, the healthcare professional is in control, but emotions are presented as just as controllable as inanimate objects that can be easily moved from one location or container to another. Within these metaphors, the person's mind is additionally presented as a container consisting of compartments that can be kept totally separate from one another (cf. Kövecses 2000).

A more nuanced view is expressed in the following post:

Example 7.39

It unfortunate to say that with time you develop a hardness that means you will be less attached to your patients.[. . .]

You will occasionally find a patient whose story shines brightly and burns a hole in your hard shell. You will feel better for remembering that patients are people, not diagnoses [. . .]. The patient will either get better—reminding you that there is hope for all of us, or die—causing you to cry with the family (even if its apart from them). The important thing is to remember that either outcome has made you a better doctor, but that trying to make that connection for all your patients will simply leave you emotionally exhausted and running late all day.

On the whole you will find a balance [. . .]

Once you develop the hard shell its not always easy to open the door without allowing the shell to crack "(it's like trying to cut a

> window in an egg shell" I once heard a consultant say). It will never be easy to close the door at will once you've opened it for a patient. But if you can strike that balance you can truely make a difference to the patient and family experience, and you can remind yourself why you became a doctor
>
> [O]

This contributor metaphorically describes the ability not to be affected by patients' stories as a 'hardness' and 'hard shell'. This is presented as necessary, but also as something that it is 'unfortunate' to have to acknowledge. However, in contrast with some of the previous examples, this post also recognises that doctors cannot control their emotions at all times. Here emotions are presented as forces that are hard or impossible to control, rather than as objects that can be placed in locations where they have no effect on the person, as in the previous two examples. The writer in Example 7.39 describes the powerful emotional effects of some patients' stories in terms of openings in the doctor's hard exterior, i.e. as holes burnt in a metaphorical shell, or doors opening that can crack the shell and cannot easily be closed again. In addition, while 'hard shell' suggests the thick shell of an animal (e.g. a tortoise), the simile attributed to the consultant mentions an egg shell, which is thin and fragile.

On the one hand, these metaphors emphasise the need to avoid constant and intense emotional involvement. On the other hand, they recognise the doctors' own humanity. In addition, even the experience of strong emotions is presented as potentially positive for the person's professional development. Finally, the notion of 'balance' is used metaphorically in Example 7.39 to summarise the point that, while emotional involvement can be problematic, it will and possibly should occur some of the time. Another forum contributor also argues for a compromise position by suggesting that, while emotions should not interfere with one's professional judgement and mental life, they have 'shaped [him] to become a better person and a better doctor'.

Similar metaphors to the ones in this particular thread are used elsewhere in our data for the same issues. The metaphor of the healthcare professional as an egg with a delicate protective shell is used by several other online writers in other contexts, as in the following extract:

Example 7.40

> My partner describes me as being like an egg . . . Capable of withstanding great force from the correct angles, but once the shell is broken it takes a lot to put me back together again. So I prefer to think of myself as having a hardened exterior, to protect the soft heart within
>
> [O]

Here the metaphor is used to suggest that allowing oneself to become emotional can be traumatic ('once the shell is broken it takes a lot to put me back together again'), but also to point out that avoiding involvement does not mean that the person is insensitive ('to protect the soft heart within').

In another contribution, the loss of control caused by emotional involvement is described as becoming 'entangled' in ways that affect one's ability to do one's job (cf. Restraint metaphors in Chapter 4). Another writer summarises their argument against emotional involvement with patients as follows:

Example 7.41

> This is a <u>slippery slope</u> and will end up <u>violating</u> the professional <u>boundaries</u>
>
> [O]

The conventional metaphorical expression 'slippery slope' suggests irreversible loss of control, and the result, according to this particular writer, is unprofessional behaviour.

Finally, some healthcare professionals in our data use different metaphors to argue in favour of emotional involvement with patients. One person describes compassion as 'the most important drug' in a doctor's 'medical bag'. Several different people positively evaluate emotional involvement by means of Openness metaphors. The following extract, for example, occurs as part of a discussion of compassion in caring for patients:

Example 7.42

> Courage is needed not only to decide to <u>set</u> a <u>wall</u>, but even more to decide to <u>open</u> yourself to others.
>
> [O]

This kind of metaphorical description relies on the conventional conception of a person as a container, and of someone's emotions and 'true' self as at the centre of the container: intimacy and meaningful communication are only possible if the outer surface of the container is open (Kövecses 2000: 90–92). The reference to 'courage' in Example 7.42 suggests that openness inevitably involves vulnerability. In Chapter 8, we will show a similar use of Openness metaphors to evaluate positively the willingness of patients in hospices to talk explicitly about dying and associated emotions. Here, however, the writer suggests that healthcare professionals are generally not willing to be 'open' themselves, and the various metaphors that involve compartmentalisation emphasise this.

Overall, the use of a variety of metaphors for the advantages and disadvantages of emotional involvement reflects the centrality and sensitivity of this issue in healthcare practice, and in the personal and professional lives of healthcare professionals.

7.6 Conclusions

In this chapter, we have discussed and compared the metaphors that patients and healthcare professionals use in our data to describe members of the other group, express what healthcare professionals do for patients, and discuss two particularly sensitive topics: interactions with healthcare professionals in the patient data, and emotional involvement with patients for healthcare professionals.

Overall, the metaphors we have identified tend to be evaluative, and to highlight similar problems and challenges from the different perspectives of the members of the two groups. A general issue that is often highlighted by the metaphors used in both datasets is the degree of agency, control and power that is associated with each party in the relationship, and the asymmetries that are inherent in institutional healthcare settings. With very few exceptions (e.g. a nurse described as the patient's 'tool'), patients' metaphors tend to present healthcare professionals as active and in control of what happens or does not happen to patients. Some metaphors suggest a grudging acceptance of this imbalance of power, on the grounds that action on the healthcare professionals' part is preferable to inaction, even if the price is the loss of the patient's individuality (e.g. 'you get on the conveyor belt'). Other metaphors express frustration when the imbalance of power results in perceived inaction ('put in a holding pattern like a 747 circling Heathrow'), lack of adequate care ('not to be given the armour to fight in') or loss of privacy ('like my body was no longer mine and all the doctors were going to get access to it'). When patients attribute supernatural powers to healthcare professionals (e.g. 'magic nurse' and 'the Doc will wave his magic wand'), however, the imbalance of power and expertise is presented more positively, or even affectionately. Such metaphors are often humorous, and seem to emphasise trust and appreciation.

In the healthcare professionals' data, metaphors are sometimes used to critique the asymmetries of power and control in the relationship with patients, and particularly the ways in which these asymmetries are interpreted or exploited by some healthcare professionals. We have mentioned one particularly prolific and passionate contributor to the professionals' online forum (Ulysses) who uses a series of metaphors provocatively in order to expose attitudes and imbalances of power that, in his view, undermine good care (e.g. the consultant as king and the patients as 'royal subjects').

A related issue, which many of the metaphors highlight, is to do with the extent to which people are treated as human beings in healthcare, and the atomistic approach to medicine that results if they are not. Ulysses' claim that some doctors view patients as machines to be fixed (e.g. 'A spot weld here, a bit of panel beating there') is a critique of what he perceives as the dehumanisation of patients, and is consistent with some mechanical metaphors used by both patients and other healthcare professionals (e.g. patients being placed on a 'conveyor belt'). Metonymies are also used to suggest that some healthcare professionals do not see patients as whole human beings (e.g. 'We see only a duodenal ulcer'). The debate about whether or not patients are 'work' similarly involves the claim that patients may be dehumanised if they are only seen as a component of one's job.

While many healthcare professionals' metaphors suggest a keen awareness of imbalances of power and the risk of dehumanisation, some of the patients' metaphors show that, in practice, they do often end up feeling deprived of both individual humanity and control. This is suggested, for example, by some of the mechanical metaphors for the systems that healthcare professionals operate in (e.g. 'into the sausage machine we go'). The patients' perceptions expressed by these metaphors contrast with the stated goals of the UK's National Health Service, which emphasise patient choice and individualised treatment and care.

More specifically, many of the metaphors that patients use to talk about communication with healthcare professionals convey a particularly negative perception of these interactions. Some of these metaphors emphasise the inability to exercise any control at all because of healthcare professionals' approach to communication (e.g. 'doctors push you to do what is easier for them and you find yourself agreeing', 'you probably sit there like a bunny in the headlights'). Other metaphors express the perception of being patronised (e.g. 'like a naughty schoolgirl'). Violence metaphors for communicative behaviour also suggest an antagonistic perception of the patient's interactions with healthcare professionals and the healthcare system (e.g. 'I will fight for Avastin'). Even if the patient is presented as active by some of these metaphors, they are placed in a position of disadvantage which can only be overcome with great effort and determination.

Interestingly, but perhaps not surprisingly, the metaphors used by patients do not seem to recognise the humanity and potential vulnerability of healthcare professionals themselves. As we have shown, a topic of considerable debate in the professionals' section of our corpus is the issue of emotional involvement with patients, and the personal consequences that this can have for mental well-being and life outside work. Different views are expressed by means of the contrast between the need for 'detachment' and 'compartmentalisation', on the one hand, and the value of 'attachment' and 'openness', on the other. A more nuanced view is conveyed by metaphors involving 'shells' that may be hard enough to protect the healthcare professional's mental life most of the time, but that can also break and deeply affect the person's emotional state. These different metaphors frame the issue in different ways. They involve different views of emotions (i.e. entities versus forces), different assumptions about the professionals' ability to control their own emotions, and different evaluations of emotional involvement in healthcare practice. In particular, the metaphors used to argue against emotional involvement tend to place healthcare professionals in a position of control, but also describe the mind as a physical space and emotions as objects that can be positioned in locations where they have no effect. This supports the idea of being able to feel no emotions in certain situations, but may also present an unrealistic view of the amount of emotional self-control that doctors and nurses can exercise. The metaphors used to argue in favour of emotional involvement, on the other hand, acknowledge the inevitability of emotional reactions and the humanity of healthcare professionals, but may also suggest standards that not everyone can aim for. Finally, the various 'shell' metaphors seem to capture both the need to protect oneself and the vulnerability of healthcare professionals themselves.

Healthcare professionals' metaphors also express different views of their goals in relation to patients. The contrast between metaphorically 'fighting for patient survival' versus 'accompanying' them on their 'uncertain journey' involves not just different kinds of agency, but also different approaches to decision-making and to what counts as professional success or failure. In the 'fighting for patient survival' metaphor, a patient's death is a professional defeat, while in the 'uncertain journey' metaphor, it is a natural part of life. In addition, on a few occasions, healthcare professionals use metaphors to suggest how their relationship with patients benefits them as professionals or as people: e.g. descriptions of patients as 'best teachers' and 'ghosts [that] help us to make better decisions in the future'; and references to patients whose stories 'burn(s) a hole' in the HPs [healthcare professional]' 'hard shell', making them 'better doctors'.

Finally, the patients in our online data repeatedly use humorous metaphors to describe healthcare professionals and what they do (e.g. 'vampire', 'Wizard of Onc', 'Head Booby Hunter'). This arguably helps to reduce the perception of power differentials in the relationship, as well as to defuse unpleasant or distressing situations (blood tests, discussion of test results), while still recognising healthcare professionals' superior knowledge and abilities. These humorous metaphors also strengthen the bonds of intimacy and complicity among contributors to the patients' online forum (see also Chapter 10). Since all our online data is from publicly accessible sources, it is not surprising that we did not find any comparable humorous metaphors in the professionals' section of our corpus.

In almost all cases, however, metaphors for the relationship between patients and healthcare professionals are strongly evaluative, and reveal the challenges that have to be faced on both sides. The majority of the metaphors also show how each group inevitably tends to focus on their own issues and concerns, and runs the risk of dehumanising the members of the other group: some healthcare professionals may see patients as symptoms, body part or diseases, but patients also tend to see doctors and nurses only as professionals rather than people with their own emotions, problems and vulnerabilities. In this sense, the metaphors we have analysed suggest that a greater awareness of the individuality and humanity of the members of the other group seems to be needed on *both* sides, to the benefit of all.

More generally, the metaphors we have discussed in this chapter show a plurality of views on a number of central topics, in both the patient data and the health professional data. In particular, the metaphors used by patients suggest different perceptions of the imbalance of power and control in the relationship with healthcare professionals. These and other differences need to be taken into account in a truly person-centred approach to healthcare.

In the next chapter, we turn to how healthcare professionals use metaphors for the more specific topic of patients' deaths.

Notes

1. These labels do not of course refer to mutually exclusive categories.
2. The expression 'off to see the Wizard' also seems to allude to the lyrics of one of the songs in the main musical adaptation of the original novel: 'We're off to see the Wizard'.
3. The use of quotation marks around the verb 'see' in Example 7.15 suggests that it is intended as not just referring to visual perception, but to fully considering the person one is looking at. This use of 'see' can be related to the conventional conceptual metaphor UNDERSTANDING IS SEEING (Lakoff and Johnson 1980: 48).

References

Dirven, R. (1999). Conversion as a conceptual metonymy of event schemata. In G. Radden and K. Panther (Eds.), *Metonymy and cognition* (pp. 275–288). Amsterdam: Amsterdam: John Benjamins.

Goatly, A. (1997). *The language of metaphors: Literal metaphorical*. London: Routledge.

Grady, J. (1997). *Foundations of meaning: Primary metaphors and primary scenes*. Unpublished PhD thesis, University of California, Berkeley, CA.

Harvey, K., and Koteyko, N. (2013). *Exploring health communication: Language in action*. London: Routledge.

Kearney, M. K., Weininger, R. B., Vachon, M. L. S., Harrison, R. L., and Mount, B. M. (2009). Self-care of physicians caring for patients at the end of life: 'Being connected . . . a key to my survival'. *Journal of the American Medical Association*, *301*(11), 115–164.

Koller, V. (2004). Businesswomen and war metaphors: 'Possessive, jealous and pugnacious?' *Journal of Sociolinguistics*, *8*(1), 3–22.

Kövecses, Z. (2000). *Metaphor and emotion: Language, culture, and body in human feeling*. Cambridge: Cambridge University Press.

Kövecses, Z. (2015). *Where metaphors come from: Reconsidering context in metaphor*. Oxford: Oxford University Press.

Lakoff, G., and Johnson, M. (1980). *Metaphors we live by*. Chicago: University of Chicago Press.

Lakoff, G., and Johnson, M. (1999). *Philosophy in the flesh: The embodied mind and its challenge to western thought*. New York: Basic Books.

Littlemore, J. (2015). *Metonymy: Hidden shortcuts in language, thought and communication*. Cambridge: Cambridge University Press.

Seale, C., Charteris-Black, J., MacFarlane, A., and McPherson, A. (2010). Interviews and internet forums: A comparison of two sources of qualitative data. *Qualitative Health Research*, *20*(5), 595–606.

Semino, E. (2008). *Metaphor in discourse*. Cambridge: Cambridge University Press.

Stefanowitsch, A. (2006). Corpus-based approaches to metaphor and metonymy. In A. Stefanowitsch and S. T. Gries (Eds.), *Corpus-based approaches to metaphor and metonymy*. Berlin: Mouton de Gruyter.

Stevenson, F. A., Kerr, C., Murray, E., and Nazareth, I. (2007). Information from the Internet and the doctor-patient perspective—a qualitative study. *BMC Family Practice*, *16*(8), 47.

Websites

Sage and Thyme, University Hospital of South Manchester. Retrieved from www.sageandthymetraining.org.uk

8 Health Professionals' Metaphors for Good and Bad Deaths

8.1 Introduction

Although death itself is a predominantly biological event, death and dying carry (changeable and dynamic) social, cultural and political significance (Cottrell and Duggleby 2016). One type of significance is the evaluation of particular kinds of death as 'good' or 'bad'—a distinction that, as we outline in this chapter, is central to the practice of end-of-life care. With this in mind, we included questions about quality of death in our semi-structured interviews with hospice-based healthcare professionals (as described in Chapter 3) and looked specifically for explicit references to this in our healthcare professional online data with the help of corpus tools (more on this later). The responses we received, and the references we identified, are the subject of this chapter. We begin here with two introductory excerpts from our healthcare professional interview data:

Example 8.1

> I guess as a professional I'd like to see them comfortable and not suffering any form of distress or agitation that the patient comfortable, the family erm at peace with the journey as it's going and where things have got to erm and that you know they can go through a natural normal grief. That to me would be a good death.
>
> [Interviewee 9]

Example 8.2

> a lady who'd suffered a lot of anxiety in her life and had a difficult relationship with her husband, and did battle with everyone. Nothing was ever right, nothing was good enough, nothing, you couldn't physically get her comfortable. You couldn't kind of get in a good place to meet her psychologically erm . . . I think she felt that being comfortable was being patronised and that made it really difficult to offer her any support. And she had quite a traumatic death in that

> she [. . .] died very fearful and very anxious and wouldn't accept any pain relief.
>
> [Interviewee 7]

Both our interviewees and the online contributors noted repeatedly that a 'good/bad' death is highly individual, subjective and therefore somewhat difficult to pin down. While recognising this, healthcare professionals in our interviews were generally able to provide examples of what they considered good (Example 8.1) or bad (Example 8.2) when it came to dying. These examples showed a remarkable degree of consistency in the metaphors used to evaluate deaths as good or bad; the two preceding examples are representative in this sense.

In section 8.2, we provide a brief overview of some of the literature in healthcare practice and linguistics on (quality of) death, which helps to shed light on this and other patterns we identified. We then outline the specific methods used for the analysis in this chapter in section 8.3, before focusing specifically on how good and bad deaths are constructed metaphorically in our data.

Throughout this chapter, we consider the results from interviews separately from the results from the online forum posts and focus more on the former. Our interviewees were a fairly homogeneous group of UK-based healthcare professionals working in hospice or palliative care, while the online corpus includes a much more diverse group. We had the opportunity to explore the topic at hand explicitly with our interviewees, but not with the online forum contributors, who simply (and luckily for us) happened to mention quality of death spontaneously. These, as well as differences inherent in the two genres (see Chapter 3), inevitably resulted in richer relevant data in the interview subcorpus. That said, in our final analysis section we consider how the metaphor patterns we found in the interviews play out in the healthcare professional online data. Throughout the analysis, we also comment, where appropriate, on similarities and differences with the findings of an analysis of narratives of 'good' and 'bad' deaths that was conducted previously (Semino et al. 2014).

8.2 Evaluating Dying and Death

The concept of the 'good death' emerged in the UK at the beginning of the hospice movement in the late 1960s and remains key in contemporary discourses on death, dying (Costello 2006; van Brussel and Carpentier 2012; Cottrell and Duggleby 2016) and palliative care (Low and Payne 1996; Smith 2000), with modern hospice care in the UK explicitly aiming to facilitate a good end-of-life experience. There is also increasing recognition in the public sphere that talking explicitly about death and dying is necessary for making death as good as possible. A prime example of this is the mission statement of the 'Dying Matters' coalition—a

UK network of organisations that aim 'to promote public awareness of dying, death and bereavement' (http://www.dyingmatters.org/overview/about-us)—which explicitly links 'talking about dying' with a good death experience. This emphasis is also reflected in governmental policies such as the Department of Health's End of Life Care Strategy for England and Wales, launched in 2008, which outlines a good death as:

- Being treated as an individual, with dignity and respect;
- Being without pain and other symptoms;
- Being in familiar surroundings; and
- Being in the company of close family and/or friends.

(Department of Health 2008: 9)

The strategy also describes the implementation of these principles through:

- Identification of people approaching the end of life and initiating discussions about preferences for end of life care;
- Care planning: assessing needs and preferences, agreeing a care plan to reflect these and reviewing these regularly;
- Coordination of care;
- Delivery of high quality services in all locations;
- Management of the last days of life;
- Care after death; and
- Support for carers, both during a person's illness and after their death.

(Department of Health 2008: 11)

While there is research to support these principles, as outlined in the document itself, it is also generally acknowledged that certain aspects remain subject to unresolved, sometimes ethical, debate. For example, Seymour et al. (2002) note that it is difficult to know what constitutes the best interest of dying people and that it is questionable whether it is even possible to preserve autonomy beyond the point at which dying people are able to make their wishes explicit. Similarly, there are questions about the extent to which the principles can be generalised across contexts and cultures (e.g. Cipolletta and Oprandi 2014; Kastbom et al. 2017).

What it means to have a 'good' death, especially in the context of cancer deaths, has been studied from several different perspectives, including of course many that do not deal explicitly with metaphor. Payne et al. (1996) conducted interviews with patients and staff in a palliative care unit to compare their views of a 'good' death. Patients' descriptions were found to be heterogeneous, and included 'dying in one's sleep, dying quietly, with dignity, being pain free and dying suddenly' (Payne et al. 1996: 307;

see also Vig et al. 2002). Staff's descriptions showed greater uniformity and emphasised 'adequate symptom control, family involvement, peacefulness and lack of distress' (Payne et al. 1996: 307; see also Steinhauser et al. 2000). They also characterised 'bad' deaths in terms of 'uncontrolled symptoms, lack of acceptance and being young' (Payne et al. 1996: 307; see also Low and Payne 1996; Cottrell and Duggleby 2016).

Taking a critical linguistic perspective, Carpentier and van Brussel (2012) point out how the notions of a 'good' or 'bad' death have changed over time, echoing some of the issues we hinted at in the introduction to this chapter, and stress the political nature of the 'discourse of death'. They argue that the current (Western) construction of a good death relies heavily on notions of 'control, autonomy, dignity, awareness, and heroism' (2012: 100) and reflects an individualistic social context, which values independence, self-mastery and self-care. Carpentier and van Brussel (2012) also note that in this context death is never absolutely good, but given its inevitability, there is still an evaluative hierarchy that allows certain types of deaths to be better than others. The authors describe this as one particular, 'medical-revivalist' discourse, which, though dominant (see also Seale 2004), should not be understood as shared by all (van Brussel and Carpentier 2012; see also Goldsteen et al. 2006). After all, what is considered to make for a good death is not the same around the world, nor is it even necessarily shared by those in the same geographical location. Cipolletta and Oprandi (2014), for example, point out that, while patient autonomy is considered important in places like the Netherlands, Switzerland and Australia, it is seen as less so in Italy and Sweden (although see also Kastbom et al. 2017 on attitudes in Sweden). Even within a nation, especially a multicultural one like the UK, the dominance of one view over others could lead to the marginalisation of minority groups (Walter 2003), or of anyone who might prefer a death that involves 'reliance on others for decision making and [. . .] avoiding information because "ignorance is bliss"' (Seale 2004: 967) (see also Cottrell and Duggleby 2016).

In linguistics, and specifically in research on metaphor, studies of death and dying have tended to focus on death as a concept or event, rather than on the process and period leading up to it, as we outlined in Chapter 2. Linguistic approaches to metaphors for death draw primarily from Conceptual Metaphor Theory. They are often based on decontextualised or literary examples, and focus on conventional conceptual metaphors such as DEATH IS SLEEP, DEATH IS DARK, DEATH IS A JOURNEY (Ritchie 2013), DEATH IS DEPARTURE (Lakoff 2008), DEATH IS THE END OF THE JOURNEY or DEATH IS REST (Kövecses 2010). These conceptual metaphors, often manifest in linguistic examples of euphemisms for death such as 'passed away', and tend to involve a very general evaluation of death as negative by default, based on the assumption that being alive is preferable to being dead. Similarly, while some studies of quality of death touch on metaphor implicitly, often advocating a conscious, sensitive and effective use of metaphor, especially on the part of professionals interacting with patients (e.g. Czechmeister 1994; Reisfeld and Wilson 2004), to the best of our knowledge no studies have focused explicitly on what metaphors are used to describe a good versus a bad death.

As we outlined in Chapters 1 and 2, evaluation and framing are prominent functions of metaphor and are relevant in this chapter, as in Chapters 5 and 6. Different framings can have consequences for how patients experience the end of their lives and/or for how they are treated by healthcare professionals (cf. Thibodeau and Boroditsky 2011; van Brussel and Carpentier 2012). For example, if a good death is framed in terms of peacefulness and acceptance, a healthcare professional will want to guide dying patients and their families towards these attitudes—potentially even if patients might prefer a different approach, or if real acceptance is almost impossible to achieve (cf. Scarre 2012). As Walters put it most poignantly:

> The rhetoric of palliative care sets great store by the autonomy of the individual patient and the fulfilling of the latter's wishes about how and where (if not when!) she chooses to die. In reality, however, this freedom can sometimes be compromised by the pressure of control towards what professionals consider to be a 'good death'.
>
> (2004: 406)

We will now outline our methods for the particular analyses in this chapter, before turning to the metaphors used by healthcare professionals to describe and frame good and bad deaths in our corpus.

8.3 Methodology for the Retrieval of Relevant Metaphors

As we outlined in Chapter 3, we asked the 16 UK-based healthcare professionals taking part in our interviews directly about quality of death, because of its centrality to their professional practice. These questions came towards the end of each interview and were expressed as: 'How would you describe a good death? How would you describe a bad or difficult death? Can you provide any examples from your experience?' (see our interview guide in Appendix 1). We manually identified metaphors in the stretches of text that our interviewees produced in response[1] (beginning with the question and ending with the interviewer-led introduction of a new topic), using our standard method for metaphor identification described in Chapter 3. The responses amounted to 10,646 words, 5,305 of which were descriptions of good deaths and 5,341 of bad deaths. We identified 167 relevant metaphors in interview descriptions of good deaths (i.e. 31.5 per 1,000 words), and 223 relevant metaphors in interview descriptions of bad deaths (i.e. 41.8 per 1,000 words).

We then needed to scale up this targeted identification of metaphors for quality of death, for our healthcare professional online data. We therefore identified stretches of text in the healthcare professional online corpus that dealt spontaneously with different types of death. To do this, we utilised a version of our online healthcare professional data to which two layers of annotation had been added: each word was given a part-of-speech tag and a semantic tag, formatted in such a way that both words and tags were searchable using the concordance tool of AntConc (Anthony 2014), a software with similar functionality to Wmatrix. AntConc allows for slightly different manual searches from Wmatrix, which is why we made use of it for the work here.

Using AntConc's regular expression search function, we ran queries for two-word sequences consisting of any adjective (denoted by the tag 'JJ' in the part-of-speech tagger CLAWS) followed by any word with 'L1–Dead' as its first USAS (UCREL Semantic Analysis System) tag, i.e. any word in the semantic field of death. 'Good death' and 'bad death' are themselves examples of the kinds of phrases this search specifies, and using the annotation allowed us to find all relevant instances without deciding in advance what specific lexical items to search for. This resulted in 429 concordance lines of examples, including combinations such as 'cardiovascular mortality', 'assisted dying', 'premature death', 'tragic loss', 'calm death', 'bad death' and 'happy death'. We manually checked all 429 concordance lines, discarding two categories of irrelevant results immediately: (a) all references to assisted dying and its variations (as 'assisted', while an adjective, does not have the evaluative function we were looking for), and (b) all technical terms (e.g. 'cardiovascular mortality'). This narrowed the number of relevant examples to 81. We explored the extended co-text of these 81 examples, further discarding any that were not descriptions or discussions of quality of death (such as reported speech, quotations or book/article titles). This left 50 concordance lines that genuinely suggested something about quality of death, which, with their extended co-texts (120-character view), amounted to 3,230 words of text. We identified metaphors in these stretches of text using the method described in Chapter 3.

We then returned to AntConc's regular expression search function to search for two-word sequences consisting of the USAS tag 'L1– Dead' as the first tag, i.e. a word in the semantic field of death, followed by a general adverb (denoted by the tag 'RR' in CLAWS). This retrieved combinations such as 'die badly', 'dying well', 'die alone', 'die soon', 'dies eventually' and so on—that is, verbal equivalents to the nominal 'good death', 'bad death', etc. This search resulted in 117 concordance lines. Replicating the process just outlined, we narrowed our results by discarding any examples that were technical medical terminology or obviously not about quality of death (e.g. 'cadavers greyly'). This left us with 42 concordance lines. We explored the co-text of these 42 examples and discarded any examples that were uttered in the context of euthanasia/ assisted dying or did not, in fact, include in situ descriptions of quality of death (such as reported speech or quotations or book/article titles). This left us with 16 examples, which with co-text amounted to 1,411 words of running text. We identified metaphors in these 1,411 words using the method described in Chapter 3. Thus, in total, we analysed for metaphor the extended co-text of 66 instances of either JJ + L1– or L1– + RR, a total of 4,641 words of online data.

Finally, for the sake of completeness, we also looked at the collocations of 'death' and 'deaths' in both the complete interviews and the complete online data for healthcare professionals (i.e. not just the stretches of text dealing with quality of death), using AntConc. As outlined in Chapters 2 and 3, a collocation analysis identifies those words that regularly co-occur (within five words) with the word(s) under study, in this case 'death(s)'. Looking at collocation patterns and how they might differ between the two data types gives us a good indication of what differences, if any, there are in how death is talked about in them. The mutual information (MI) score, a measure of effect size, and a minimum frequency of three were used for this analysis.

8.4 Analysis of Healthcare Professionals' Descriptions of Death and Dying

*8.4.1 Collocations of Death**

In our healthcare professional online data, the top 50 collocates of 'death(s)' (MI scores between 6.64 and 9.96) generally indicate medical terms and precise procedures (e.g. 'cellular', somatic', 'certifying', 'certificate(s)', 'bureaucracy', '(re)defin(ing)', 'biological', 'stem', 'brain', 'recorded'), temporal proximity of death ('hasten', 'impending', 'timing', 'unexpected'), socio-cultural aspects of death ('taboo', 'hindu', 'café') and causes of death ('cause', 'injured'). Some also suggest quality of death—'impressive', '(un)natural', 'serene', 'experiencing', '(un)dignified', 'peaceful'—but these items have MI scores in the lower part of the range (6.64–7.55), indicating somewhat weaker collocations.

In our interview data, by contrast, four of the top five collocates of 'death(s)' (MI scores between 11.51 and 12.35) are suggestive of quality of death ('perfect', 'bad', 'preferred', 'good'), and we additionally have collocates such as 'difficult' (MI = 10.70) and 'hard' (MI = 8.86), which also indicate quality. A few collocates represent the examples that healthcare professionals gave ('her', 'person', 'example', 'respondent'); a few indicate conversational features, i.e. are related to the genre of the data ('hmmm', 'like', 'cos' and various contractions); and many of them are verbs, adverbs and modal verbs that qualify and hedge statements ('suppose', 'perhaps', 'maybe', 'might', 'would', 'could').

It is interesting to note that, as indicated by the difference in MI-score range of the top 50 collocates for the two genres, the top 50 collocate types in the interviews are represented by 758 tokens (i.e. individual instances), but only 327 tokens in the online data. In other words, the top 50 collocates are used more frequently in the interview data than in the online data, even though the interview corpus is only about a quarter of the size of the online corpus.

These results suggest that healthcare professionals speak/write about death in our interviews differently from online. The MI scores indicate stronger collocations with descriptors of quality in the interview corpus than in the online corpus, and the more frequent use of the top 50 collocates in the interviews suggests greater homogeneity in that genre. This is as we would expect given the differences in the type of data; the greater variety of medical backgrounds of the online contributors; the fact that we asked interviewees directly about quality of death; and the tendency of medical professionals not to use the online medium to discuss patients, carers or specific cases (as we indicated in Chapter 3). Interviews also involved a more everyday, non-technical discourse, typically with non-categorical statements, while the top collocates in the online data are technical or semi-technical terms and do not necessarily relate to the quality or experience of dying. This is partly explained by the face-to-face nature of the interviews, but it also seems to mirror what Steinhauser et al. (2000) noted: physicians focus most on the biomedical aspects of death and dying. An interesting exception to this is the metaphor 'peaceful', which is among the top 50 collocates in the online but not the interview corpus.

We now turn to a more detailed analysis of the stretches of text that focus on quality of death.

8.4.2 Overview of 'Good' and 'Bad' Death Descriptions

In contrast to the focus of the Conceptual Metaphor Theory literature at least, in our interviews a patient's actual death is often mentioned only briefly and almost as an afterthought, as it is seen as an obligatory and predictable part of the good/bad death description. Instead, the *process* of dying is more the focus; and that process is not evaluated relative to life, but relative to alternative ways of dying. There is also an explicit awareness of the pitfalls of using euphemisms for death, so our interviewees tended to avoid them. In the online data, we did find repeated conventional euphemistic references to death, such as 'passing', 'pass away', 'fade from this world', 'suffer a loss', 'life's last journey' and so on. While some contributors apparently favoured these expressions, others also explicitly critiqued such language.

In discussing good and bad deaths, most healthcare professionals (in both the online and interview data) emphasised that what constitutes a good death is a matter of perspective ('it's so dependent on everybody's experiences' —Interviewee 3; 'Who is to say what a "good death" is' —Online data), and that it was therefore essential to give patients options, and to try to fulfill their wishes ('it has to go back to what's right for that individual patient' —Interviewee 11). Both the interviewees and the online contributors also noted that most people wished to die at home, but interviewees emphasised the ways in which hospice care can actually provide patients and their families with a better overall experience. Online contributors also tended to praise hospice care, when it was mentioned, and to contrast dying at home (mostly seen as positive) with dying in hospital (seen as negative). However, online contributors also tended to describe two different types of bad deaths: those that were bad for the patient and/or family, and those that were difficult for themselves to witness. By contrast, our interviewees tended to focus much more on the patient and family perspective. The good deaths that our interviewees described were often a result of successful intervention on their part, while bad deaths were often described as the result of interventions that were less successful due to external circumstances, or of situations where there was no opportunity for intervention (see also Semino et al. 2014). Online contributors did not go into this type of detail in their discussions of good and bad deaths.

Despite acknowledging the extremely subjective and personal nature of evaluating a death as good or bad, most interviewees were able to give concrete examples of both, especially after our prompt questions. The examples tended to include: a description of the patient's background, often including family circumstances and relationships; an account of any interventions by the hospice staff; a brief reference to the patient's death; and some reflections on what made that particular patient's death 'good' or 'bad'. The online data, as would be expected, included very few examples of narratives of specific cases. When examples were given, they tended to be from the contributors' personal rather than professional experiences (with some exceptions). Healthcare professionals writing online tended to speak at a higher level of generality, and to position their discussions of quality of death within broader political and policy debates. One such debate, frequently used by the online contributors to orient their discussion, was assisted dying. The concept of assisted dying (as well as 'euthanasia' and 'assisted suicide') is even more politicised than the concepts of good/bad deaths, and tends to involve markedly different ethical and/or legal issues. For these reasons, we have chosen not to discuss examples that are focused on this debate further in our analysis here.

8.4.3 Metaphors for a 'Good' Death in the Interviews

In this section and the next one, we focus more on the results from our semi-structured interviews than on the online data because of the relative richness of the former. In response to the 'good death' question, interviewees typically introduced a difficult situation that had the potential to result in a 'bad' death, which was then addressed by professional intervention in the hospice and altered to such an extent that the patient could eventually have a 'good' death. Interviewees' explanations of what this 'good' death entailed included a number of recurring metaphors: having 'reached' a 'stage' of 'acceptance', being 'at peace', being 'symptom/pain free' and having 'controlled' symptoms. A key contributor to achieving these states was having 'open' conversations with family members (as we also indicated in Chapter 4) and 'preparing' for the 'end'. We classified these metaphors in our manual analysis as:

- Movement and Location (e.g. 'reached the stage of') (NB: we later grouped these under Journey metaphors);
- Acceptance/Exchange (e.g. 'accept', 'acceptance');
- Peace (e.g. 'peace', 'peaceful');
- Freedom (e.g. 'pain free');
- Control (e.g. 'symptom controlled');
- Openness (e.g. 'open discussion').

Extended excerpts using these metaphors for a good death are presented in Examples 8.3 to 8.7.

Example 8.3

for me I suppose it's a good death . . . it's about peacefulness you know and having peace being peaceful being comfortable you know being at peace with yourself but also with the your surroundings erm being as comfortable and pain free, I think pain free is to the a the crucial element to it

(Interviewee 3)

Example 8.4

she was able to accept that it was the end so I think that's what you would call a good death. Where both the patient and the family have reached the stage of saying this is now where where it needs to end.

(Interviewee 14)

Example 8.5

> I think part of it being able to let probably to <u>let go</u> and also maybe having that permission from their family that they can <u>let go</u> as well where their symptoms are under <u>control</u>.
>
> (Interviewee 2)

Example 8.6

> when the whole team works together like that and then a patient has a symptom <u>controlled</u> erm death which both the patient and the family are <u>prepared</u> for then that that's sort of what I would say is a sort of good example.
>
> (Interviewee 5)

Example 8.7

> and difficult conversations about the fact that you er it may be that you know that they aren't going to get any better, so what would be their preferred option given that that's situation. So it's having those kind of <u>open</u> discussions with them to try and erm <u>give</u> them the options
>
> (Interviewee 8)

Most of these are highly conventional metaphors, which tell us that a good death is characterised both by the presence of 'peace', as opposed to 'struggle'/'war', and by the absence of negative physical sensations (like pain or other symptoms). The latter are implicitly presented as potential restraints by means of the adjective 'free' (Example 8.3). Sometimes, when the complete absence of such symptoms cannot be guaranteed, the objective becomes to have them under control (Examples 8.5 and 8.6). A 'good' death was associated with being able to appropriately reduce the patient's symptoms and help them and their families prepare for and accept death. Similar views were found by Low and Payne (1996) among nurses and social workers and by Cottrell and Duggleby (2016) in a systemic review of 39 articles on a 'good death' from 1992 to 2014. Interestingly, in our data there is also a complex interaction between these various factors expressed through metaphor.

For instance, 'peace' at the end of life is contingent not only on the absence of negative symptoms, but also on the patients' and families' attitudes, specifically their acceptance of the prospect of death (Examples 8.1 and 8.4). In this sense, both Peace metaphors and Acceptance/Exchange metaphors (which include expressions such as 'give', 'provide' and 'receive') contrast with the Battle or Violence scenario described as leading to a bad death (see later discussion). However, as the Movement metaphor 'reached' in Example 8.4 shows, the attitude of acceptance is not a given, but needs to be obtained through a mental 'journey'. This resonates with what Seale (1998: 92) described as the socially valued 'inner-directed heroics of the self', or the effortful emotional progress from denying, to fighting, and finally accepting death (also echoing Kübler-Ross' (1969) stage theory of grief, discussed in Chapter 9). Similar patterns have been noted and critiqued by various scholars (for a summary see Cottrell and Duggleby 2016); Zimmerman, for example, questions the justification behind the requirement of acceptance, and suggests that arriving at that attitude not only facilitates the dying process 'but also renders care easier' (2012: 217).

The mental 'journey' towards 'acceptance' is helped by 'preparation' and explicit conversations in which the patient and his or her family acknowledge to themselves and to one another that the patient is dying, enabling them to plan ahead (Example 8.7). These explicit conversations are referred to by Openness metaphors as well as by the verb 'address'. The metaphorical use of 'open', with its associations of open doors and arms, helps to convey a positive evaluation of these explicit conversations, and they are assumed to be necessary for controlling one's death, i.e. articulating wishes and making decisions regarding one's death.

In addition to this mental shift, another type of 'journey' is referred to in these examples via Movement and Location metaphors: life itself. Death is described as the 'end' of life's journey, 'where' the living need to 'let' the dying 'go' and vice versa. To some extent, these Movement and Location metaphors provide useful vocabulary for talking about death euphemistically, as in Example 8.5. In addition, however, they also help to integrate the deaths that our interviewees consider to be 'good' into the conventional LIFE IS A JOURNEY conceptualisation. In this way, the frequent use of these metaphors in descriptions of a good death, in contrast with their absence in descriptions of a bad death (see later discussion), implicitly normalises these 'good' deaths. They are evaluated as very much in line with the usual LIFE IS A JOURNEY conceptualisation of everyday experience. Of course, death is the natural end to life, but these metaphors suggest that perhaps only the good death described by the professionals is in fact such a natural end. This evaluation may or may not be shared by patients and carers, and it may affect how professionals approach their work (cf. Zimmerman 2012; Cottrell and Duggleby 2016).

In fact, professional practice, training and identity seem to be implicit in other aspects of good death descriptions as well. The various Control metaphors in Example 8.6, for instance, denote a kind of control by proxy. Control is exercised by medical professionals, but is in accordance with patients' wishes. From a professional identity perspective, it is understandable why our interviewees consider control to be such a crucial aspect of a good death (and why its counterpart, 'uncontrolled', is often implicated in bad deaths): this control is the active manifestation of their role; it is what they can actually do (cf. Low and Payne 1996; Costello 2006). Unsurprisingly, we also saw professional roles and practices foregrounded in the narratives that the interviewees told in response to the good death question (Semino et al. 2014): good death narratives were narratives of successful professional/hospice intervention. As we will show in the following, this framing is not prominent in the online data, which may be related to the fact that online contributors are, for the most part, not palliative care practitioners, may not have been contributing from within their workplace and are therefore less likely to be invested in this aspect of dying.

We now turn to the metaphors for bad deaths. As we will show in the next section, the difference between good and bad deaths was, in fact, often expressed via contrasting metaphors.

8.4.4 Metaphors for a 'Bad' Death in the Interviews

Our interview questions about 'bad' deaths were arguably more challenging for the interviewees to answer than those about good deaths. Responses to our 'bad' death questions inevitably involved situations where professional intervention was unsuccessful, and since the goal of hospice care is to provide the best possible death, a 'bad' death resulting from unsuccessful intervention is a challenge to the professional identity or *face* (Goffman 1967) of hospice staff. Interviewees often managed this 'face threat' by explaining frustrated interventions in terms of problems that were outside hospice staff's control. In a few cases, the interviewees mentioned lack of adequate resources, or unfortunate circumstances (e.g. patients being admitted at particularly busy times), but more often a bad death was described as the result of the attitude of the people involved: the patient or their close relatives. This kind of reasoning is, of course, rhetorically delicate, as it involves implicit or explicit criticisms of vulnerable people. The metaphors used to describe 'bad' deaths in our interviews helped to communicate these evaluations while avoiding explicit criticisms of dying patients and their relatives.

In contrast with the good deaths discussed in the preceding section, bad deaths are described as involving a lack of 'acceptance' on the part of patients and family members: not only non-acceptance of death but also a 'pushing away' of professional help or 'support'. These patients were described as seeing death as an opponent against which to 'struggle', 'battle' or 'fight' (also Example 8.2) in order to 'keep going'. External circumstances and various life choices were also described as contributing to a bad death. Patients' problems within their families were sometimes 'highlighted'; at other times they remained 'in the background' or in a 'place' inside the patient that hospice staff were not allowed to 'reach'. These therefore could not be 'addressed' or 'controlled'. Longer excerpts showing these metaphors in context are presented in the following three examples:

Example 8.8

> there can be a lot of anger and concern, which has been highlighted because someone is dying. So I think . . . dying you know where we can't get the symptoms completely under control erm dying perhaps where they didn't really want to die but circumstances they've landed up there erm and somebody who really still hasn't reconciled themselves and they want to keep fighting fighting fighting and therefore they want all the stops pulled out to keep them going. So those are the sorts of deaths that are that are difficult.
>
> (Interviewee 14)

Example 8.9

> so they are the deaths that I think that are psychologically difficult where somebody where somebody not only doesn't want to address it, cos people can die OK not having addressed it and be OK. But it's where they've not addressed it but actually there's a lot of fear in the background or a lot of battling in the background. And so you'd get this kind of horrible overlay of pretending it's not going on, but actually they're really scared and you can't quite reach into the scared place to support them, because they won't let you, but you know it's there. So I find those deaths really . . . difficult, where the conversations that needed to happen haven't happened where the support's been pushed away
>
> (Interviewee 7)

Example 8.10

> and we couldn't control his pain erm and we'd got a syringe driver going [. . .] and we were going up and up and up in the strength of medication and we could not get him settled we just could not get him settled and that was you know watching his mum watch him like that was really hard erm she was upset, we were upset
>
> (Interviewee 16)

These examples, which are typical of the stretches of text describing bad deaths, contain metaphors drawing on a wider variety of semantic domains and show greater complexity in terms of how they are combined than the descriptions of good deaths in the previous section. These extracts include:

- Vision metaphors (e.g. 'highlighted');
- (Negated) Control metaphors (e.g. 'can't get [. . .] under control', 'couldn't control');
- Violence metaphors (e.g. 'fighting', 'battling', 'pushed away');
- (Negated) Peace metaphor (e.g. 'having peace');
- Hiding/Invisibility metaphors (e.g. 'in the background', 'overlay').

These main groups co-occur with:

- Movement and Location metaphors (e.g. 'landed up there', 'keep . . . going');
- Building/Construction metaphors (e.g. 'support');
- Container metaphors (e.g. 'reach into the scared place', 'internally').

Several of these metaphors describe the circumstances that lead to a death being bad and help to express, less threateningly, the interviewees' challenges, practices and frustrations, as well as their evaluations, not just of the death, but also of the vulnerable individuals involved. Violence metaphors in Examples 8.8 and 8.9 ('fighting', 'battle') represent a coherent and consistent counterpart to metaphors of 'peace' and 'acceptance' identified in descriptions of good deaths. There seem to be two types of 'battles' that can lead to a bad death: those that refer to a way of living one's life in general, and those that refer to attitudes towards death itself. The use of Violence metaphors to describe these attitudes and ways of life allows the healthcare professionals to offer a negative evaluation of vulnerable individuals indirectly, by exploiting the connotations of literal meanings of the vehicles of the metaphors. In fact, another set of metaphors, related to music, are used by a different interviewee to mitigate a similar statement about how the imminence of death makes problems within families worse: 'where there is some tension or discord and it almost gets amplified' (Interviewee 1). On the surface, it may appear inappropriate to imply criticism of patients and their families, but Scarre (2012) argues that normally there is insufficient recognition of the fact that personality traits and characteristics also contribute to the quality of death. In this light, the indirect rhetorical strategy here can be seen as progressive or adaptive on the part of the healthcare professionals, and indicative of their wealth of experience.

A further counterpart to patterns we demonstrated in the context of good death descriptions are the metaphors describing things being 'in the background' or 'overlaid' and difficult to 'reach' in Example 8.9. These contrast with the idea of 'openness' in good deaths. Hospice staff, in line with the aims of the hospice movement as outlined earlier, see it as part of their role to enable patients to discuss their most intimate feelings and fears, and to discuss explicitly with them and/or with their families the fact that they are dying. Cases where this does not happen are negatively evaluated, and these metaphors help to express that. The combination of the notions of openness as 'good' and of hidden/in-the-background as 'bad' presents another strong and coherent professional framing.

The absence of control in two different senses is also an important factor potentially leading to bad deaths; again, this represents a counterpart to the existence of control in good deaths. It is seen as detrimental to the situation if the patient has no control over their own destiny (e.g. 'landed up there'), as opposed to having wishes that are fulfilled, as in good deaths. In Example 8.8, the patient's agency or ability to control is effectively reduced to mental processes of unfulfilled volition (repetition of 'want'). Similarly, it is also important for the professionals to have proxy control over the situation, executing patients' wishes when they are unable to act for themselves; the absence of this leads to a bad death (Example 8.10) (cf. Costello 2006). There is also a similar kind of complex interaction between the different metaphor patterns here as we described for good deaths. Metaphorical violence (as an attitude both towards death and towards other people) impedes 'acceptance' and prevents the interviewees from doing their job ('control', 'settle'); these in turn prevent a good death. The kinds of antagonistic attitudes described are often a result of things being 'in the background', or not being 'addressed', i.e. the absence of 'open' conversations. This interrelationship is the exact converse of the good death scenario, and is also consistent with the dominant medical-revivalist discourse of a good death (Walter 2003; Seale 2004; van Brussel and Carpentier 2012).

The greater variety of source domains we noted in these examples needs to be considered hand in hand with the higher relative number of metaphor vehicles in bad death descriptions that we noted in section 8.3 (31.5 per 1,000 words for good, and 41.8 per 1,000 words for bad deaths). As we outline in Demjén et al. (2016), based on a log-likelihood calculation, the difference between metaphor token frequencies in good and bad death responses in interviews is statistically significant ($LL = 7.69$, $p < 0.01$). The dense clusters of different source domains in bad death descriptions (compare Example 8.8 with Example 8.3 for instance) also indicate an increased level of complexity and creativity in metaphor use. Just in Example 8.8, for instance, there are examples of Vision metaphors, negated Control metaphors and Violence metaphors, which combine with Movement and Location metaphors ('landed up there', 'keep going', 'stops pulled out'). On the one hand, this may simply be consistent with Cameron's (2017) hypothesis that metaphor 'favours the negative'. However, Gibbs et al. (2002) note that metaphors are more frequent in descriptions of intensely emotional topics, and Ortony and Fainsilber (1987) find that a higher percentage of novel or creative metaphors are involved in such cases. The higher frequency of metaphors in bad death descriptions could therefore indicate that bad deaths are more emotional, sensitive or difficult to talk about, even for professionals. In further support of this, Semino et al. (2014) noted that narratives of bad deaths tended to use the second-person pronoun 'you', while good death narratives used 'we'. Both pronouns can include the healthcare professionals and their teams. However, 'you' is also a more generic referent than 'we' (it can be used to mean 'me, you, and anyone else in a similar situation'). It therefore allows interviewees to distribute responsibility for bad deaths more broadly, by signalling that anyone in a similar circumstance would have acted the same. Semino et al. (2014) argued that the additional rhetorical work done around bad deaths may partly be related to the fact that the very existence of bad deaths is a potential challenge to the professional identities of those working in hospice and palliative care.

It is also worth noting the absence of conventional LIFE IS A JOURNEY metaphors, or other Movement metaphors that would easily integrate into that concept. Although there are Journey metaphors, they are negated or non-realised, as in 'want all the stops pulled out to keep them going' in Example 8.8. The word 'want' emphasises the desirability but also the non-reality of a situation consistent with the normal LIFE IS A JOURNEY metaphor. As we pointed out in the previous section, linguistic manifestations of LIFE IS A JOURNEY help to integrate or normalise the types of deaths that our interviewees consider to be good. Their absence in bad death descriptions suggests that such deaths are perhaps seen as less 'natural'.

In addition to metaphors being used in the descriptions of bad deaths themselves, they were also used by interviewees to describe the after effects of a patient's death.

Example 8.11

I see her daughter professionally and she carries that distress still two years later and I think will carry it . . . maybe always and it will I suspect colour her vision of how her death might be or how her father's death might be in the future

(Interviewee 13)

Example 8.12

And when I do a lot of staff support it's often because the nursing staff have been erm paralysed or overwhelmed by seeing somebody so fearfully dying and struggling against

(Interviewee 7)

The emotional consequences of a bad death for family members (and sometimes for healthcare professionals themselves) are expressed in terms of Altered Vision and Burden metaphors (Example 8.11), as well as the inability to move or be in control (Example 8.12). Burdens carry negative evaluations, as do Lack of Movement metaphors in a LIFE IS A JOURNEY context, where progress is movement forward (cf. Demjén 2011). There is also a sense in which the 'badness' of a bad death goes beyond the actual event, and can have long-term negative consequences. Similar discussions about the effects of a death on those left behind happen in good death descriptions as well, but they tend to rely on Movement metaphors that are consistent with a desirable LIFE IS A JOURNEY scenario, such as 'going through a normal grief'. This seems to support our interpretation of the differences in metaphor frequencies between good and bad death descriptions in the interviews: bad deaths are more emotional and sensitive, making them more difficult to process. One interviewee made this explicit by saying that it is harder to remember examples of a good death because 'when they're good, I let them go'. It is worth noting that these examples are similar to healthcare professionals writing online about the effects of seeing deaths on themselves and 'those left behind'.

In the next section, we reflect on how these findings relate to what we found in the online data specifically.

8.4.5 Metaphors for 'Good' and 'Bad' Deaths Online

As we outlined in section 8.3, descriptions of good and bad deaths in the online data had to be obtained in a very different way from the direct elicitation of the interviews. The interviews involved a fairly homogeneous group of participants being asked explicit questions about good and bad deaths, while online a much more diverse group just happened to mention quality of death on occasion. As a result, and given the differences between writing online and speaking face-to-face in an interview conducted in a professional setting, the descriptions of good and bad deaths online tended to be much shorter, less detailed and less focused on how a good death can be achieved or on healthcare professionals' own role in that process. For these reasons, we consider the two datasets in separate sections and do not attempt any kind of quantitative comparison between metaphors for good/bad deaths in the online and interview data.

That said, based on our collocation analysis in section 8.4.1, which was not focused on metaphor, we were able to suggest that the online healthcare professional data seemed to be more heterogeneous than the interview data (for various reasons). In general terms, the same can also be said for heterogeneity of metaphor choices: there seemed to be less consistency in metaphors used online to describe good and bad deaths. The spontaneous discussions online touched on a wider range of aspects of good/bad deaths—the causes of death, its speed (sudden, slow) and the extent to which it was natural versus unnatural (often in the context of euthanasia (unnatural) versus illness (natural))—than our interviewees did. The lower consistency in the metaphors used online means there are fewer distinct metaphor patterns.

Nevertheless, traces of some of the patterns from the interview data are present in the online data too: a good death as 'peaceful', 'supported', 'calm', 'prepared' and 'pain free'; a bad death as 'violent', 'struggling' and 'tormented'. There is also the occasional mention of 'acceptance', and the related 'facing' of death with courage facilitating a good death, as in Example 8.13 (NB: as in previous chapters, original spellings are retained in quotations from the online data).

Example 8.13

> peace, acceptance, faith, hope, help, and courage to face what is before them

Overall, the framings for a good and a bad death in the online data that are most consistent with the interviews draw on Violence and Acceptance metaphors ('torment', 'pain free', 'peaceful', 'acceptance'). However, other than pointing out the need for accepting death, there seems to be much less focus on what the 'desired' attitude for patients/families is, and how this can be facilitated. This is again likely a result of the shared background of interviewees in hospice or palliative care, which emphasises the psychosocial aspects of dying, while online contributors had more diverse backgrounds.

An interesting difference between the interviews and online contributions is an additional use of Violence metaphors in the latter. While in interviews Violence metaphors tend to be used for attitudes and behaviours of patients or carers, online they are also used frequently to refer to treatments that the contributors see as unnecessary once a patient is dying ('invasive', 'aggressive interventions', 'sabotaged', 'destroyed', 'tortured', 'heroic measures'). This is the most variously lexicalised metaphor pattern in health professionals' descriptions of a bad death online, and it is interesting because it potentially attributes blame for the bad death to healthcare professionals, albeit as a collective group rather than as individuals. Of course, this contrasts with the potential distribution of blame for bad deaths by means of pronouns and metaphors in the interviews.

There are some additional metaphors and non-figurative expressions in the online data that are worth noting. Length and speed of a death are repeatedly mentioned, usually with Distance metaphors and non-figurative references, respectively. 'Long', 'prolonged' and 'protracted' deaths are generally seen as bad (Example 8.14)—often, though not exclusively, from the perspective of the family or the healthcare professional. Consistently with these Distance metaphors, a slow death is generally presented as a bad death (although some contributors also question this framing), while a rapid death is good ('we cope well with rapid death but badly with slow death'); a sudden death can be either. As the following examples show, dying is ideally 'long' enough to allow patients time to say goodbye and have religious rites performed, but not so 'long' that it results in discomfort or negative effects on the families or health professionals:

Example 8.14

he had a <u>protracted</u> illness, and died uncomfortably.

Example 8.15

those few days can be crucial to the dying patient, <u>giving</u> them the opportunity to <u>spend</u> time with relatives and have any religious rites that they may want performed.

Another complete, partly figurative scenario involves bad deaths being ones where the patient is alone or 'abandoned', while a good death is metonymically described as occurring 'in someone's arms' (potentially literally) or with someone 'around'. This partly mirrors a framing that we also found in interviews (e.g. 'surrounded by friends and family'). However, in interviews this was only mentioned in the context of good death descriptions, potentially suggesting that this particular way of distinguishing between good and bad death is important among the healthcare professionals in our online data, but perhaps less central to the hospice professionals we interviewed.

A number of other aspects of death are also talked about repeatedly in non-figurative ways in the online data, specifically dignity and faith (e.g. Example 8.13). These are not given much attention in our interviews. Dignity and its variants, and religion and faith, are only mentioned a total of three times each in response to our good/bad death questions (although spiritual care and comfort as part of what hospices offer *is* discussed, mostly in other parts of the interviews). In fact, while in the online data religious faith is mentioned as contributing to a good death, its few mentions in the interviews relate to potential problems it can cause.

Overall, while interviewees could be criticised for presenting too unified a view, online contributors demonstrate more variety. In fact, our findings from the online data resemble much more the variety that was found in Low and Payne's (1996) and Payne et al.'s (1996) studies.

8.5 Conclusions

In this chapter, we looked at the metaphors used by 16 UK-based palliative healthcare professionals, as well as multiple online contributors, to describe 'good' and 'bad' deaths. We began by looking at the (not necessarily metaphorical) collocations of 'death(s)' in our interview and online corpora and showed that the interviews were more homogeneous and focused more strongly on quality of death than the online data did. This was not surprising, since our interviewees shared similar professional backgrounds, and we spoke to them in similar professional settings and asked them explicitly to describe and give examples of good and bad deaths.

We then moved on to the metaphors used to describe quality of death in the interviews with healthcare professionals, commenting where appropriate on how any patterns played out in the online data. Towards the end of the chapter, we also discussed the findings from the online data in more detail, showing how online references to quality of death made use of a wider variety of metaphor vehicles and addressed more aspects of the dying process.

Interviewees generally constructed a good death as being 'at peace' and 'free' of negative symptoms. In addition, interviewees described 'accepting' death as the 'end' of one's 'journey', after having had 'open' conversations with healthcare professionals and family members, as important in achieving a good death. These patterns were echoed in the online healthcare professional corpus. Some of the metaphors our interviewees used also helped to normalise the deaths that they considered to be 'good' by integrating them into the LIFE IS A JOURNEY conceptual metaphor. By contrast, a bad death in the interviews involved opposing conceptualisations and were not aligned with LIFE IS A JOURNEY: a lack of 'acceptance' of death and a 'pushing away' of professional help; and problems 'in the background' or in a 'place' inside the patient that hospice staff are not allowed to 'reach'. As opposed to 'peace', there was a 'struggle', 'battle' or 'fight' against death in an effort to 'keep going'. Such Violence metaphors, in particular, helped our interviewees express indirect negative evaluations of patients' attitudes and life-styles in a context where explicit criticism would not be appropriate. Violence metaphors were also prominent in the online data, but contributors tended to use them to describe treatments they saw as unnecessary and contributing to a bad death ('invasive', 'aggressive interventions', 'sabotaged', 'destroyed'). Online contributors additionally used Distance metaphors to distinguish between good (just long enough) and bad deaths (too short or too long), while also commenting on the importance of faith and dignity.

We briefly noted that bad death descriptions in our interviews contained more frequent and more creative metaphors than good death descriptions and that the relative frequency and creativity of metaphorical expressions can be indicative of the intensity of emotion that speakers feel towards their subject or topic. The higher frequency of metaphors in bad death narratives could therefore indicate that bad deaths are more emotional, sensitive or difficult to talk about, even for professionals. They may, in fact, be *particularly* difficult to talk about for such professionals, because the very existence of bad deaths is a potential challenge to the professional identities of those working in hospice and palliative care. Semino et al. (2014) suggest that the interviewees constructed particular professional roles and identities through these good and bad death descriptions, which helped define, elaborate on and justify their role in end-of-life care. This was most likely cued by the situational context, as we interviewed people in their role as hospice managers, and mostly conducted the interviews in their workplaces. In fact, the metaphors in these examples not only evaluate different ways of dying but also support the interviewees' general arguments for the role of hospices and hospice staff in facilitating good deaths and avoiding bad deaths. This echoes Steinhauser et al.'s (2000) finding that social and professional roles shape views on a good death more than other factors (in their case, age and gender).

Overall, we found much more detail and consistency in metaphor framing in our interview data than online. Although the differences in data type and data collection methods go some way towards explaining this, the degree of consistency in interviews was remarkable. As we have pointed out in other chapters, the point here is not about the specific types of metaphorical expressions or source domains, but the ways in which they are used and the framing effects they might have. The metaphors for good deaths had opposite counterparts in the bad death descriptions, suggesting consistent, coherent scenarios. What seems to emerge then—despite explicit verbal recognition that, when it comes to dying, what counts as 'good' or 'bad' is highly individual and subjective—is in fact a stable and unified view of what counts as and leads to each of these kinds of death. And this consistency of framing in the interview data mirrored the consistency we found when investigating the narratives that our interviewees produced in response to our good/bad death questions (Semino et al. 2014).

The consistent framings we noted are, of course, also inextricably linked with the dominant socio-cultural and professional contexts of our interviewees (Steinhauser et al. 2000). Hospice professionals are expected to subscribe to the medical-revivalist view of a good death (Zimmerman 2012), so such a unified view could be an indicator of well-trained professionalism. However, the degree of consistency could also be signalling a hegemony of dying in hospice care (cf. van Brussel and Carpentier 2012). Others have, for example, questioned the uncritical promotion of the acceptance of death by pointing out the impossibility of combining 'tranquillity with staring into the abyss of nothingness' (online contributor quoting Geoffrey Scarre; see also Scarre 2007). Although we only noted metaphor consistency in our interview data, healthcare professionals online, despite their different backgrounds, are also exposed to some of the same ideologies, with potentially similar consequences. As one online contributor commented, a professional development seminar on dying well 'unnerved some who felt that we would now be under tremendous pressure to die well and leave everybody uplifted'.

The discrepancy between a unified, consistent professional view—a potential hegemony of dying—and the more heterogeneous lay view noted by Payne et al. 1996 and Cottrell and Duggleby (2016), among others, could also potentially be a source of tension in or dissatisfaction with end-of-life care. A uniform view potentially precludes alternative perspectives. For example, a recently widowed woman comments in our online corpus that the last two days of her husband's life were 'stolen' from them by the well-meaning but unwelcome intervention of strangers in a hospice 'who decided they knew what would help'. Similarly, not everyone may share a positive view of an open awareness of impending death, as one of the patients in our online data notes: "I myself am not ready to know what difficulties I will face at the end or the heartache I will cause my family—sometimes ignorance IS bliss.'

Citing cultural variation in end-of-life preferences, Seale and Geest (2004) and Goldsteen et al. (2006) also question the need for 'open' conversations. Indeed, it could be argued, from a different perspective, that open and explicit conversations might be described as potentially harrowing and possibly unwelcome or unnecessary intrusions. While the existence of a unified 'front' is understandable and arguably even necessary in the circumstances, it is important to be aware that it may limit the range of 'acceptable' choices and attitudes that are open to patients and families (e.g. Walters 2004; Costello 2006; Zimmerman 2012). In other words, it is important to ensure that any dominant professional formulations do not prevent those with alternative views from voicing their wishes and receiving the end-of-life care that *they* believe will lead to a good death.

Having discussed metaphors for professional views on quality of death, in the next chapter we turn to the metaphors used by bereaved carers writing online.

Note

1. We manually analysed the responses of all our interviewees, not just those that were part of our 90,000-word sample. However, one interviewee declined to answer these questions, so there are no responses included from him.

References

Anthony, L. (2014). *AntPConc (3.4.3)* [Computer Software]. Tokyo, Japan: Waseda University. Retrieved from www.laurenceanthony.net/

Cameron, L. (2017). Using metaphor for peace-building, empathy and reconciliation. In E. Semino and Z. Demjén (Eds.), *The Routledge handbook of metaphor and language* (pp. 426–442). Abingdon: Routledge.

Carpentier, N., and van Brussel, L. (2012). On the contingency of death: A discourse-theoretical perspective on the construction of death. *Critical Discourse Studies*, *9*(2), 99.

Cipolletta, S., and Oprandi, N. (2014). What is a good death? Health care professionals' narrations on end-of-life care. *Death Studies*, *38*(1), 20–27.

Costello, J. (2006). Dying well: Nurses' experiences of 'good and bad' deaths in hospital. *Journal of Advanced Nursing*, *54*(5), 594–601. doi:10.1111/j.1365-2648.2006.03867.x

Cottrell, L., and Duggleby, W. (2016). The "good death": An integrative literature review. *Palliative and Supportive Care*, 14(6), 686–712.

Czechmeister, C. A. (1994). Metaphor in illness and nursing: A two-edged sword: A discussion of the social use of metaphor in everyday language, and implications of nursing and nursing education. *Journal of Advanced Nursing*, *19*, 1226–1233.

Demjén, Z. (2011). Motion and conflicted self metaphors in the Sylvia Plath's Smith journal. *Metaphor and the Social World*, *1*(1), 7–25.

Demjén, Z., Semino, E., and Koller, V. (2016). Metaphors for 'good' and 'bad' deaths: A health professional view. *Metaphor and the Social World*, *6*(1), 1–19.

Department of Health. (2008). *End of life care strategy promoting high quality care for all adults at the end of life*. London: DH. Retrieved April 2017, from www.gov.uk/government/uploads/system/uploads/attachment_data/file/136431/End_of_life_strategy.pdf

Gibbs, R. W., Leggitt, J. S., and Turner, E. A. (2002). What's special about figurative language in emotional communication? In S. R. Fussell (Ed.), *The verbal communication of emotions: Interdisciplinary perspectives* (pp. 125–149). Mahwah, NJ: Lawrence Erlbaum.

Goffman, E. (1967). *Interactional ritual: Essays on face-to-face behavior*. Allen Lane: The Penguin Press.

Goldsteen, M., Houtepen, R., Proot, I. M., Abu-Saad, H. H., Spreeuwenberg, C., and Widdershoven, G. (2006). What is a good death? Terminally ill patients dealing with normative expectations around death and dying. *Patient Education and Counseling*, *64*(1–3), 378–386. doi: 10.1016/j.pec.2006.04.008

Kastbom, L., Milberg, A., and Karlsson, M. (2017). A good death from the perspective of palliative cancer patients. *Supportive Care in Cancer*, *25*(3), .933–939

Kövecses, Z. (2010). *Metaphor: A practical introduction* (2nd ed.). New York: Oxford University Press.

Kübler-Ross, E. (1969). *On death and dying*. London: Tavistock Publications.

Lakoff, G. (2008). *The political mind: Why you can't understand 21st-century politics with an 18th-century brain*. New York: Viking.

Low, J. T. S., and Payne, S. A. (1996). The good and bad death perceptions of health professionals working in palliative care. *European Journal of Cancer Care*, *5*, 237–241.

Ortony, A., and Fainsilber, L. (1987). The role of metaphors in descriptions of emotions. Paper presented at the *Proceedings of the 1987 workshop on Theoretical issues in natural language processing*, Las Cruces, New Mexico.

Payne, S. A., Langley-Evans, A., and Hiller, R. (1996). Perceptions of a 'good' death: A comparative study of the views of hospice staff and patients. *Palliative Medicine*, *10*, 307–312.

Reisfeld, G. M., and Wilson, G. R. (2004). Use of metaphor in the discourse on cancer. *Journal of Clinical Oncology*, *22*, 4024–4027.

Ritchie, L. D. (2013). *Metaphor*. Cambridge and New York: Cambridge University Press.

Scarre, G. (2007). *Death*. Stocksfield: Acumen.

Scarre, G. (2012). Can there be a good death? *Journal of Evaluation in Clinical Practice*, *18*(5), 1082–1086.

Seale, C. (1998). *Constructing death: The sociology of dying and bereavement*. Cambridge: Cambridge University Press.

Seale, C. (2004). Media constructions of dying alone: A form of 'bad death'. *Social Science & Medicine*, *58*(5), 967–974.

Seale, C., and Geest, S. (2004). Introduction: Good and bad death: Introduction. *Social Science & Medicine*, *58*, 883–885.

Semino, E., Demjén, Z., and Koller, V. (2014). 'Good' and 'bad' deaths: Narratives and professional identities in interviews with hospice managers. *Discourse Studies*, *16*(5), 667–685.

Seymour, J. E., Bellamy, G., Gott, M., Ahmedzai, S. H., and Clark, D. (2002). Good deaths, bad deaths: Older people's assessments of the risks and benefits of morphine and terminal sedation in end-of-life care. *Health, Risk & Society*, *4*(3), 287–303.

Smith, R. (2000). A good death: An important aim for health services and for us all. *BMJ*, *320*, 129–130.

Steinhauser, K. E., Clipp, E. C., McNeilly, M., Christakis, N. A., McIntyre, L. M., and Tulsky, J. A. (2000). In search of a good death: Observations of patients, families, and providers. *Annals of Internal Medicine*, *132*(10), 825–832.

Thibodeau, P. H., and Boroditsky, L. (2011). Metaphors we think with: The role of metaphor in reasoning. *PLoS ONE*, *6*(2), e16782.

van Brussel, L., and Carpentier, N. (2012). The discursive construction of the good death and the dying person: A discourse-theoretical analysis of Belgian newspaper articles on medical end-of-life decision making. *Journal of Language and Politics*, *11*(4), 479–499.

Vig, E. K., Davenport, N. A., and Pearlman, R. A. (2002). Good deaths, bad deaths, and preferences for the end of life: A qualitative study of geriatric outpatients. *Journal of the America Geriatrics Society*, *50*(9), 1541–1548.

Walter, T. (2003). Historical and cultural variants on the good death. *British Medical Journal: International Edition*, *327*(7408), 218–219.

Walters, G. (2004). Is there such a thing as a good death? *Palliative Medicine*, *18*(5), 404–408.

Zimmerman, C. (2012). Acceptance of dying: A discourse analysis of palliative care literature. *Social Science & Medicine*, *75*, 217–224.

9 Family Carers' Metaphors for the Emotions Associated With Bereavement

9.1 Introduction

Many of the family carers represented in our online data continue to be active on the forum after the person they cared for has died. From that point onwards, their posts tend to revolve around their experiences of bereavement and grieving, with a particular focus on emotional states and changes. The following extract is taken from a post by a recently widowed woman:

> *Example 9.1*
>
> At least on here you get a chance to let your feelings out and also to realise that we aren't going mad we are just extremely sad at losing our better halves and the person who made us whole. [. . .] Fathers day is causing a few problems for my kids as well. We have planned to go to the cemetery in the morning and then we have booked to go for a meal with my Mum and Dad in the afternoon. I just hope we all keep it together for my Dad's sake as much as anything. It is his Father's day as well.

At the beginning of the extract, this writer spells out the importance of the online forum at this point in her life. The forum gives her an opportunity to express her feelings freely ('you get a chance to let your feelings out') and to reassure herself that these feelings are not an indication of mental illness ('to realise that we aren't going mad'). Many other bereaved contributors express similar attitudes towards the forum, and this particular extract clearly shows how bereaved carers use their posts to share their experiences and to support one another emotionally (see Young 2007 for similar observations on the positive function of offline bereavement groups). In this case, the writer spells out the problems her own family is experiencing in advance of Father's Day in response to another contributor who had reported similar problems. Special days (including also birthdays, anniversaries, Christmas, etc.) are well-known to be difficult following a bereavement, and indeed, in the first sentence of the extract, both the pronouns 'you' and 'we' are used to refer generically to all bereaved contributors to the forum.

We have chosen this example to open this chapter, because its author talks about the emotional aspects of bereavement and grieving not just via a literal reference to a particular emotion ('extremely sad') but via several metaphorical expressions:

- 'losing our better halves' and 'person who made us whole' for the consequences of the death of a partner for one's sense of self;
- 'let your feelings out' for the verbal communication of emotions;
- 'keep it together' for the attempt not to become emotional in a context where this could be upsetting for others.

In the rest of this chapter, we discuss in detail the variety of metaphors that bereaved carers use in our online data to talk about their emotional experiences following the death of the person they cared for (usually a spouse or a parent). In section 9.2, we provide some background on models of bereavement and grieving and on metaphors for emotions. In section 9.3, we briefly outline our methodology for this chapter, and in section 9.4 we present our findings in two main parts: metaphors for the individual felt experience of grief, and metaphors for the social implications of bereavement. In section 9.5, we reflect on the implications of our findings for studying metaphors for emotions, on the one hand, and, on the other hand, for understanding the challenges and needs of bereaved carers as reflected in our data.

9.2 Background: Bereavement and Grieving, and Metaphors for Emotions

9.2.1 Models of Bereavement and Grieving

Grief is a normal reaction to the death of a person or other major event that can be described, metaphorically, as a 'loss'. However, it is increasingly recognised that there is no single paradigm for dealing with the kind of irrevocable loss caused by a person's death (Machin 2009). Rather, the manifestations of grief vary from person to person, but will often include physical, cognitive, behavioural and emotional elements. For a close personal bereavement, grief is likely to continue for a long time and may recur in a modified form, particularly in association with anniversaries, further losses or other reminders, such as Father's Day in Example 9.1.

People are likely to feel changed by the experience of grieving, but most, in time, find that they are able to function well and eventually enjoy life again. Typically, patterns and expressions of grieving are influenced by religious beliefs and practices, norms and conventions that change over time, and variables such as age, gender and social status.

Much of the Western concept of grief has been heavily influenced by the work of Sigmund Freud. During the First World War, he published an influential essay on mourning and melancholia (Freud 1917/1961), in which he differentiated between clinical depression and grief and proposed a mechanistic stage model of grief, involving:

- Acknowledging the loss;
- Feeling the pain;
- Doing 'grief work' (cognitive processing), i.e. withdrawing emotional attachment from the deceased ('letting go') to allow the formation of new relationships.

Freud's work largely conceptualised grief as an intra-psychic phenomenon that was experienced as emotionally painful and that required active and sustained cognitive engagement over an extended period of time. In his view, this ultimately led to a resolution of grief and an ability to form new relationships by severing the person's relationship with the deceased. Subsequent theorists elaborated upon these ideas to propose various stage models of grief, such as the psychiatrists Bowlby (1969), Kübler-Ross (1969) and Parkes (1996).

In recent years, theorists have increasingly moved away from such stage models of grief and rejected the notion of 'grief work' as described by Freud. Instead, there is greater emphasis on an individual's personal narrative and on the disruption that bereavement causes to this narrative and to significant relationships. Within this kind of approach, the notion of grief work is replaced with that of 'continuing bonds', i.e. the reconstruction of a personal narrative for both the deceased and those who live on (Klass et al. 1996).

An alternative theory of loss relies on a particular psychological model of stress and coping (Lazarus and Faulkman 1984). Within this approach, nothing is inherently stressful, but the experience of stress depends on our appraisal of problematic situations. More specifically, a distinction is made between focusing on the emotional aspects of the situation versus focusing on the problem and how to deal with it. Drawing on this model of stress, Stroebe and Schut (1999) propose a 'dual process' theory of loss, where emotion-focused coping is balanced by problem-focused coping.

Overall, it is generally agreed that there is no single theory that fully explains the experience of loss or accounts for the emotions, experiences and cultural practices which characterise bereavement and grieving. Within broad cultural constraints, individuals manage bereavement in different ways, reflecting the diverse range of human responses and cultures. In the UK, there are a number of accepted ways to behave after bereavement, but most are traditionally characterised by stoicism and emotional restraint, especially in public. By contrast, bereavement support services tend to emphasise the importance of emotional expression, acknowledgement of the reality of the loss and sharing of thoughts and feelings with others. The importance of communication in this latter kind of approach to grief raises, for us, the issue of how metaphors are utilised by people experiencing bereavement to put into words the emotions that they feel, and to talk about their perception of the social consequences of bereavement.

9.2.2 Metaphor and (Negative) Emotions

Emotions are notoriously difficult to define. For the purposes of this chapter, we take a broad view of emotions as affective states that are intrinsically 'valenced' in nature—that is, they can be placed somewhere on a scale from positive (e.g. happiness) to negative (e.g. sadness) (Manstead 2007). This is in fact consistent with the representation of emotions in the USAS (UCREL Semantic Analysis System) semantic tagset of Wmatrix, where the symbols + and – are appended to tags for emotions to distinguish between positive and negative emotional states. For example, the tag E4.1 (Happy/Sad) has two variants: E4.1+ (Happy) and E4.1– (Sad). In this chapter, we focus particularly on the negative end of the scale of valence, because of our concern for the experience of grieving.

When people talk about their emotions and feelings,[1] they can label or name them by means of literal terms such as 'sad', 'happy' or 'angry', or express them by means of figurative language, including particularly metonymies and metaphors. Metonymy is involved when an emotional state is suggested implicitly by mentioning a concrete reaction or behaviour that is associated with that emotion. For instance, 'tears' may be used as a metonym for sadness, as in this example from our carer online data: 'Oh dear, here come the tears again'. Metaphor is involved when an emotional state is referred to via a different kind of state, entity or process which it can be perceived to resemble. An example of this occurs when one of the bereaved carers in our data says 'in my shatter wreck state', invoking both an inanimate physical entity (a wreck) and a physical process (shattering) as concrete equivalents for the non-physical emotional experience.

In a classic study from a Conceptual Metaphor Theory perspective, Kövecses (2000) argues that figurative language, and metaphor in particular, is by far the most common way of talking about emotions. This is explained in terms of metaphor's ability to convey complex, subjective experiences vividly and concisely: metaphors for emotions do not just express the emotion itself, but also convey additional information about it in terms of its intensity, cause, control and duration. As Grossen and Norrick (1990: 111) note, '[w]hen emotion is felt, metaphor is the vehicle to express it, and when an emotion or emotional reaction is desired, metaphor is employed to call it forth'. Kövecses (2002) argues that the most fundamental conceptual metaphor for emotions is EMOTION IS A (PHYSICAL/NATURAL) FORCE, with different specific expressions suggesting different kinds of external forces (e.g. 'That was a terrible blow' and 'Waves of depression came over him'; Kövecses 2000: 25). This general metaphor highlights the main ways in which emotions tend to be viewed and experienced: they seem to happen to us out of their own volition, are somewhat unpredictable and intense and are therefore perceived as needing to be kept under some degree of control, depending on the situation.

According to Kövecses (2000), other conventional conceptual metaphors for emotions generally include THE BODY AS CONTAINER OF THE EMOTIONS (e.g. 'the sight filled her with fear'), EMOTION AS OPPONENT (e.g. 'to struggle with depression') or CAPTIVE ANIMAL (e.g. 'his joy broke loose') and EMOTION AS A DIVIDED SELF (e.g. 'to be beside oneself') (examples adapted from Kövecses 2000; see also Crawford 2009; Lakoff and Johnson 1999; Lakoff 2016). Negative emotions, and particularly sadness, have been found to be expressed in English via a specific set of metaphors, including SAD IS DOWN (e.g. 'He brought me down with his remarks'), SAD IS DARK (e.g. 'He is in a dark mood'), SADNESS IS AN ILLNESS (e.g. 'She was heart-sick') and SADNESS IS A BURDEN (e.g. 'He staggered under the pain') (Kövecses 2000: 25, underlining as in original; see also McMullen and Conway 2002; Charteris-Black 2012; Demjén 2011, 2015). Using corpus linguistic methods (searching for source- and target-domain vocabulary in a large corpus), Stefanowitsch (2006) tested and broadly confirmed the range of conceptual metaphors suggested by Kövecses (2000), but refined Kövecses' claims about prevalence/frequency and typical linguistic realisations.

In addition to being linked with particular emotions, specific conceptual metaphors account for different aspects of emotions, such as their intensity, cause and duration, as well as whether, how and to what extent they are controlled by the person experiencing the emotion. For example, emotional control is often expressed via FORCE, OPPONENT, CAPTIVE ANIMAL, FLUID IN A CONTAINER, or INSANITY metaphors (e.g. 'she kept her emotions in check'; 'his emotions ran away with him'; 'she couldn't hold back her feelings'; 'he was overwhelmed'). Intensity, on the other hand, is usually expressed via CONTAINER metaphors (e.g. 'she was overflowing with joy'), HEAT/FIRE metaphors (e.g. 'She was burning with shame/embarrassment') or NATURAL/PHYSICAL FORCE metaphors (e.g. 'I was swept off my feet') (examples adapted from Kövecses 2000). In addition, as we have indicated in Chapter 2 and Chapter 8, the relative frequency and novelty of metaphorical expressions can also be indicative of the intensity of the emotions described (Gibbs et al. 2002; Ortony and Fainsilber 1987). Cameron (2017) specifically suggests that a high frequency or density of metaphor tends to correlate with negativity, including negative emotional valence (see also Demjén 2015).

Finally, Young (2007) discusses the metaphors used by the members of a community-based bereavement writing group in a US college town. Young identifies a number of recurring patterns of metaphor, such as expressing the emotional consequences of death in terms of breakage (e.g. a ripped page) or erasure (e.g. a sand sculpture washed out by the tide), and describing grief as a natural force, such as whirlwinds and storms. Young additionally shows how the sharing of these metaphors within the group helped members to bond with one another, and to identify and deal with particularly difficult and stigmatised aspects of death and grief, such as abuse and suicide (see also Spall et al. 2013).

9.3 Methodology for the Identification of Relevant Metaphors

As with the case studies presented in previous chapters, the instances of metaphor use that we discuss in this chapter were identified by means of a multi-pronged approach to our data. First, we picked out metaphors for emotions associated with bereavement and grieving from the 2,415 metaphorical expressions we identified in the carer online data via our main approach discussed in Chapter 3. Second, we analysed all similes expressed by means of 'like' and 'as if' in our online carer data, and picked out all those that are used to express relevant emotional experiences. This was based on the analysis of the sample corpus, where we observed that similes played an important part in the expression of (negative) emotions. Third, we analysed the complete concordance of the semantic field E4.1– (Sad) in the online carer data, which consisted of 1,625 lines. For each concordance line, we considered both the expression that was tagged as belonging to the semantic field and the immediately preceding and following co-text to identify any metaphorical descriptions of emotional experiences associated with bereavement.

In the rest of this chapter, we present the main patterns of metaphor use that we identified by analysing in detail all of these concordance lines from the online carer data.

9.4 Analysis of Metaphors for the Emotions Associated With Bereavement

In this section, we make a broad distinction between, on the one hand, metaphors for the individual felt experience of grief and, on the other hand, metaphors for the emotional aspects of the social consequences of bereavement. The family carers in our online data use a range of metaphors for both types of emotional experiences. As we will show, these metaphors do not just reflect conventional conceptualisations of emotions, but also reveal the challenges, needs, evaluations, expectations and pressures of the carers contributing to the online forum from which our data is drawn.

9.4.1 Metaphors for the Individual Felt Experience of Grief

A range of different metaphors are used in our data to express different aspects of the individual experience of grief. We will consider particularly the metaphorical description of grieving as Physical Fragmentation, External Force, Journey and Movement more generally.

Grieving as Physical Fragmentation

Metaphors related to different types of physical fragmentation are used to describe the feelings that bereaved carers experience while living without the person who has died (see also Young 2007). In the terms we used in Chapter 4, these metaphors fall under the broader Wholeness group, as they involve loss of wholeness, or of physical integrity. This can apply either to the person him/herself or to their perception of their own lives or circumstances. In Example 9.2, for instance, the expression 'your whole world is falling apart' suggests a sense of intense emotional distress and disorientation while trying to 'keep busy':

> *Example 9.2*
>
> I am in the process of organising at present and none of it feels real it keeps you busy but somewhere in between you feel like your whole world is falling apart.

The following examples rely on the conventional metaphorical conceptualisation of a couple as forming a single whole, so that it is the bereaved person him/herself who is presented as having fragmented:

> *Example 9.3*
>
> I remember the desperate days when you realise you are only half a person.

> *Example 9.4*
>
> I was more upset because it is OUR car and I don't want to have to part with it unless I really have to. Silly I know but it is just like losing another part of you.

Although conventional in English, all these expressions emphasise the finality and irreversibility of the change caused by a loved one's death and the impact this has on the identity or self of the one left behind. In Examples 9.3 and 9.4, the change involves particularly the perception of one's own individual identity. In all three examples, the writers also switch from an 'I' perspective to using the second-person pronoun 'you'. This switch presents their personal experiences as generalisable—inherent in the generic meaning of 'you' as 'one'—and, because of the specificity of the experience described, shared especially by others on the forum. The address function of the pronoun 'you', which is simultaneously involved, additionally invites active engagement and potentially interaction (e.g. expressions of sympathy and mutual understanding), thereby contributing to solidarity and community building.

The following extracts involve more extended and creative metaphors where an improvement in the person's life following bereavement is described in terms of regaining or maintaining physical wholeness. In Example 9.5, this applies to the person's 'world', while in Example 9.6 it applies to the person himself:

Example 9.5

Yes world fell apart but slowly bits of the puzzle are put in place and the picture emerges.

Example 9.6

Funny, today I was saying [. . .] that I feel guilty because today I feel like I am not missing her enough [. . .] or feeling upset enough. Does that sound terrible? I know I am, but it's almost like my body is putting up a wall to stop me falling apart.

In Example 9.5, the idiomatic metaphorical expression 'world fell apart' is followed by the description of a different metaphorical scenario in which a state of physical fragmentation is specified as a 'puzzle' and reversed ('put in place'). The metaphorical 'picture' that 'emerges' seems to suggest some form of return to normality, though it is ambiguous whether the picture is a new or an old one. Example 9.6, in contrast, expresses what seems to be a common experience of guilt when one's emotional state begins to improve. The simile 'like my body is putting up a wall to stop me falling apart' presents the avoidance of extreme negative emotions in terms of a metaphorical wall that prevents the person's physical fragmentation. Interestingly, agency in the process of preventing physical fragmentation is attributed to the person's 'body', which is implicitly separated from the person's own self ('me'). This split-self description can be seen as a way of attempting to reduce the guilt involved in feeling better in the first place. We return to 'split-self' metaphors later.

In fact, one characteristic that is shared by all the different Physical Fragmentation metaphors is that the bereaved person is never presented as the agent in the processes that are being described. Even Example 9.5, which is relatively optimistic, includes a passive structure with no explicit reference to an agent ('bits of the puzzle are put in place') and an intransitive structure with an inanimate metaphorical agent ('the picture emerges'). This suggests a sense of lack of control of one's own emotions, which perhaps reflects lack of control over the circumstances more generally, something that is also conveyed by several other metaphorical patterns in our data (cf. Parkes 1996).

Grieving as an Attack by an External Agent

As we mentioned earlier, in English (and other languages) emotions can be conventionally described both as objects and as forces that act on the person experiencing the emotion. In our online carer data, different aspects of grieving are presented metaphorically in terms of different kinds of entities that act forcefully on the bereaved person (see also Young 2007). In all cases, this involves presenting the emotion as something external and other than oneself, although the specific kind of force involved varies from case to case.

Some instances involve objects that can cause physical damage to the body, as in the following simile:

> *Example 9.7*
>
> am two years out now—it's true, it does get easier. Not better, but definitely easier. But it still <u>hits like a sledgehammer</u> sometimes.

Others suggest an animate or human agent:

> *Example 9.8*
>
> can put my head in the sand as I do but pineing for you keeps <u>catching</u> me <u>up</u> and <u>biteing</u> me on the bum

> *Example 9.9*
>
> The loneliness <u>gets</u> you when your not expecting it to, its like you <u>let down</u> your <u>guard</u> and its there

Yet others involve different kinds of natural forces:

Example 9.10

> Once you are satisfied all the essential things have been organised you will probably find the loss <u>hits</u> you <u>like an avalanche</u>, that's what I experienced.

Example 9.11

> God I miss her she was so wonderful. It <u>hits</u> me in <u>waves</u> of emotion (I thought that phrase was one of those poetic inventions, but <u>it is like waves battering you on the beach and knocking you over and holding you under</u>.

Example 9.12

> sorry you are finding things so tough. I feel calm and strong at the moment with just <u>waves</u> of grief that sometimes resemble a <u>tsunami</u>.

All of these metaphors suggest that the emotional experience of grief involves repeated cycles in which the emotion is felt less intensely for a while and then, suddenly and unpredictably, much more intensely. The extracts that involve highly forceful entities emphasise the intensity and uncontrollability of the moments when grief is felt (e.g. 'sledgehammer', 'avalanche', 'tsunami'). In contrast, the expressions in Examples 9.8 and 9.9 involve less overtly powerful forces (e.g. 'biting me on the bum'), but emphasise the sense of threat (and potentially of pain) that results from the constant presence of an opponent that is ready to strike when the person is particularly vulnerable ('you let down your guard'). While all the different examples involve conventional metaphors for emotions, some writers use these metaphors creatively to express their own individual experiences (see Ortony and Fainsilber 1987; Gibbs et al. 2002). In Example 9.8, where the writer addresses his deceased wife directly, the idea of emotions as external forces is combined with the conventional idiom 'put one's head in the sand' to produce a scenario in which something like an animal can bite the person's bottom without being seen. In Example 9.11, the writer explicitly reassesses the conventional expression 'waves of emotion' and extends it creatively in a lengthy and detailed simile that emphasises the intense negativity of the emotions that he experiences from time to time.

In all the different cases discussed in this section, the bereaved person is presented as helpless and unable to control their negative emotions. However, the online forum seems to give contributors an opportunity not just to disclose their own emotional experiences (see Suler's 2004 notion of 'benign disinhibition' online) but also to reassure one another that those experiences are shared and therefore not something to be ashamed of. For example, the writer in Example 9.9 uses the generic 'you' to generalise her own experiences; the writer in Example 9.7 explicitly validates somebody else's experience with references to her own ('it's true'); and the writer in Example 9.10 tells someone else what they should expect on the basis of his own past experience ('you will probably find'). This sense of commonality among bereaved contributors to the forum can also be expressed via Journey metaphors, to which we turn next.

Grieving as a Journey

Like many other experiences in our corpus and in English generally, grieving is described metaphorically in our online carer data as a 'journey':

> *Example 9.13*
>
> I am guessing from your reply that you have just begun this journey of grief.

> *Example 9.14*
>
> Be gentle with yourself and understanding of your grief in the future, as it can be a difficult journey.

This use of 'journey' is of course consistent with what Lakoff and Johnson (1980) call the LIFE IS A JOURNEY conceptual metaphor, and more specifically with the idea that different parts of life can themselves be described as journeys within the broader lifetime's journey. As we noted in Chapter 6, Journey metaphors tend to frame experiences in terms of processes involving longer periods of time, with different stages, options/choices, change and potential difficulties. This applies to the preceding examples: in contrast with the metaphors we discussed in the previous section, Examples 9.13 and 9.14 are not used to express the momentary felt experience of grief, but to capture the long-term process of living with grief.

As we saw in Chapter 6, one of the possible uses of Journey metaphors is to present people who have similar experiences as being on the same metaphorical journey. In our online carer data, this applies to grieving too:

> *Example 9.15*
>
> It is 18 weeks now since my wonderful [husband] died and having read your posts I have in effect read my own journey. I am much further down the road than most of you and still finding myself in limbo most of the time. I have no motivation and can see no point in doing

> anything. [. . .] When people ask me how I spend my days I just say 'I have no idea' and this is because I am just muddling through life at the minute. [. . .]. Hopefully you will all start to feel better soon but it does take time and each of you will reach milestones at different times even though you are all travelling the same road. I wish you all well.

As well as suggesting a sense of commonality among people 'travelling' on the same 'journey' or 'road', this writer exploits metaphorically other aspects of journeys. The expression 'muddling through' suggests difficulties or confusion, slow positive change and lack of control and purpose. The notion of 'reach[ing] milestones at different times' suggests that there are standard stages to go through but allows for the fact that it takes people different amounts of time to feel better. Moreover, the religious metaphor in 'finding myself in limbo' conveys an unwelcome sense of lack of certainty and activity at that point in the person's life.

Although the destination of the journey of grief is not usually spelt out, it is often implied to be the time when grief is no longer felt. The positive nature of this destination can then be combined with the notion of continued linear progression as the default way of reaching a desired destination. This can lead to an expectation of continued, if gradual, improvement in one's emotions over time. Carers turn to the forum when this expectation does not seem to be met:

> *Example 9.16*
>
> Yes it is like going one step forward and a few steps back but I am hoping that we will all get there in the end.

> *Example 9.17*
>
> I know I'm further down the line than you in the grieving process but at the moment I feel as if I've taken ten steps backwards.

In the default Journey scenario, one aims to reach the destination as quickly and efficiently as possible. Hence, movement forward is typically used metaphorically to suggest positive change, and movement backward is used to suggest negative change, or lack of positive change. In the preceding examples, this notion is applied to grieving, so that forward movement stands metaphorically for feeling better, while backward movement stands metaphorically for re-experiencing negative emotions after feeling better for a while.

In other words, the particular framing imposed by the Journey metaphor presents the cyclical nature of emotions associated with grieving as not simply unwelcome, but also as something that, in principle, the person should avoid. This does not adequately allow for the way in which most people experience the grieving process, and can potentially lead to disappointment or even a sense of personal failure when one feels worse than expected. In other words, the Journey framing can facilitate a negative evaluation not just of the emotion itself, but of the fact that the emotion is being re-experienced in the first place. As we also showed in Chapter 6, Journey metaphors cannot therefore be seen as involving positive or neutral framings of difficult experiences by default, whether that be an illness or a bereavement.

Grieving as Other Types of Movement

Some aspects of the experience of grieving are expressed in our corpus by means of metaphors that suggest different kinds of movement. These metaphors differ from prototypical Journey metaphors in that they do not involve movement along a path from a starting point to a destination.

In some cases, grieving is described in terms of the inability to find a direction or destination for one's attempts to move:

> *Example 9.18*
>
> i feel like there's <u>nowhere</u> to <u>turn</u> or to <u>run</u> but i expect everyone feels similar

> *Example 9.19*
>
> A shrink would say I'm trying to <u>run from</u> grief and that would be true, I'm lucky that I can do this, ain't got a gang of kids to feed, but <u>where</u> will I <u>run to</u> next?

Both examples implicitly assume the metaphorical view of a successful, purposeful life as being able to move forward towards a destination. Against this view, having 'nowhere to turn or to run' suggests helplessness, confusion and potentially despair. The metaphorical use of 'run' can more specifically suggest a scenario in which one has to move urgently away from something unpleasant or dangerous, such as an opponent. This is particularly obvious in Example 9.19, where the writer presents grief itself as the place or entity that she is trying to run away from. In this context, wondering 'where' to 'run to next' suggests that the person feels unable to find an alternative way to be or feel.

A different kind of non-goal-directed movement is exploited metaphorically in uses of the verb 'wallow' such as the following:

Example 9.20

> Hi there, I lost my husband almost a year ago now. [. . .] I found that I just wanted to wallow in my own grief but was unable to do that because I do have a very loving family and a great support network.

Example 9.21

> Hi [. . .], your right I am fed up wollowing in misery, I have two sons to be proud of, a lovely home and plenty of good friends and neighbours.

When used literally, 'wallowing' suggests circular, on-the-spot movement, and is usually applied to animals rolling in dirt or mud. This may explain why its metaphorical use not only is associated with negative emotions, but also tends to negatively evaluate as self-indulgent the experience of the negative emotion itself. This negative evaluation is present in both of the preceding examples, as both writers seem to suggest that it is selfish, or, at the very least, inappropriate, to focus on one's grief when one has loving people in one's life. This use of 'wallow' is therefore similar to the 'forward/backward' examples in the previous subsection insofar as it imposes a negative framing on the (continued) individual experience of grief, and suggests that bereaved people should be able to control their negative emotions in view of other, more positive, aspects of their lives.

Finally, in the following example, the alternation between different emotions in the process of grieving is described as a 'roller coaster':

Example 9.22

> The roller coaster just never stops long enough for me to get off and sometimes it spins out of control. At those times I like to be on my own so that I can cry freely.

The metaphorical use of 'roller coaster' in relation to the emotions is highly conventional, and presents changes in mood in terms of rapid and uncontrollable up-and-down movement. This in turn relies on the conventional metaphorical representation of negative versus positive emotions in terms of the opposition between Up and Down. When 'roller coaster' is used metaphorically in this way, however, the focus is not on fun and exhilaration, but rather on the extreme nature of mood changes and the perception of lack of control over one's emotions and reactions. The latter aspect is explicitly emphasised in Example 9.22 by the reference to the person's inability to 'get off' and the expression 'spins out of control' (see Chapter 4 for other examples of 'roller coaster' metaphors). The final sentence of the extract expresses a common experience on the online forum: the feeling that crying in public, or generally becoming emotional in public, has to be avoided. In the next section, we consider a range of metaphors for this social dimension of bereavement.

9.4.2 Metaphors for the Social Experience of Bereavement

The bereaved carers in our online data also talk metaphorically about the emotional aspects of the social consequences of bereavement, and particularly the experiences of communicating their grief, becoming emotional and living with grief. These metaphors highlight specifically the attempt to control the external manifestations of grief (Kövecses 2000), and reflect the perception on the part of many of the carers in our data that it is socially unacceptable or undesirable to become emotional in public or to manifest the full extent of one's grief, even to family and friends (see Walters et al. 1995 for a critical discussion). In particular, in the following we consider metaphors to do with Release, Physical Fragmentation and Physical Separation from others and oneself.

Expressing Grief as Release

One of the conventional ways of representing emotions, in English and other languages, is as substances or entities that exist inside the body, so that the expression or manifestation of emotions is metaphorically conceived in terms of movement from inside the body into the open. This can be presented as involving different degrees of control on the part of the person who experiences the emotion:

> *Example 9.23*
>
> I also can see that they [forum posts] are a mechanism by which you can release some of your anguish but you may not have realised how much they encapsulate so much of what those of us who similarly grieve are suffering. Thank you for sharing your heart with us all.

In Example 9.23, the writer talks about the function of the online forum for another bereaved carer. The metaphorical use of 'release' suggests that the addressee's anguish is an entity or substance that is contained inside the body, and that the expression of anguish involves allowing this entity or substance to come out. The metaphorical use of 'mechanism' to describe the forum posts presents them as the means through which anguish can be expressed in a controlled manner and in a context where this is acceptable. Indeed, the rest of the quote emphasises that the addressee's posts are helpful to others who are in a similar situation. The phrase 'sharing your heart' relies on a conventional metonymic association between the heart and emotions, and also suggests that communicating one's subjective states involves moving something from inside to outside the body. Here, however, the metaphorical use of 'sharing' conveys both a sense of control and a positive evaluation of the person's communicative behaviour as altruistic, in contrast with a possible view of expressing negative emotions as self-indulgent. In fact, Example 9.23 is one of many instances in our data in which the forum is described as providing an opportunity to express negative emotions in a way that contrasts with conventional expectations of stoicism and is helpful for both writer and readers. In such cases, this positive function seemed to be due primarily to the fact that others on the forum experience, or have experienced, the same emotions, rather than to the anonymity that the forum provides.

Other metaphorical expressions involving movement from inside to outside the body are very conventional (e.g. 'get it [grief] out of my system' and 'letting my feelings out'), but are similarly used by bereaved carers in our online data to convey a degree of control over when, where and how to manifest their grief. In most cases, this controlled manifestation of grief happens either on the forum or when the person is alone.

Expressing Grief as Physical Fragmentation

In the previous section, we showed how the individual felt experience of grief is talked about metaphorically by some of the bereaved carers in our data in terms of Physical Fragmentation. Another aspect of bereavement that is sometimes expressed through Physical Fragmentation metaphors is the experience of becoming visibly emotional as a result of grief:

> *Example 9.24*
>
> I'm thinking of boxing all the little mementos up and putting them together in place which I can look at, and <u>fall apart</u> when I want to rather than every other minute of the day!

This conventional metaphorical use of 'fall[ing] apart' implies that emotional control corresponds to physical wholeness or integrity, so that loss of control of one's emotions corresponds to physical fragmentation. In fact, Physical Fragmentation metaphors tend to be used to talk about the attempt to control one's emotional reactions so that they only take place, and become visible, in appropriate circumstances (see 'when I want to' in Example 9.24).

Not surprisingly, therefore, this kind of Physical Fragmentation metaphor often occurs in the context of intentions and hopes for upcoming celebrations or anniversaries that might trigger strong emotions. In Example 9.1, a recently widowed woman is concerned about her father being able to enjoy a Father's Day meal even though it is going to be difficult for herself and her own children to control their own grief on that day. She therefore expresses the hope that 'we all keep it together'. In Example 9.25, a different writer attempts to encourage another forum member in advance of a difficult anniversary.

Example 9.25

> on this very difficult day I would like to send love and hugs to you and your family. [. . .] I hope that you can get through this day without completely falling apart.

As well as using a Physical Fragmentation metaphor ('falling apart'), this writer employs 'get through' metaphorically to indicate the experience of something emotionally difficult (see Chapter 6).

Overall, these Physical Fragmentation metaphors describe the external manifestation of strong negative emotions in terms of an irreversible and catastrophic physical process. Even though these metaphors are highly conventional in English, they suggest a negative evaluation of the external manifestation of grief. This reflects both a general sense that one should be able to control one's emotions in public and the belief that the external manifestation of grief is socially inappropriate, as it might cause distress and/or embarrassment to others as well as oneself. In this sense, these metaphors both reflect and reinforce culture-specific normative assumptions about emotions generally and bereavement in particular, and may generate feelings of guilt and inadequacy when bereaved people are unable, or in some cases unwilling, to control their own emotional reactions.

Living With Bereavement as Physical Separation From Others or Oneself

Finally, a number of bereaved contributors to the online forum express their experiences of social situations in terms of metaphors of Physical Separation from other people. The following two extracts are taken from different posts by the same contributor to the online forum:

Example 9.26

> Had a nice bbq at my mum and dad's. It was fun and we had lots of good food. I still feel like I am sitting on the edge though.

Example 9.27

> I still feel like I am on the outside looking in when i try to join in with some fun things but I assume that will get better.

It is well-known that a sense of intimacy with others is conventionally expressed metaphorically in terms of Physical Closeness, as in the case of expressions such as 'close friend' (Grady 1997). In addition, the oppositions between inside versus outside and centre versus periphery can be used metaphorically to express (lack of) involvement and belonging (e.g. 'people on the outside of society' and 'Del Monte was at the centre of the most cultured circles in Rome', from the Oxford English Corpus). The preceding two examples rely on these conventional associations to suggest that bereavement makes one feel alone and estranged even when engaging in potentially pleasurable activities with people one knows well.

A different contributor uses similar Physical Separation metaphors to talk about her experience of family events after bereavement:

Example 9.28

> I found I was taking part in family events but my mind was wandering (and still does) to other places. I retreated inside myself and wanted to be left alone but at the same time wanted people around me.

This extract includes two Journey metaphors that result in physical separation from others. These metaphors capture two different aspects of the person's difficulties at family events: 'my mind was wandering [. . .] to other places' describes the experience of thinking about other things instead of focusing on people and activities around her; and 'I retreated inside myself' suggests the inability to engage with others socially and emotionally. Both expressions also involve 'split-self' metaphors (Lakoff 1996; Emmott 2002; Demjén 2015). In 'my mind was wandering' there is a split between the person's mind and her body; in 'retreated inside myself', the same person is both the agent and the destination of the metaphorical movement. In the latter case, the expression is also followed by a statement of internal conflict between a desire for loneliness and a desire for company after bereavement.

A metaphorical split in the person's self is conveyed even more strongly in cases where bereaved carers explicitly express a sense of separation from themselves, rather than from others:

Example 9.29

> I personally am going through the motions of life and Christmas at the moment. I feel like I am 'watching' someone else's life unfolding like a black and white movie.

Here the simile 'like a black and white movie' is embedded inside the broader simile 'like I am "watching" someone else's life'. The quote marks around 'watching' seems to function as a signal of figurativeness, and 'unfolding' is also used metaphorically to suggest change and the passage of time. The broader simile involves a split in the person's self between the person living the life and the person watching someone else living their life. The person's 'real' self is positioned in the passive role of spectator, while the 'movie' in the embedded simile suggests that what is being watched is fictional rather than real. In this context, 'black and white' can emphasise a sense of unreality or temporal distance, as well as suggest low emotional intensity, or lack of positive emotions. The use of the metaphorical idiom 'going through the motions', which is common among bereaved carers in our data, emphasises the idea that the person's life has lost authenticity, and now involves a contrast between appearance and (emotional) reality.

Overall, the different Physical Separation metaphors show how the bereaved carers in our data feel that they have to continue living as they did previously, for their own sake and others', but find that many activities, and particularly social events, lack the significance, sense of purpose and enjoyment that they had before.

9.5 Conclusions

Our analysis in this chapter has implications both for metaphor studies and for an understanding of the emotional aspects of bereavement as described by the carers in our data. There is indeed increasing recognition that the needs of lay carers require greater attention, including particularly in end-of-life care (e.g. Grande et al. 2009).

As far as metaphor studies are concerned, we have found more evidence for well-known conventional metaphorical descriptions of emotions (e.g. as external forces), but we have also identified some patterns that have not been widely discussed in relation to negative emotional experiences. This applies particularly to Physical Fragmentation metaphors for the lived experience of grief and for changes in identity after bereavement (e.g. 'like losing another part of you'; but see Demjén 2015 for a discussion of Physical Fragmentation metaphors for depression). Our analysis in section 9.4.2 also suggests that the social implications of negative emotions need to be included in accounts of metaphors for emotions more systematically than they have been to date. Finally, our findings are consistent with earlier studies that emphasise the role of creative metaphors in conveying the intensity of individual emotional experiences, as in 'it is like waves battering you on the beach and knocking you over and holding you under' (Example 9.11; see also Ortony and Fainsilber 1987; Gibbs et al. 2002).

The metaphor patterns we have analysed in relation to different aspects of the experiences of bereavement and grieving highlight the difficulties, needs and (culturally based) assumptions of the contributors to the online forum. More specifically, different metaphors have different evaluative implications both for the experience of emotions and for the manifestation of emotions after bereavement.

The metaphors that are used to express the lived experience of grief emphasise the intensity of those experiences and the helplessness that people feel in relation to their own feelings of grief. Metaphors to do with External Forces express both intensity and lack of control over when and how grief is felt (e.g. 'hits like a sledgehammer'). Physical Fragmentation metaphors capture the finality and irreversibility of the change that has been caused by a loved one's death, and particularly the loss of identity that results from the death of a partner (e.g. 'you are only half a person'). The metaphors of grief as a Journey capture the fact that it is a lengthy, continuous process, and can express a feeling of companionship with others in the same situation (e.g. 'all travelling the same road'). On the other hand, the Journey framing can also generate expectations of linear incremental change towards feeling better, which leads to negative self-evaluation when re-experiencing intense grief (e.g. 'one step forward and a few steps back'). As we have mentioned, this view of grieving has been criticised as inadequate, but, on the basis of our data, it seems to persist, and to lead to unrealistic expectations and to feelings of guilt and personal failure. A negative evaluation of continued grief, and of the person who is grieving, is also suggested by metaphorical uses of 'wallowing', which implies self-indulgence and lack of sufficient appreciation of the remaining positives in one's life.

Metaphors used for the social aspects of bereavement reveal the different ways in which the death of a family member impacts upon daily life, relationships with others and one's sense of self. The external manifestation of grief (whether by talking about it or becoming emotional) is described through metaphors to do with Release and Physical Fragmentation. In most cases, emphasis is on the need to control one's negative emotions, to avoid causing embarrassment and distress to others, especially during celebrations and family events (e.g. 'I just hope we all keep it together for my Dad's sake'). This perception of the importance of control is consistent with Physical Separation metaphors for the inability to enjoy other people's company at social occasions (e.g. 'I still feel like I am sitting on the edge'). These metaphors reflect the culture-specific assumption that it is inappropriate to show negative emotions in public, and that it is therefore up to the bereaved person to control their emotions and reactions in the presence of other people. While traditions and cultural norms around death and grieving can provide comfort and purpose, feelings of guilt and personal failure may arise when someone is not able to exercise control in the way that they think is expected of them.

Overall, therefore, the metaphors we have discussed in this chapter point out a number of beliefs which arguably limit the range of post-bereavement reactions and behaviours that carers themselves regard as socially acceptable in the cultural context that is reflected in our data. This applies particularly to the view of grieving as a linear, incremental process towards the absence of grief; and to the assumption that manifesting one's grief in public is an indication of personal failure or weakness, and therefore needs to be avoided at all costs. In this context, the benefits of the online forum for bereaved carers are very much in evidence. Given that contributors often do not feel it is appropriate to show their grief even to close family and friends, writing about their emotions on the forum seems to be the main alternative to simply suffering on one's own. The forum provides the opportunity to disclose one's emotions without embarrassment or guilt, not just because it is possible to remain anonymous, but because other contributors are in a similar situation. As we have suggested, bereaved carers support each other emotionally and express a strong sense of community and companionship with other contributors.

Note

1. We use the terms 'emotion' and 'feeling' interchangeably.

References

Bowlby, J. (1969). *Attachment and loss* (Vol. 1). Harmondsworth: Penguin.

Cameron, L. (2017). Using metaphor for peace-building, empathy, and reconciliation. In E. Semino and Z. Demjén (Eds.), *The Routledge handbook of metaphor and language* (pp. 426–442). London and New York: Routledge.

Charteris-Black, J. (2012). Shattering the bell jar: Metaphor, gender and depression. *Metaphor and Symbol*, *27*(3), 199–216.

Crawford, E. L. (2009). Conceptual metaphors of affect. *Emotion Review*, *2*, 129–139.

Demjén, Z. (2011). Motion and conflicted self metaphors in the Sylvia Plath's Smith journal. *Metaphor and the Social World*, *1*(1), 7–25.

Demjén, Z. (2015). *Sylvia Plath and the language of affective states: Written discourse and the experience of depression*. London: Bloomsbury.

Emmott, C. (2002). 'Split selves' in fiction and in medical life stories: Cognitive linguistic theory and narrative practice. In E. Semino and J. Culpeper (Eds.), *Cognitive stylistics: Language and cognition in text analysis* (pp. 153–181). Amsterdam: John Benjamins.

Freud, S. (1961). Mourning and melancholia. In J. Strachey (Ed. and Trans.), *The standard edition of the complete psychological works of Sigmund Freud* (Vol. 14, pp. 243–258). London: Hogarth Press (original work published 1917).

Gibbs, R. W. Jr, Leggitt, J. S., and Turner, E. A. (2002). What's special about figurative language in emotional communication? In S. R. Fussell (Ed.), *The verbal communication of emotions: Interdisciplinary perspectives* (pp. 125–149). Mahwah, NJ: Lawrence Erlbaum.

Grady, J. (1997). *Foundations of meaning: Primary metaphors and primary scenes*. Unpublished PhD thesis, University of California, Berkeley, CA.

Grande, G., Stajduhar, K., Aoun, S., Toye, C., Funk, L., Addington-Hall, J., Payne, S., and Todd, C. (2009). Supporting lay carers in end of life care: Current gaps and future priorities. *Palliative Medicine*, *23*(4), 339–344.

Grossen, B. R., and Norrick, N. R. (1990). Metaphoric emotions, emotional metaphors. *Grazer Linguistische Studien*, *33–34*, 111–119.

Klass, D., Silverman, P., and Nickman, S. (Eds.). (1996). *Continuing bonds*. London: Taylor & Francis.

Kövecses, Z. (2000). *Metaphor and emotion: Language, culture, and body in human feeling*. Cambridge: Cambridge University Press.

Kövecses, Z. (2002). Emotion concepts: Social constructionism and cognitive linguistics. In S. R. Fussell (Ed.), *The verbal communication of emotions: Interdisciplinary perspectives* (pp. 109–124). Mahwah, NJ: Lawrence Erlbaum.

Kübler-Ross, E. (1969). *On death and dying*. London: Tavistock Publications.

Lakoff, G. (1996). Sorry, I'm not myself today: The metaphor system for conceptualizing the self. In G. Fauconnier and E. Sweetser (Eds.), *Spaces, worlds and grammar* (pp. 91–123). Chicago: University of Chicago Press.

Lakoff, G. (2016). Language and emotion. *Emotion Review*, *8*(3), 269–273.

Lakoff, G., and Johnson, M. (1980). *Metaphors we live by*. Chicago: University of Chicago Press.

Lakoff, G., and Johnson, M. (1999). *Philosophy in the flesh: The embodied mind and its challenge to western thought*. New York: Basic Books.

Lazarus, R., and Faulkman, S. (1984). *Stress, appraisal and coping*. New York: Springer Publishing Company.

Machin, L. (2009). *Working with loss and grief: A new model for practitioners*. London: Sage.

Manstead, A. S. R. (2007). Emotion. In R. F. Baumeister and K. D. Vohs (Eds.), *Encyclopedia of social psychology* (pp. 285–291). Thousand Oaks, CA: Sage.

McMullen, L. M., and Conway, J. B. (2002). Conventional metaphors for depression. In S. R. Fussell (Ed.), *The verbal communication of emotions: Interdisciplinary perspectives* (pp. 167–181). Mahwah, NJ: Lawrence Erlbaum Associates.

Ortony, A., and Fainsilber, L. (1987). The role of metaphors in descriptions of emotions In *Proceedings of the 1987 workshop on Theoretical issues in natural language processing*, Association for Computational Linguistics, Las Cruces, New Mexico.

Parkes, C. M. (1996). *Bereavement* (3rd ed.). London: Routledge.

Spall, B., Read, S., and Chantry, D. (2013). Metaphor: Exploring its origins and therapeutic use in death, dying and bereavement. *International Journal of Palliative Nursing*, *7*(7), 345–353.

Stefanowitsch, A. (2006). Words and their metaphors: A corpus-based approach. In A. Stefanowitsch and S. T. Gries (Eds.), *Corpus-based approaches to metaphor and metonymy* (pp. 63–105). Berlin: Mouton de Gruyter.

Stroebe, M., and Schut, H. (1999). The dual process model of coping with bereavement. *Death Studies*, *23*, 197–224.

Suler, J. (2004). The online disinhibition effect. *Cyber Psychology and Behavior*. *7*(3), 321–326.

Walters, T., Littlewood, J., and Pickering, M. (1995). Death in the news: The public invigilation of private emotions. *Sociology*, *29*(4), 579–596.

Young, E. (2007). Figures of grief: Metaphors from a bereavement writing group. *Omega*, *56*(4), 359–367.

10 Patients' Humorous Metaphors for Cancer Online

10.1 Introduction

To introduce the final analysis chapter of this book, there is perhaps nothing more apt than the Monty Python catch phrase: 'and now for something completely different'.

> *Example 10.1*
>
> Since my bowel cancer operation in January I have met a Russian Schitt called Bagov schitt. Bagov schitt has become very attached to me, but I think he could be a spy because he leaks things occasionally. Bagov needs constant attention and can be a real drain on me, to be honest I want to get rid of him as soon as I can. At least Bagov Schitt is not a pain in the bum.
>
> [Sam][1]

The preceding is characteristic of the types of examples we will focus on in this chapter: a patient with colorectal cancer writing online makes light of an unpleasant and embarrassing (potentially even taboo) side effect of having a colostomy bag—occasional leaks. He personifies the stoma bag and uses humorous puns, drawing on the literal and metaphorical meanings of the words 'leak' and 'drain'. The nonce expression 'Bagov Schitt' allows the patient to avoid mentioning the stoma bag explicitly: it can instead be inferred through the combination of the literal and metaphorical meaning of 'attached' and the phonological similarity of 'Schitt'–'shit', and 'Bagov'—'bag of'. The specific personification as a Russian spy has connotations of secrecy, underhandedness and untrustworthiness. This allows the patient to communicate a negative evaluation of living with a stoma bag without explicitly saying that he might be struggling with his situation. The humorous tone probably makes all this easier to talk about, and in fact, by joking about it, 'Sam' might already be feeling better.

Although this is certainly 'something completely different', we briefly discussed humorous uses of metaphor in some of the previous chapters of this book: in Chapter 5 we commented on the humorous potential of some

Violence metaphors, and in Chapter 7 we discussed the role of humour in how patients sometimes describe their healthcare professionals. Here we focus wholly on humorous metaphors (and humorous uses of metaphors) and the aspects of patient experience that they are used to describe.

Example 10.1 is just one of many instances of patient humour on a thread entitled 'For those with a warped sense of humour WARNING- no punches pulled here' (henceforth 'Warped') within the larger forum from which we have drawn our online data for patients and carers in this book. Laughing at cancer can be problematic (Chapple and Ziebland 2004), as demonstrated by the warning in the title of the thread (and the disclaimer in the first post; see next excerpt). Disease and death are still among the topics considered taboo or improper to discuss in a number of situations (Dohan and Levintova 2007; Norrick and Bubel 2005). At the same time, there seems to be an increasing trend of discussing the funny side of the cancer experience in certain public domains. In August 2015, for example, the Edinburgh Festival Fringe saw Beth Vyse, Alastair Barrie and Adam Hills base their comedy routines around personal cancer experiences. There also seems to be a proliferation of greeting cards for cancer that take a humorous tone, such as those by LA-based designer Emily McDowell (http://slate.me/1P0BE52), or PostTea's 'Inappropriately Appropriate' Cancer Cards range (http://etsy.me/2fAFV0y), 'based on the principle that "laughter is the greatest medicine"', and sporting messages such as 'I've heard your oncologist is a rubbish hairdresser'.

To do justice to the nature of the humorous phenomena in question, in this chapter we consider the complete Warped thread, instead of just the sections that were included in the online patient corpus. Based on the number of posts, Warped is among the longest 15 of approximately 30,000 threads on the online forum of the UK-based cancer charity from which we have drawn our data. It contains 2,544 posts contributed by 68 unique participants over 13 months. Of these participants, 39 self-identify as patients, many have various forms of colorectal cancer, and they contribute around 90% of the 530,055 words on the thread. The title designates the thread as a space specifically for irreverent verbal play, implying perhaps that such humour might not be appropriate for everyone or everywhere on the forum. The specific purpose of the thread and the potential dangers are made even more explicit in the first post:

> I set up this thread as explained below with a lovely dear lady called Sunshine May. We had a lot of chat on here and the silliness got me and her and lots of others through some hard times. Sunshine left the site when there was some criticism of warped and she deleted all her posts when she left. [. . .] If you are feeling sensitive please don't read this thread as you may feel offended. . . . and we need a place to say what we need to say without worrying about offending people so you have been warned!!!! This is for those of us who cope by being irreverent and silly and able to laugh at all the bad stuff.
>
> [HoneyBee]

In what follows, we discuss why patients may be using metaphors humorously on Warped (even at the risk of causing offence) and the ways in which they do so. We begin with some definitions and a brief overview of relevant literature in humour studies, metaphor and health communication. We then give a more detailed introduction to the Warped thread and its contributors, and outline how corpus methods helped us identify the humorous metaphors that are the focus of this chapter—after all, humour does not have a single identifiable form. In our analysis, we then examine three characteristically humorous uses of metaphors: personifications of cancer and treatment paraphernalia, participants' figurative references to one another, and co-created fantasy scenarios involving metaphor. We discuss how these seem to enable patients to discuss aspects of their experience that are embarrassing or taboo; maintain a coherent identity in the face of rapid change; facilitate a sense of empowerment in circumstances where people are likely to feel powerless; and contribute to bonding, cohesion and a sense of community at a time when people might feel isolated.

10.2 Preliminary Considerations

Humour is 'a type of mental play involving a lighthearted, nonserious attitude toward ideas and events' (Martin 2007: 1). Three theories of humour remain the most influential: Incongruity Theory (e.g. Kant 1951 [1790]), Superiority Theory (also known as Aggression or Disparagement Theory; e.g. Hobbes 1840) and Release or Relief Theory, generally associated with Freud (1905), among others. The Incongruity Theory of humour says that humour is a result of a resolution or ending that is in some way inconsistent with a particular set-up. This theory accounts for the structure of numerous jokes. The Superiority Theory of humour argues that humour results from the pleasure we take in others' mistakes or discomfort. Slapstick comedy and jocular teasing are good examples of this, but the theory can also account for self-deprecating humour, where someone makes fun of their own mistakes or failings. Finally, in the Release Theory account, humour comes from a release of excess nervous energy that has resulted from danger/fear, the breaking of social taboos, or the like. The dramatic principles of *comic relief* or *catharsis* embody this theory. In practice, these three theories are not mutually exclusive and can be integrated into explanations for why something is funny. For example, Spiegel (2015) argues that fart jokes are 'universally funny' precisely because they satisfy all three of these theories.

The two phenomena in question in this chapter—metaphor and humour—actually have something in common: both combine two disparate ideas to create new meanings and effects (e.g. Attardo 1994; Coulson 2000; Krikmann 2009; Kyratzis 2003; Mio and Graesser 1991; Ritchie 2013). At the same time, of course, not all humorous utterances are metaphors, and not all metaphors are humorous. Kyratzis (2003) and Krikmann (2009) follow Pollio (1996) in arguing that *humorous metaphors* generally emphasise or foreground the boundaries or differences between the two domains they bring together. They do this by drawing attention to a conventional metaphor's literal meaning along with its contextual meaning, for example. Compatible approaches explain metaphor humorousness as stemming from:

- An incomplete resolution of incongruity (e.g. Oring 2003), allowing a simultaneous appreciation of both ideas that were juxtaposed (Attardo and Raskin 1991; Dynel 2009b);
- A large discrepancy between the semantic domains that make up the source and target (e.g. Attardo 2015; Dynel 2009b; Mio and Graesser 1991); this discrepancy can be in the form of a status difference between semantic domains, if one is serious like life-threatening cancer, for example, and the other trivial like a stubbed toe (Attardo 2015; Dynel 2009b).

Both of these again help to foreground the differences between two ideas. This, however, does not account for all humorous uses of metaphor, nor for why some metaphors might meet these criteria and not be humorous (cf. Dynel 2009b; Krikmann 2009). A variety of additional factors can also make metaphors humorous:

- Humour that is already inherent in the source domain (Attardo 2015; Dynel 2009b);
- Excessive detail or exaggeration in the metaphors (Attardo 2015);
- The mixing of potentially clashing metaphors (Attardo 2015; Dynel 2009b);
- Distortions or twists of existing and familiar metaphorical idioms (Ritchie 2013);
- An already established humorous or 'play' frame (Apter 1982), which colours how any metaphor is interpreted.

In this chapter, we focus on *humorous metaphors* and metaphor used in humorous utterances as examples of (written) verbal behaviour within one particular forum thread. In fact, online fora are known to foster such verbal play (Daisley 1994; Georgakopoulou 2011; Vandergriff 2010), potentially as a result of the disruption of everyday hierarchies (North 2007) and the possibility of remaining relatively anonymous. This kind of *conversational humour* (Dynel 2009a) is interwoven into conversations and is always co-constructed by a number of participants reacting to each other (Chovanec 2011; Dynel 2011; Coates 2007). In fact, this is another overlap between metaphor and humour: both can be seen as developing dynamically in interaction (cf. Gibbs and Cameron 2008).

But the question remains: why use humorous metaphor at all, especially given the potential risks in this particular context? In the following analysis sections, we discuss why Warped contributors might do what they do, but the general functions of humour and metaphor are also worth bearing in mind. Metaphor and humour are both multifunctional, but both are generally thought to contribute to group bonding. In the case of humour, this happens by virtue of *laughing together* (Attardo 1994; Hübler and Bell 2003), but also because humour facilitates social or discourse control, and helps to convey some social norms, establish common ground and defuse unpleasant situations (Attardo 1994). Group-specific ways of using metaphor are also thought to contribute to bonding, persuasion and community formation (Cameron and Deignan 2006; Gibbs and Cameron 2008; Goatly 1997), among others. Both metaphor and humour also involve a certain amount of ambiguity, which can give the speaker the opportunity to retract the force of their utterance—a sort of deniability. For this reason, they are useful when discussing sensitive or embarrassing topics such as illness and death.

Although, to date, we have not been able to find studies examining the use of humorous metaphors specifically in the context of illness, a number of studies suggest that humour in itself can be beneficial (see Tanay et al. 2014 and references therein for a summary). Kuiper et al. (1993), for example, show that it contributes to the regulation of negative emotion or *affect* by facilitating re-appraisals and emotional distancing from stressful situations like illness (see also Martin 2007). Similarly, McCreaddie and Wiggins (2008: 589), reviewing 88 studies, argue that for healthcare professionals it acts as a stress moderator by providing a more 'palatable' outlet for frustration and because 'if something is ridiculous then it cannot be serious or threatening'. According to Watson (2011) this is also the function of healthcare professionals' use of gallows humour. Studies investigating patients' use of humour, usually in interactions with healthcare professionals or in more formal settings such as focus groups, show that humour helps patients (and carers) when they receive a cancer diagnosis (Tanay et al. 2014) and with subsequent difficult healthcare interactions (Chapple and Ziebland 2004). McCreaddie and Payne (2014: 341) note that cancer patients believe humour is 'integral to their health-care experiences with health-care staff as well as other patients and impacts upon how they cope and assert their identity at a time of challenge and crisis' (see also McCreaddie et al. 2010).

Generally speaking, then, joking and laughing about cancer can help turn serious, threatening and unpredictable life circumstances into objects of non-serious play, thereby reducing their psychological impact (Martin 2007). Little is known, however, about the use of humour when patients interact among themselves, probably because of the difficulties of gathering appropriate data (a notable exception from the hospice context is Langley-Evans and Payne (1997)). As illustrated in the first post, quoted earlier, Warped contributors state explicitly that the humour on Warped helps them cope with cancer. And they do this repeatedly. Contributors talk about the 'advice, laughs and hugs' helping them through the 'shittest times' in their lives and about being made to laugh at a time when they 'didn't think it was possible'. However, unsurprisingly, contributors do not explain in detail exactly how the specific discursive strategies are helpful. This seems to be fairly characteristic even of the aforementioned studies:

there is often little discussion of how humour might help people cope with illness, and it is this gap that we hope to begin to address here. Examining closely the usage of systematically selected patterns of humorous metaphor, we focus on the possible interpersonal functions and psychological effects that might be helping Warped contributors cope with cancer.

10.3 Introduction to Humour on Warped

Contributions to Warped generally touch on everyday topics like contributors' pets, Jehovah's Witnesses at the door, gardening, needing to buy new clothes, jobs and annoying colleagues, and getting drunk, as well as aspects of the patients' lives related to their illness. They describe, for example, things that were different before they had cancer, how other people react to their cancer, the physical consequences of the illness and its treatment, the use of stoma bags and so on. All of this is done in line with the humorous tone of the thread: a play frame which is explicitly established in the title and first post (cf. Apter 1982).

Contributors themselves orient to the humorous nature of the thread in various ways. They describe it explicitly as 'warped', 'sick', 'gallows', 'dark', 'toilet' and 'bum'[2] humour (see Concordance 10.1). And while newcomers to the larger forum often establish their right to participate by first posting about their own cancer experience, newcomers to Warped tend to begin by expressing an appreciation of, or by engaging in, the type of humour expected on Warped: 'so I hope i've passed the warped test and can join you haha' [Sue2].

A good proportion of the 68 contributors to Warped post on a regular basis. Figure 10.1 demonstrates this clearly by showing the frequency and regularity of posts by each author. Each horizontal row represents one contributor. The posts of each contributor are marked by a circle, if the contributor is a patient, or a plus sign if they are not a patient, along their row. From left to right, this represents the passage of time. The more densely packed the circles or crosses are in a row, the more frequently that contributor posts on Warped. There is one participant, a woman with colorectal cancer, whose contributions play a defining role. We have called her HoneyBee (marked with an arrow in Figure 10.1). HoneyBee sets up the thread, explains its purpose in the first post (quoted earlier) and remains the most frequent and prolific contributor throughout the data collection period. She also initiates a number of the humorous metaphor uses discussed in this chapter, whether within the thread or in one of her blog posts hosted on the same charity website. That said, the examples we discuss in the following are not only from HoneyBee. Other participants take up, recycle, adapt and repurpose HoneyBee's metaphors in the interconnected and intertextual manner typical of social networking sites (Seargeant and Tagg 2014), and they also propose their own humorous metaphors (e.g. the 'Bagov Schitt' example at the start of this chapter).

In the next sections, we briefly outline how we identified the specific patterns of humorous metaphor use we focus on here, before examining more closely the discursive strategies and possible psychological effects that these patterns appear to reflect.

Concordance 10.1 Extracts from a Concordance of ‘humour’ in ‘Warped’

ll . . . good to have you here . . . I always had a gallows	humour	. . . good job i got cancer then so can use it properly e
Well, do n’t say we did n’t warn you about the warped	humour	. . . . Be warned ! ! ! ! ! ! (You need to read
nny ‘s birthday, a bottle of coke (for comedy toilet	humour	) and a bar of chocolate. . . . can it get any better ? ?
hy not try one of our themed ranges ? The Toilet	humour	range proving popular this month with those that want a
2011 3:50 PM” words=“15”> lol tomregarding your sick	humour	im sorry but i laughed too thats just brilliant !
this is, you would think we all had warped senses of	humour	or something . . . . . Anyway, the more the merrier
going in round the back (snigger) sorry, awful bum	humour	) The site is only closed overnight in case you are won
tune next week. . . . apologies for the ‘gallows ‘	humour	. . . actually, no apologies- that is why we did warped
s me snigger everytime and I know I have stupid toilet	humour	but am I the only one that thinks doing a blog sounds f
phew, a baggy invasion . . . no let up from the toilet	humour	then eh ? You might sympathise with the little pu
hy warped came into existence. Rare cancer and warped	humour	. . . needed somewhere to hang out with like minded peopl
laughing. . . . I suppose that as we find toilet	humour	so funny in this country, I should have guessed that i
inks up these shit games, must be someone into toilet	humour	big time. LM, I am fishing a canal tomorrow and
date=“19 Mar 2012 4:54 PM” words=“90”> Love the toilet	humour	Val and I forgot to say to winnie (new name for Sam)
e coloured maggs your using. Back to the toilet	humour	, I seem to remember as a child being removed by my mot
es, because not everyone appreciates the dark side of	humour	like what we do, whether it is anal or otherwise. <br
here is always the chance that I will need some warped	humour	on here again. . . . In the meantime. I love you a
will never forget, where else could we engage in bum	humour	without offending people ! I want to say thanks t

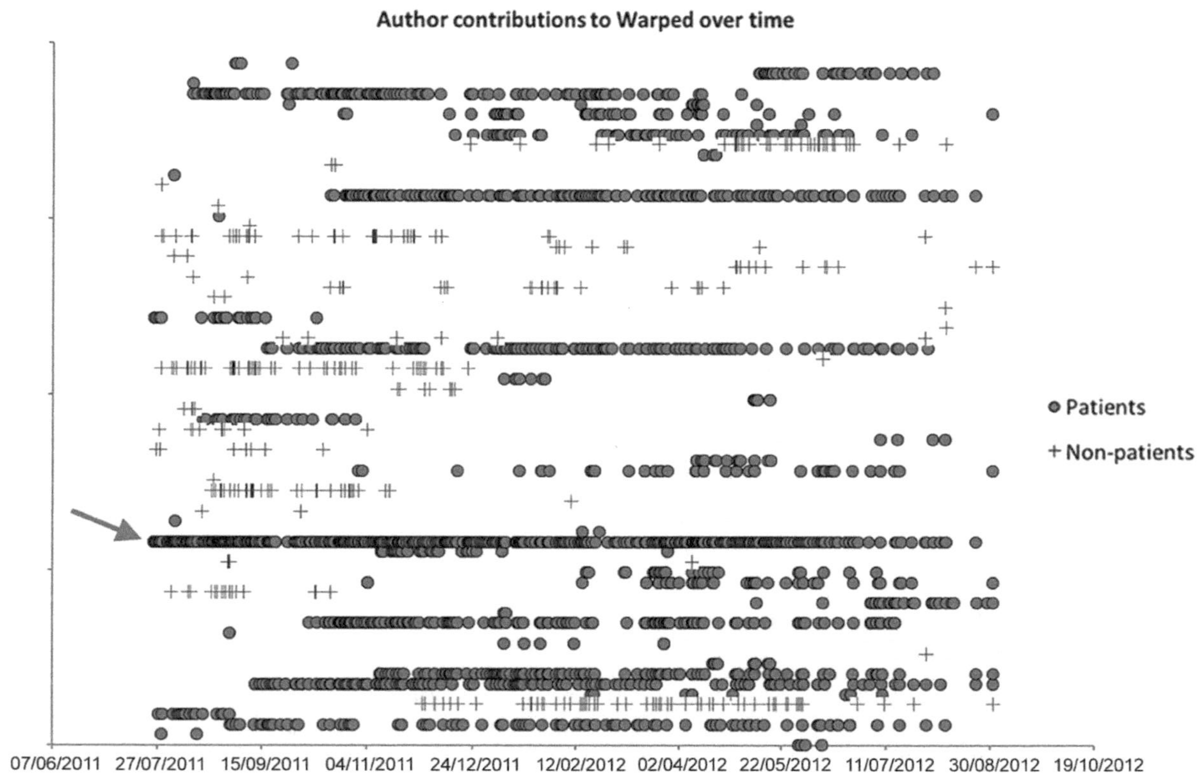

Figure 10.1 Contributions to Warped Over Time

10.3.1 Key Semantic/Grammatical Categories on Warped

We repeatedly came across humorous uses of metaphor from Warped in our overall analysis of the corpus (as discussed in Chapters 4, 5 and 7), and, given the potential risks of using humour in the context of cancer, we decided to investigate these in more detail by examining the whole Warped thread. This involved an elaboration on our general method and an extension to the data outlined in Chapter 3. We performed a keyness analysis (see Chapters 3 and 4) of the Warped thread, which led us to identify the patterns of humorous metaphors that we focus on here. The reference corpus consisted of 450,000 words of patient, and 500,000 words of carer contributions[3] to the online forum within which Warped was one thread, but did not contain any parts of Warped. The log-likelihood cut-off was 10.83 (99% chance of non-randomness, $p < 0.01$, 1 d.f.). Tables 10.1 and 10.2 below show key parts-of-speech and semantic tags that are relevant for this discussion.

Some of these key parts of speech and semantic domains suggest that Warped has a more conversational/informal tone than the rest of the online forum: e.g. UH (Interjections) and some items under Z99 (Unmatched), S1.2.6– (Foolish), G2.2– (Unethical), and X9.1– (Inability/unintelligence). Others, like the affectionate sign-offs 'xxxxx' and 'cwtches' in the POS category NNU and SEM category Z99 and the frequent address of each other on the thread using names, handles and titles (under NP2, NNB and Z99), suggest a more interactive style (Biber 1999; see also Seale et al. 2010). These are particularly interesting findings, since the reference corpus consists of the same kind of data as Warped, produced under the same kinds of conditions of anonymity, reduced inhibition (Suler 2004), round-the-clock availability and accessibility. Despite these similarities, the language of Warped is more informal, more affectionate and more explicitly interactive. As already outlined, this can be a consequence of the humorous tone (Attardo 1994; Dynel 2009a).

Unsurprisingly then, a number of the key features of Warped also include lexical items linked to humour. There are signals of humour (e.g. 'kidding', 'cheeky', 'silliness', 'naughty', 'mischief', 'haha', 'funny') and potential reactions to humour ('haha', 'hehe', 'hee hee', 'lol', 'laugh', 'funny', 'snigger'). The first group includes examples that suggest self-deprecation ('no wonder I spend so much time on naughty step' [Pretzel]) and examples where participants gently tease each other ('What's that? hooray you say? cheeky lot. . . ' [HoneyBee]). The second group—reactions to humour—demonstrates that the thread is fulfilling the mission stated in its first post: it includes more overt markers of laughter than the rest of the cancer forum.[4]

Aside from linguistic features indicating humour generally, a number of the key parts of speech and semantic categories of Warped also include humorous uses of metaphor. Among key parts of speech, the category NNB includes the use of titles: 'Mr', 'Mrs', 'Uncle' and 'Dr', as well as 'Corporal', 'Wing Commander', 'Colonel', 'Captain' and 'Commandant'.

Table 10.1 Selected Key Parts-of-Speech (POS) on Warped

POS Tag	*Description*	*Freq. 1*	*% 1*	*Freq. 2*	*% 2*	*LL*[1]	*Log Ratio*	*Examples*
UH	interjection (e.g. oh, yes, um)	5,646	1.12	5,602	0.6	1,049	0.89	oh, ha, hi, eh, yes, hello, no, haha, oooh, blah
NNU	unit of measurement, neutral for number (e.g. in, cc)	2,318	0.46	2,552	0.27	312	0.74	Xxxx,[1] xxxxx, hmmm, xxxxxx, http, xxxxxxx, xxxxxxxx, hmmmm
NP2	plural proper noun (e.g. Browns, Reagans, Koreas)	284	0.06	135	0.01	183	1.95	Rolos, Roobs, Hodgkins, PMs, Waltons, Archers, Malverns
NNB	preceding noun of title (e.g. Mr., Prof.)	234	0.05	191	0.02	69	1.17	Mr_Crab, Mrs_PF, Mr, Mrs_NH, Mrs, Mr_G, Uncle_Bulgaria, Mr._Crab, Mrs_Doyle, Dr
FO	formula	581	0.11	747	0.08	41	0.51	bl**dy, sc, a&e,[2] b*****d
FU	unclassified word	466	0.09	604	0.07	31	0.5	yay, hee, la, non, ai, er, grrr, em, *, da

1 As representations of kisses
2 As representations of character codes that made it into the corpus

Table 10.2 Selected Key Semantic (SEM) Tags of Warped

SEM Tag	*Description*	*Freq. 1*	*% 1*	*Freq. 2*	*% 2*	*LL*[1]	*Log Ratio*	*Examples*
Z99	Unmatched items	13,719	2.71	14,937	1.61	1,917	0.75	haha, xxxx, hils, xxxxx, Scranton, im, cwtches, xxxxxx, pube, joycee, warpies, rolos, hehe, warpy, Roobs, ive, womble, Dunc, FB, xxxxxxx, nobhead, Nin, hahaaaa, manflu, warpees, hols, macland, norty, eachother, xxxxxxxx
B5	Clothes and personal belongings	2,437	0.48	1,165	0.13	1,559	1.94	bag, pants, wear, bags, clothes, dress, wearing, knickers, shoes, dressing
O4.4	Shape	1,531	0.3	806	0.09	882	1.8	warped, baggy, lines, line, straight corner, cross, baggies, flat, shape
E4.1+	Happy	2,662	0.53	2,776	0.3	428	0.82	fun, happy, laugh, funny, lol, snigger, laughing, smile, sense_of_humour, joke
B4	Cleaning and personal care	908	0.18	668	0.07	326	1.32	shower, loo, bathroom, wash, washing, hoover, toilet, wheelie_bin, hoovering, clean, toothbrush
N3.2+	Size: Big	1,042	0.21	1,029	0.11	196	0.89	big, fat, large, massive, growing, grow, Hefty, grown
S1.2.6–	Foolish	522	0.1	383	0.04	188	1.32	silly, stupid, loony, bonkers, daft, ass, silliness, wanker, nutter, sillies, stupidly
G2.2–	Unethical	496	0.1	436	0.05	125	1.06	naughty, shame, trick, wrong, mischief, unfair, evil
S7.1+	In power	1,135	0.22	1,426	0.15	89	0.55	managed, boss, manage, Invincibles, won, order, invincible
G3	Warfare, defence and the army; weapons	269	0.05	231	0.02	71	1.1	gun, shot, shoot, armed, war, bombing, shooting
A5.2–	Evaluation: FALSE	261	0.05	228	0.02	66	1.07	lie, kidding, drivel, make_up
S1.2.4–	Impolite	135	0.03	112	0.01	39	1.15	rude, offended, cheeky
X3.5	Sensory: Smell	83	0.02	53	0.01	37	1.52	smell, smelly, smells
X9.1–	Inability/ unintelligence	106	0.02	101	0.01	22	0.95	idiot, arsehole, idiots
X3.2+	Sound: Loud	86	0.02	81	0.01	18	0.96	loudly, loud, noisy

1 Log-likelihood.

As we show later, these titles are used (a) metonymically in reference to people the contributors know in their everyday lives (and often find annoying), (b) metaphorically in reference to contributors themselves, as well as (c) in reference to cancer personified (e.g. 'Mr Crab'). Among the key semantic categories, the following stand out: B5 (Clothes and personal belongings), B4 (Cleaning and personal care), X3.5 (Sensory: Smell), X3.2+ (Sound: Loud) and G3 (Warfare, defence and the army; weapons). These groups consist to a large extent of (a) references to potentially embarrassing/taboo bodily functions, (b) personifications of paraphernalia required as part of cancer treatment and (c) metaphorical references to conflict, war and violence.[5] Because the parts of speech and semantic categories including these metaphors were overused statistically significantly and were involved in the production of humour, they arguably capture the humorous metaphor use that is most characteristic of Warped. We therefore narrow our focus in the rest of this chapter to a detailed analysis of the functions that these items perform.

10.4 Humorous Metaphor (Use) and Its Functions

In this section, we examine three distinctive types of humorous metaphors that emerged from the quantitative analysis. The discussion is organised by the main functions that these different types of metaphors appear to perform, i.e. the ways in which and the reasons why they might help Warped contributors cope with having cancer.

Given the literature discussed in section 10.2, it is worth outlining at the beginning the ways in which the metaphors we discuss might be considered humorous. As already mentioned, all interactions on Warped happen within a humorous frame (cf. Apter 1982), which means that potentially any metaphor can be seen as humorous, with the proviso that humorous and non-humorous discourse are often interwoven and even the same utterance can sometimes be read as both serious and humorous (Dynel 2011). More specifically, however, the personification of cancer and treatment paraphernalia and contributors' address of each other using military titles are incongruous and emphasise the differences between the two ideas they bring together. In the case of military references for each other, for example, this is achieved by the status difference between the semantic domains involved (Attardo 2015; Dynel 2009b): cancer patients are often physically weakened and sometimes helpless, while soldiers are strong and engaged in strenuous physical activity. In the case of personified treatment paraphernalia, on the other hand, the boundary between source domains is potentially emphasised through the simultaneous attention to the literal meaning of the words. The boundary between illness/inanimate object and person is also emphasised further in more creative/novel examples by attributing anthropomorphic mental states and intentions to these entities. However, in a number of cases, as we show in the following, humour comes not necessarily from the metaphors themselves, but from the way in which they are used in a particular co-text and context.

We begin the discussion with a few examples detailing experiences that are potentially embarrassing or taboo. We then discuss: examples that enable contributors to maintain a coherent sense of identity in the face of rapid change; examples that potentially facilitate a sense of self-empowerment; and, finally, a group of examples that, as their main function, seem to contribute to solidarity, bonding and a sense of community. It should be noted, however, that such functions are not exclusive to any particular type of humorous metaphor use: as is the case with most language use, humorous metaphor tends to perform multiple functions at once.

10.4.1 Talking about Embarrassing or Taboo Topics

One of the perhaps simplest functions of humour on Warped—as expressed through humorous metaphor, but also other tropes (see Demjén 2016)—is to allow contributors to talk about embarrassing or taboo aspects of their illness experience in a socially acceptable way. This of course builds on humour's general ability to facilitate the exploration of 'things which are difficult or taboo' (Coates 2007: 32). One effect of the colostomies and stoma bags that colorectal cancer patients might receive as part of their treatment is reduced control over bodily functions, such as passing gas or defecation. These taboo subjects are repeatedly mentioned on Warped and are a considerable source of punning and mirth (cf. Spiegel 2015), as in these cases of personification of colostomy bags:

Example 10.2

Naughty baggy is sounding his disapproval at my fruity breakfast

[Sam]

Example 10.3

I got up at 4am 'cos silly baggy was full of wind and i nearly floated off.

[Sue2]

Example 10.4

Here is a puzzle for you. . . . baggy is constipated. . . . Sunday best bum has diarrhoea. eh? what?

[HoneyBee]

By jokingly talking about socially taboo topics and behaviour, contributors can minimise face loss and embarrassment, but still communicate information indirectly (cf. Attardo 1994); they can describe to each other what having a colostomy bag entails. In addition, in the preceding examples, the stoma bag is endowed with anthropomorphic attitudes ('silly', 'naughty') and bodily functions of its own ('constipated'), making them *humorous metaphors*. This personification allows patients to attribute the embarrassing aspect of their illness experience to the baggy: *it* makes funny noises and is constipated, not the contributor. This strategy allows contributors to avoid embarrassment even more successfully, as they discursively absolve themselves of responsibility for the taboo behaviours.

10.4.2 Maintaining a Coherent Identity

Other examples of humorous metaphors also allow contributors to relieve themselves of responsibility for things that they cannot control anyway. In the following cases, this is not about the inability to control bodily functions, but about uncontrollable changes in habits and behaviours:

> *Example 10.5*
>
> It's just one of the evil Mr Crab's funny little jokes that we now have to spend our lives thinking not just "What shall I have for tea?" but "What shall I have for this random nameless meal—that I am having at an odd time because I couldn't face food till now—that won't kill me?" I am pretty sure that my own evil Mr Crab has taken control of my stomach-to-brain signals. He gets hungry in the night, and demands steak and chips. I don't eat meat!! Bastard.
>
> [Valerie]

> *Example 10.6*
>
> I'm just jealous because I can't have booze. It says so in the Little Red Chemo Book, but I can tell without that that Mr Crab would kill me if I tried.
>
> [Valerie]

> *Example 10.7*
>
> a party pooper Mr Cancer who sometimes buggers up one's plans.
>
> [HoneyBee]

These examples all describe changes resulting from cancer, like being hungry at strange times, wanting food that one previously did not want and not being able to have or do what one does want, in terms of malicious things that cancer does. Such changes can come on quite suddenly and unpredictably, and there is not much that the person can do about them. The elaborate personification allows patients to attribute these uncontrollable changes to 'someone' else, thereby relieving themselves of the responsibility for the behaviours: it becomes the behaviour of Mr Crab/Cancer. This potentially allows contributors to maintain a coherent sense of self—a consistent identity—in the face of big changes which may come on very quickly and which might make them appear to be different people. Similarly, personifying and externalising the illness allows patients to create a distance between themselves and their cancer. This can be particularly useful in a healthcare context (and society) where people can become equated with their disease.

To some extent, the examples in this and the previous section could be seen as demonstrating a form of psychological agency or power. Contributors have very consciously and explicitly chosen to adopt a humorous attitude, so while they may not be able to control the embarrassing side effects of stoma bags or the changes cancer brings about, they can exercise agency in how they react to these aspects of their experience. In fact, some even go so far as to talk about the benefits of having cancer using humorous metaphors:

Example 10.8

lets face it, once you become aquainted with Mr Cancer and his mates arsehole colleauges are a walk in the park

[HoneyBee]

Example 10.9

If baggy had farted lots then [HoneyBee] would have shot across the pool . . . jet propulsion!

[Smelly]

By demonstrating 'an alternative interpretation of the stressor' (Heath and Blonder 2003: 99), a strategy that stroke survivors with lasting disabilities have also been found to adopt, these examples position contributors as potential beneficiaries, rather than victims, of their illness (we discuss similar examples in Semino and Demjén 2017). This re-appraisal of something potentially restrictive as helpful—even bestowing an advantage—allows contributors to re-establish their autonomy in the face of things they cannot control.

There are also other patterns of humorous metaphor use on Warped that construct patients as empowered in ways that we have discussed elsewhere in this book. It is to these examples that we now turn.

10.4.3 Empowering Patients in Relation to Cancer

In previous chapters, particularly Chapters 5 and 6, we discussed empowering uses of different metaphors and described this as the process through which linguistic choices reflect and facilitate high degrees of agency, validation, positive evaluation and control (where this is desired), with positive implications for identities, emotions and relationships desired (see also Semino et al. 2017). The examples in this section are in line with examples we have discussed elsewhere, but pertain specifically to the power relationship between patients and their cancer. In the first few examples, Warped contributors undermine the authority or power of cancer, thereby increasing their own power in relation to it, while from Example 10.15 onwards they begin to exert power over the illness.

There are two main ways in which Warped contributors undermine the power of cancer. First, as in Examples 10.10 and 10.11, they describe things that might make existence difficult for the personified illness:

Example 10.10

With all those songs you listen to, I'm surprised Mr Crab hasn't left screaming NO!NO!NO! holding his fingers in his ears.

[Lakedweller]

Example 10.11

sorry Mr Crab was in a bad mood last night it is hoped the chemo will teach him a lesson he much deserves

[Pretzel]

Although Example 10.10 also gently teases the patient who listens to apparently terrible music, both examples suggest that there are things that can deter cancer; even something as simple as music. This in itself downplays the power of cancer. However, in the second example, cancer is also talked about as if it was a person of inferior status, such as a child who can be taught a lesson by someone (or something, in this case) more powerful (chemotherapy). This attributed inferior status—the second way in which the power of cancer is undermined—is even more apparent in the following examples:

Example 10.12

My baggy has been sulking all weekend

[HoneyBee]

Example 10.13

baggy did behave on the plane, so gold star to him for that eh.

[Sue2]

Example 10.14

sausages [intestines] and baggy were very badly behaved

[HoneyBee]

The diminutive term 'baggy' suggests a friendly, possibly even affectionate relationship between the patient and the personified entity, but references to 'behaving' and 'sulking' (and indeed 'naughty' in Example 10.2) also cast the baggy in a childlike, perhaps teenage, role. This simultaneously casts the contributor in the role of a parent, and gives them a certain amount of power and authority (in addition to the same face-saving potential as Example 10.4).

A counterpart to downplaying the power of cancer involves Warped contributors displaying more overt power over cancer using mockery/sarcasm:

Example 10.15

wine gives me tummy cramps. Which, I suspect, is yet another by-product of Mr Crab. The gift that keeps on giving!

[Valerie]

Example 10.16

Ah, sweet memories of Mr. Crab—not

[Spiral]

The sarcasm in some of the examples is considered an 'aggressive' form of humour (Dynel 2008; Martin 2007; Norrick 2003) and can signal resistance to the target. Contributors denigrate cancer (the butt of the remark) and, in this way, are able to assert virtual authority over a potentially life-threatening and uncontrollable illness (cf. McCreaddie and Wiggins 2008). This kind of metaphorical aggression towards the illness becomes very explicit in the following examples:

Example 10.17

cheers everyone, and a kick up the arse for Mr C!

[Smelly]

Example 10.18

Boot to Mr Crab. Hugs to everyone else

[HoneyBee]

In Chapter 5, we discuss examples similar to these in the context of Violence metaphors. Such examples are empowering uses of the much criticised Violence metaphor, as they construct patients as active and determined within the metaphorical scenario. Not only do these examples express aggressive intent towards the personified cancer, thereby positioning contributors as more powerful; that aggression is also enhanced by the juxtapositioning with explicit affection towards other contributors. This shows a kind of collective power (potentially also facilitating solidarity and bonding) that is even more apparent in the following:

Example 10.19

come on girl we're all here growling at Mr. Crab and chasing him off xx

[Sue2]

Empowerment therefore stems not only from seeing the positive sides of the illness, downplaying its power by positioning it as of inferior status, and up-playing patients' own power in relation to it, but also from a sense of community. As Martin puts it:

> [t]his type of humor enables members of an in-group to enhance their feelings of group identity and cohesiveness [. . .] by actively seeking to humiliate, embarrass, or ridicule [the target] in some way and thereby enhancing one's own status relative to theirs.
>
> (Martin 2007: 18)

10.4.4 Displaying Solidarity, Support and Collective Power

The previous analysis sections have mostly focused on the potential functions of humorous metaphors in relation to individuals. Yet some of our examples involve explicit expressions of affection towards each other, and in the quantitative analysis we showed that affectionate sign-offs are a distinguishing feature of Warped. This suggests a significant sense of community. Providing such a sense of solidarity and support is arguably the most important function of some of the humorous uses of metaphor we identified in the Warped thread as this can reduce the sense of isolation and loneliness that some might experience during serious illness. In this section, we examine this collective or interpersonal function in more detail and return to two types of humorous metaphors we discussed earlier: those that constructed stoma bags as naughty children, thereby constructing Warped contributors as having some authority over them, and those that involved expressions of explicit aggression towards cancer.

In the following examples, 'baggy' and 'bags' are once again constructed as inferior to Warped contributors (through the use of 'behave'), potentially positioning the bags as children faced with adults. However, contributors in these examples are talking about others' rather than their own paraphernalia:

Example 10.20

DO YOU HEAR THAT BAGGY *behave yourself, Sam deserves a bloody good night out

[Sue2]

Example 10.21

Well, hope everyone's bags are behaving this morning. Poos if you wish, no poos if you wish : -)

[Smelly]

By scolding each other's stoma bags, contributors reference a shared or collective experience and express explicit solidarity. This reflects the strong sense of community among contributors and is likely to contribute to further bonding in the same way that neighbourhood parents looking out for each other's children might.

The second type of humorous metaphor we revisit here involves expressions of overt aggression. In Chapter 5, we focused in detail on such Violence metaphors and discussed their multiple functions in our data despite substantial media and academic criticism. Here we continue this discussion with examples of arguably humorous Violence that seem to also contribute to bonding and community building.

On the Warped thread, we found several examples of the types of Violence metaphors we discussed in Chapter 5, using lexical items such as 'fight', 'kick' etc. Interestingly, however, we also found many more examples where the source domain can more specifically be pinpointed as Military. In fact, this pattern is so pervasive that, as already outlined, the USAS (UCREL Semantic Analysis System) category G3 'Warfare, defence and the army; weapons' is statistically significantly overused on Warped when compared to the rest of the patient and carer online corpus (despite the fact that we identified Violence metaphors as the most frequent in this data). We now look at the function of these examples in detail.

Warped contributors, and HoneyBee in particular, sometimes use military titles as nicknames to refer to each other:

Example 10.22

Well done Flight lieutennant Tom for finding your way all the way over here from blog land. I am impressed. I would promote you but a) i think you have reached top rank already and b) I can't think of other ranks . . . and not sure what the top one is . . . I think Brigadeer is my favourite . . . what's yours commander?

[HoneyBee]

Example 10.23

I think that it might turn out to be a quick evacuation to the Ark again—that's if our Captain Joe is organised enough

[Lynnie]

Norrick and Bubel (2005) note that nicknames such as these can signal intimacy almost irrespective of what the names actually are, especially if they are used exclusively with each other; 'what counts is the relationship they encode' (Norrick and Bubel 2005: 165). The military titles can be seen as terms of endearment signalling mutual respect (they are all high ranks), especially because they are explicitly appreciated. Example 10.22, for instance, seems to be Tom's third promotion and follows his gratitude for the previous one: 'Thanks for the further promotion! Do I get shiny things to wear on my dress uniform?' The fact that multiple participants use and/or expressly appreciate the repertoire of military titles is also likely to contribute to group cohesion. This, however, could be true of any nicknames that the participants chose to use for each other. For our purposes, it is particularly interesting that they chose military titles, essentially Military (or Violence) metaphors. To make sense of the significance of this particular choice, we now examine other examples of Violence metaphors that Warped contributors use.

Fairly early on the thread, Warped contributors are established as a *camp* of officers or an army via self-referring expressions such as 'Camp Commandant' and 'regiment'. This army of 'Warped people who will not let cancer beat them/Whose weapons include humour, love and hope' [Valerie] collectively confronts cancer:

Example 10.24

Cancer is the reason we are all here, so let's all fight that as an army together, chaaaaaaaaaaaaarge.

[Sue2]

This pattern is very similar to the examples of empowering Violence metaphors we discussed in Chapter 5, but they index a collective experience through the use of plurals in 'people', 'them', 'we' and 'together'. These therefore suggest a sense of collective strength and power. A little later on, Violence metaphors begin to get used in a slightly different, and perhaps more obviously humorous, way.

Among the things that Warped contributors often discuss are impending medical check-ups. These are always tense situations, and of course everyone hopes that no evidence of disease will be found or that existing tumours will have shrunk. If the results show a recurrence or lack of improvement, people can be kept in hospital for further testing. This potential outcome is the context of the following example:

Example 10.25

> It's got to be good results Valerie or they've made a mistake. Don't forget we have a formidable fighting force in our rescue team which now has two successful missions under their belts. Tell them if they get it wrong we will all travel in Pretzel's bin to put it right.
>
> [Lakedweller]

Here the contributor continues with the construction of the Warped group as troops in confrontation, but now the enemy is the healthcare system (we discussed similar examples in Chapter 5), which might deliver 'bad' results and keep people in hospital. The Warped 'army camp' can now also run rescue missions as a team. In this way, the language of warfare combines with related notions of captivity, rescue and liberation into an elaborate metaphorical scenario (Musolff 2006) reminiscent of various kinds of 'joint fantasising' described in the humour literature (see, for example, Kotthoff 2007). These metaphors are motivational and empowering (Semino et al. 2017) and demonstrate a community spirit, since the group is engaged in a collective activity involving strength and effort within the scenario.

Another way in which these metaphorical scenarios involve collective effort is in their joint development by a number of participants over several posts. This is likely facilitated by the online environment, where previous contributions are clearly visible and which therefore makes it easy for people to return to and draw on constructions that have come before (Hübler and Bell 2003). To illustrate this and to explain the multiple elements at play in Example 10.25, we now trace the development of this extended fantasy scenario within the thread.

In early January 2012, Pretzel, one of the frequent contributors to Warped, complains about a strange noise coming from her garage. After some humorously described investigation, she identifies an old fire alarm with a flat battery in the back of the garage as the source of the noise. She decides to get rid of it by putting it in her wheelie bin, because the bin collectors are due that day. The bin collectors, however, do not turn up. This spurs a humorous, somewhat absurdist, fantasy scenario, initiated by Pretzel but expanded and developed by others, in which passing neighbours, or indeed the bin collectors themselves once they arrive, call the 'bomb squad' (G3 lexis) for fear of what might be in the bin. This fantasy scenario is based on and uses past metaphorical constructions, but it is not in itself metaphorical. In between the posts developing the fantasy scenario, another Warped contributor Suzysue metaphorically describes having to stay in hospital longer than expected as being 'still imprisoned' by 'warders'. In response, contributor Powerthru asks whether there is a way of using Pretzel's bin with the smoke alarm as a distraction, which could then get Suzysue 'evacuated' and 'liberated'. Another contributor, Lakedweller, picks up on the now-established metaphorical scenario of captivity and liberation and combines it with the fantasy scenario initiated by Pretzel, and with the already-established the army camp scenario, to create the new 'mission' of 'rescue':

Example 10.26

> We need a plan of this prison, we don't want to rescue the wrong person. If you can send this to Pretzel who must stop the bin men emptying her wheelie bin. Pretztel if you can wheel your wheelie bin around to the main entrance of the prison, this will cause the distraction with everyone being evacuated through other entrances.
>
> [Lakedweller]

From this point on in the thread, rescue with the help of Pretzel's bin is a key activity for the army camp, with the bin eventually turning into a kind of tank, as in the next example:

Example 10.27

> as there has to be one as official armourer for warped I will put some balls of wool in the armoury may come in useful for launching from the bin at those most deserving
>
> [Pretzel]

Example 10.27 was written in mid-April 2012, showing how the fantasy scenario is picked up and developed over the course of approximately four months. Pretzel's bin is even referenced briefly one more time in July 2012. Taken in combination, the military titles and other metaphors of Violence and Captivity construct a fantasy scenario where contributors are a metaphorical army, with its own (relatively high) ranks. This army has weapons and tanks (i.e. cotton wool and a bin) to fight overt enemies such as cancer and the healthcare system, but also covert ones (spies, like 'Bagov Schitt'[6]) such as the consequences of cancer and treatment paraphernalia. When one of their troops is captured and imprisoned (hospitals are constructed as prisons), they devise rescue missions. We can think of this as a Prisoners-of-War scenario within the larger Army Camp scenario established earlier on. Both of these scenarios are co-created by multiple contributors reacting to each other's posts over a long period of time. The collective power of the army allows contributors to position themselves as more powerful than their 'enemies' and to demonstrate a high degree of solidarity. They effectively become each other's heroes, subverting the usual rhetoric around cancer (Sandaunet 2008) where patients are ideally brave fighters alone against cancer. In this way, they not only live through adventures together within the scenario, but also manage to resist a dominant cultural framing of the cancer experience in real life.

The collective, co-created military scenario on Warped is related to the Violence metaphors and scenarios we discussed in Chapter 5, which are used throughout our corpus. However, on Warped, proportionally speaking, the humorous Violence metaphors contained within the G3 USAS category are more frequently empowering than in the rest of our corpus. They emphasise the collective in a way most of the examples in Chapter 5 do not.

10.5 Conclusions

In this chapter, we have shown how patients use metaphors humorously on Warped, a popular thread within the online forum which constitutes part of our online subcorpus, and have reflected on the possible functions of these humorous metaphors. After a brief overview of relevant literature in humour studies, metaphor and health communication, we outlined how corpus methods helped us identify the humorous metaphors that are the focus of this chapter. Our analysis then examined three characteristically humorous uses of metaphors: personifications of cancer and treatment paraphernalia, participants' figurative references to one another, and co-created fantasy scenarios involving Violence and Captivity metaphors. We showed how these distinctive types of humorous metaphor use seemed to enable patients to discuss aspects of their experience that are embarrassing or taboo; maintain a coherent identity in the face of rapid change; facilitate a sense of empowerment in circumstances where people might feel powerless; and contribute to bonding, cohesion and a sense of community.

Generally speaking, all of these functions potentially help patients cope with having cancer. The disclaimer that opens the thread demonstrates the participants' awareness that joking about (some aspects of) cancer is still socially unacceptable, but for this group it is necessary and appropriate: 'as writers of their own lives patients have authority to turn their tragedies into comedies' (Watson 2011: 40). Contributors are able to openly talk about embarrassing and uncontrollable aspects of their illness and its treatment, which can relieve psychological tension. They can also maintain a coherent sense of self and identity by personifying and externalising their illness and attributing to it behaviours that might be inconsistent with these identities. Some humorous metaphors also facilitate a sense of empowerment. On the one hand, by focusing on the potential positive sides of the illness, patients demonstrate a kind of psychological agency or 'positive attitude'. More concretely, through humorous metaphor use, they undermine cancer's power by mocking it and denigrating it to the status of a child, thereby positioning themselves as more powerful and authoritative. And, because in some cases they direct their utterances towards each other's rather than their own cancer, a sense of empowerment also stems from the collective, from a sense of community. This can be particularly important in the context of an illness that can leave people disempowered and lonely.

This important sense of a community also seems to be the main function of the humorous, potentially even absurd, partly metaphorical fantasy scenarios Warped contributors develop together. These scenarios emerge from a number of interacting factors: the atmosphere of explicit affection towards each other (juxtaposed with aggression towards cancer); the use of military titles and other Violence metaphors that construct contributors as an 'army camp'; the co-development of fantasy scenarios within which participants are engaged in joint activities; and the combination of all of this with Captivity metaphors. The creativity and complexity involved help to create a language and a type of humour that is specific to this particular group. This phenomenon, possibly an 'idiohumour' (cf. Fine 1977's notion of 'idioculture'), effectively helps to delineate and define the group as a distinct discourse community within the larger cancer forum. Contributors even refer to themselves as 'warpies', 'warpees' or the 'Warped family'. Ultimately, all of this helps them cope with the experience of cancer.

Is humour in the context of cancer helpful or empowering for patients? The answer to this is not always straightforward. Some studies of people with breast cancer (e.g. Carver et al. 1993; Culver et al. 2004) have found limited or no evidence of a positive psychological impact of humour in coping with the disease. However, as Martin (2007) points out, both of these studies relied on the Coping Orientations to Problem Experiences (COPE) scale as a measure of humour (regarding humour as a trait) rather than observing naturally occurring humorous behaviour. This is not surprising: as outlined earlier, it can be difficult to observe humour in action. However, this is precisely where studies of spontaneous communication on health fora such as this one are particularly illuminating. By looking at how participants use even potentially risqué humour on Warped, how they respond to each other's utterances and the explicit references to the importance of having this virtual space, we stand on more solid ground in claiming that for these people in this context laughing at cancer is absolutely essential. The participants express this best:

> I found a warped sense of humour came with the cancer, it was either laugh. . . . . . or cry, I prefer to laugh. It's a sort of "gallows humour", it gets worse every day. You begin to notice what miserable sods the "non cancer" community are, with their trivial worries and whinges. Lunacy is therapeutic, everyone should be mad.
>
> [Russ]

Notes

1. In this chapter, we indicate the author of each quote in order to give a sense of interactions on a particular thread on the online forum, and of the number of different people who use humorous metaphors. All names have been changed.
2. While toilet humour is not generally considered the same as gallows humour, 'toilet' and 'bum' humour can be seen as overlapping with gallows humour to the extent that the rectal problems Warped contributors face because of their particular type of cancer are part of their 'life-threatening, disastrous, or terrifying' illness experiences (Watson 2011: 38).
3. While there are carers who also contribute to Warped, we are treating Warped as patient discourse due to the proportion that they contribute. However, for comparison, carer data is included in the reference corpus. Carer contributions are also included in quantitative analysis, but all the examples in the qualitative analysis are patient contributions.
4. Of course these lexical items are only proxy markers, and it is well-established that laughter does not necessarily correlate with humour (Attardo 2003; Dynel 2009a).
5. Additional lexical items used in the same ways are included under O4.4 (Shape) ('baggy', 'baggie' used in reference to colostomy or stoma bags), S7.1+ (In power) ('invincible' used in reference to special underwear suitable for those post colostomy operation) and Z99 (Unmatched) ('lieutennant' and 'Brigadeer', which are non-standard spellings of military ranks).
6. Even the Bagov Schitt example at the start of this chapter is not an isolated occurrence. It is a response to a supposedly mistaken post by a different contributor which began: 'For some time many of us have wondered just who is Jack Schitt? We find ourselves at a loss when someone says, "You don't know Jack Schitt!" Well, thanks to my genealogy efforts, you can now respond in an intellectual way. Jack Schitt is the only son of Awe Schitt. Awe Schitt, the fertilizer magnate, married O. Schitt, the owner of Needeep N. Schitt, Inc.' The contributor followed this post by apologising, saying she'd mistakenly posted it on Warped, but due to its appropriacy to the topic at hand the language play was taken up by others.

References

Apter, M. (1982). *The experience of motivation: The theory of psychological reversals*. London: Academic Press.

Attardo, S. (1994). *Linguistic theories of humor*. Berlin: Mouton de Gruyter.

Attardo, S. (2003). Introduction: The pragmatics of humor. *Journal of Pragmatics*, *35*, 1287–1294.

Attardo, S. (2015). Humorous metaphors. In G. Brône, K. Feyaerts, and T. Veale (Eds.), *Cognitive linguistics and humor research* (pp. 91–110). Berlin and Boston, MA: De Gruyter.

Attardo, S., and Raskin, V. (1991). Script theory revis(it)ed: Joke similarity and joke representation model. *Humor*, *4*, 293–348.

Biber, D. (1999). *Longman grammar of spoken and written English*. New York: Longman.

Cameron, L., and Deignan, A. (2006). The emergence of metaphor in discourse. *Applied Linguistics*, *27*(4), 671–690.

Carver, C. S., Pozo, C., Harris, S. D., Noriega, V., Scheier, M. F., and Robinson, D. S. (1993). How coping mediates the effect of optimism on distress: A study of women with early stage breast cancer. *Journal of Personality & Social Psychology*, *65*(2), 375–390.

Chapple, A., and Ziebland, S. (2004). The role of humor for men with testicular cancer. *Qualitative Health Research*, *14*(8), 1123–1139.

Chovanec, J. (2011). Humour in quasi-conversations: Constructing fun in online sports journalism. In M. Dynel (Ed.), *The pragmatics of humour across discourse domains* (pp. 243–264). Amsterdam: John Benjamins.

Coates, J. (2007). Talk in a play frame: More on laughter and intimacy. *Journal of Pragmatics*, *39*(1), 29–49.

Coulson, S. (2000). *Semantic leaps: Frame-shifting and conceptual blending in meaning construction*. Cambridge: Cambridge University Press.

Culver, J. L., Arena, P. L., Wimberly, S. R., Antoni, M. H., and Carver, C. S. (2004). Coping among African-American, Hispanic, and non-Hispanic White women recently treated for early stage breast cancer. *Psychology & Health*, *19*(2), 157–166.

Daisley, M. (1994). The game of literacy: The meaning of play in computer-mediated communication. *Computers and Composition*, *2*(1), 107–119.

Demjén, Z. (2016). Laughing at cancer: Humour, empowerment, solidarity and coping online. *Journal of Pragmatics*, *101*, 18–30.

Dohan, D., and Levintova, M. (2007). Barriers beyond words: Cancer, culture, and translation in a community of Russian speakers. *Journal of General Internal Medicine*, *22*(Suppl 2), 300–305.

Dynel, M. (2008). No aggression, only teasing: The pragmatics of teasing and banter. *Lodz Papers in Pragmatics*, *4*(2), 241–261.

Dynel, M. (2009a). Beyond a joke: Types of conversational humour. *Language and Linguistics Compass*, *3/5*, 1284–1299.

Dynel, M. (2009b). Creative metaphor is a birthday cake: Metaphor as the source of humour. *metaphorik.de*, *17*, 27–48.

Dynel, M. (2011). Pragmatics and linguistic research into humour. In M. Dynel (Ed.), *The pragmatics of humour across discourse domains* (pp. 1–16). Amsterdam and Philadelphia, PA: John Benjamins Pub. Co.

Fine, G. A. (1977). Humour in situ: The role of humour in small group culture. In A. J. Chapman and H. C. Foot (Eds.), *It's a funny thing, humour* (pp. 315–318). Oxford: Pergamon Press.

Freud, S. (1905). *Der Witz und seine Beziehung zum Unbewußten [Jokes and Their Relation to the Unconscious]*. Vienna: F. Deuticke.

Georgakopoulou, A. (2011). Computer-mediated communication. In J-O. Östman and J. Verschueren (Eds.), *Pragmatics in practice* (pp. 93–110). Amsterdam: John Benjamins.

Gibbs, R. W., and Cameron, L. (2008). The social-cognitive dynamics of metaphor performance. *Cognitive Systems Research*, *9*(1–2), 64–75. doi:10.1016/j.cogsys.2007.06.008

Goatly, A. (1997). *The language of metaphors*. London and New York: Routledge.

Heath, R. L., and Blonder, L. X. (2003). Conversational humour among stroke survivors. *Humor*, *16*(1), 91–106.

Hobbes, T. (1840). Human nature. In W. Molesworth (Ed.), *The English works of Thomas Hobbes of Malmesbury* (Vol. IV). London: Bohn.

Hübler, M. T., and Bell, D. C. (2003). Computer-mediated humor and ethos: Exploring threads of constitutive laughter in online communities. *Computers and Composition*, *20*(3), 277–294. doi:10.1016/s8755-4615(03).00036-7

Kant, E. (1951 [1790]). *Critique of judgement* (J. H. Bernard, Trans.). New York: Hafner.

Kotthoff, H. (2007). Oral genres of humour: On the dialectic of genre knowledge and creative authoring. *Pragmatics*, *17*(2), 263–296.

Krikmann, A. (2009). On the similarity and distinguishability of humour and figurative speech. *Trames. Journal of the Humanities and Social Sciences*, *13*(1), 14. doi:10.3176/tr.2009.1.02

Kuiper, N. A., Martin, R. A., and Olinger, L. J. (1993). Coping humour, stress, and cognitive appraisals. *Canadian Journal of Behavioural Science*, *25*, 81–96. doi:10.1037/h0078791

Kyratzis, S. (2003). Laughing metaphorically: Metaphor and humour in discourse. In *8th International Cognitive Linguistics Conference*, Logroño.

Langley-Evans, A., and Payne, S. (1997). Light-hearted death talk in a palliative day care context. *Journal of Advanced Nursing*, *26*(6), 1091–1097.

Martin, R. A. (2007). *The psychology of humor: An integrative approach*. Burlington, MA and London: Elsevier Academic Press.

McCreaddie, M., and Payne, S. (2014). Humour in health-care interactions: A risk worth taking. *Health Expectations*, *17*(3), 332–344. doi:10.1111/j.1369-7625.2011.00758.x

McCreaddie, M., Payne, S., and Froggatt, K. (2010). Ensnared by positivity: A constructivist perspective on 'being positive' in cancer care. *European Journal of Oncology Nursing*, *14*(4), 283–290. doi:10.1016/j.ejon.2010.03.002

McCreaddie, M., and Wiggins, S. (2008). The purpose and function of humour in health, health care and nursing: A narrative review. *Journal of Advanced Nursing*, *61*(6), 584–595. doi:10.1111/j.1365E-2648.2007.04548.x

Mio, J. S., and Graesser, A. C. (1991). Humor, language, and metaphor. *Metaphor and Symbolic Activity*, *6*(2), 87–102.

Musolff, A. (2006). Metaphor scenarios in public discourse. *Metaphor & Symbol*, *21*(1), 23–38.

Norrick, N. R. (2003). Issues in conversational joking. *Journal of Pragmatics*, *35*, 1333–1359.

Norrick, N. R., and Bubel, C. (2005). On the pragmatics of direct address in conversation. *Lodz Papers in Pragmatics*, *1*, 159–178.

North, S. (2007). 'The voices, the voices': Creativity in online conversation. *Applied Linguistics*, *28*(4), 538–555. doi:10.1093/applin/amm042

Oring, E. (2003). *Engaging humor*. Urbana and Chicago, IL: University of Illinois Press.

Pollio, H. R. (1996). Boundaries in humor and metaphor. In J. S. Mio and A. N. Katz (Eds.), *Metaphor, implications and applications* (pp. 231–253). Mahwah, NJ: Lawrence Erlbaum Associates.

Ritchie, L. D. (2013). *Metaphor*. Cambridge and New York: Cambridge University Press.

Sandaunet, A-G. (2008). A space for suffering? Communicating breast cancer in an online self-help context. *Qualitative Health Research*, *18*(12), 1631–1641.

Seale, C., Charteris-Black, J., MacFarlane, A., and McPherson, A. (2010). Interviews and internet forums: A comparison of two sources of qualitative data. *Qualitative Health Research*, *20*(5), 595–606. doi:10.1177/1049732309354094

Seargeant, P., and Tagg, C. (2014). Introduction: The language of social media. In P. Seargeant and C. Tagg (Eds.), *The language of social media: Identity and community on the internet* (pp. 1–20). Basingstoke: Palgrave Macmillan.

Semino, E., and Demjén, Z. (2017). The cancer card: Metaphor and humour in online interactions about the experience of cancer. In B. Hampe (Ed.), *Metaphor: From embodied cognition to discourse*. Cambridge: Cambridge University Press.

Semino, E., Demjén, Z., Demmen, J., Koller, V., Payne, S. A., Hardie, A., and Rayson, P. (2017). The online use of 'Violence' and 'Journey' metaphors by cancer patients, as compared with health professionals: A mixed methods study. *BMJ Palliative & Supportive Care*, *7*(1), 60–66.

Spiegel, J. (2015, August 17). From the Sumerians to Shakespeare to Twain: Why fart jokes never get old. *The Conversation*. Retrieved April 2017, fromhttps://theconversation.com/from-the-sumerians-to-shakespeare-to-twain-why-fart-jokes-never-get-old-41211

Suler, J. (2004). The online disinhibition effect. *Cyber Psychology & Behavior*, *7*(3), 321–326.

Tanay, M. A., Wiseman, T., Roberts, J., and Ream, E. (2014). A time to weep and a time to laugh: Humour in the nurse-patient relationship in an adult cancer setting. *Support Care Cancer*, *22*(5), 1295–1301. doi:10.1007/s00520-013-2084-0

Vandergriff, I. (2010). Humor and play in CMC. In R. Taiwo (Ed.), *Handbook of research on discourse behavior and digital communication: Language structures and social interaction* (pp. 235–251). Hershey, PA: Information Science Reference.

Watson, K. (2011). Gallows humour in medicine. *Hastings Center Report*, *41*(5), 37–45.

Websites

Emily McDowell's cancer cards. Retrieved April 2017, from www.slate.com/blogs/the_eye/2015/05/06/empathy_cards_by_emily_mcdowell_are_greeting_cards_designed_for_cancer_patients.html

PostTea cancer cards. Retrieved April 2017, from www.etsy.com/uk/listing/233403805/ive-heard-your-oncologist-funny-cancer?ga_order=most_relevant&ga_search_type=all&ga_view_type=gallery&ga_search_query=cancer%20card&ref=sr_gallery_32

11 Conclusions

11.1 The Contribution of This Book: An Overview

This book has presented the largest and most systematic study to date of metaphors for cancer and (care at) the end of life. The timeliness, originality and significance of our study lie in the particular intersection of *topic* (cancer and the end of life), *focus* (metaphor), *data* (interviews and online fora) and *methods* (corpus and computational linguistic tools).

Topic: Cancer is among the leading causes of morbidity and mortality worldwide (World Health Organization 2017). In the UK, both the incidence of the disease and length of survival are increasing, which means that more people live longer after diagnosis and/or treatment (Cancer Research UK 2017). Therefore, it is increasingly important to understand the (often lengthy) experience of cancer, including the effects it may have on people's psychological well-being and identity. Our analyses go some way towards achieving this.

Care at the end of life and palliative care are recognised as priorities internationally, as witnessed by the 2013 call by the European Association for Palliative Care to have palliative care recognised as a human right. In this context, it is particularly important that communication with and about people receiving such care does not inadvertently heighten negative feelings and self-perceptions, but rather enhances mental well-being and quality of life. We have provided systematic evidence of current communicative practices, which can be used to validate, develop and improve practice in healthcare and beyond (e.g. media and charity communications).

Focus: Metaphor is well-known to be both frequent and important in communication and thinking, particularly in relation to sensitive and subjective experiences such as illness and dying. The framing power of metaphor means that it can both improve and worsen the experience, depending on whether the metaphors clarify or obfuscate, encourage or demoralise, empower or disempower, and so on. A case in point: Violence metaphors for cancer have been seen as particularly problematic (e.g. by Sontag 1979), while the metaphor of the 'cancer journey' has been adopted as more appropriate and helpful. We have provided systematic evidence of the frequencies, uses and functions of these and other metaphors for cancer and (care at) the end of life based on a 1.5-million-word corpus, representing three different groups in healthcare (patients, family carers and healthcare professionals) and two different genres (interviews and online forum contributions). This has led to new insights into the manifestations and workings of metaphors across topics, discourse communities and genres, and has implications for how different metaphors are viewed and used in communication by, with and about people who are ill or dying.

Data: The composition of our corpus reflects an increasing recognition of the importance of lived-experience accounts by people who are unwell and by caregivers, whether professional or otherwise (e.g. Charon 2006). Our study is, however, unique in its comparison of three participant groups in healthcare, and particularly in its inclusion of family carers on an equal footing with patients and healthcare professionals. Our choice of genres encompasses both a well-established approach to the collection of qualitative data (semi-structured interviews) and a form of computer-mediated communication that has grown exponentially in recent years (peer-to-peer online fora). We have demonstrated both similarities and differences among participant groups and across genres, which have implications for understanding different experiences, on the one hand, and different ways of accessing those experiences, on the other. We have also provided further evidence of the important role of online forum communication in the lives and experiences of members of these three participant groups, and of how these fora are used by people in different circumstances.

Method: Corpus and computational linguistic tools enabled us to collect and analyse a dataset that is too large for investigation by hand and eye alone, and to combine quantitative and qualitative approaches in the study of metaphor. We have introduced and applied an innovative, eclectic, but data-driven approach to the identification of potential metaphorical expressions, which is widely applicable in metaphor research. Thanks to this approach, we have provided frequency information about metaphor use in the corpus as a whole and in each of its subsections, and identified many individual examples for discussion in context. More generally, this approach addresses the methodological divide in healthcare research identified by Greenhalgh (2016), between the qualitative analysis of illness narratives, on the one hand, and more established quantitative epidemiological approaches, on the other. Corpus and computational linguistics provide the 'appropriate and rigorous methods' that, Greenhalgh argues, are needed for the former type of qualitative analysis to be accepted and valued by researchers and practitioners in the latter quantitative tradition.

Overall, therefore, our corpus-based analysis of metaphors in a 1.5-million-word corpus representing three main participant groups in healthcare breaks new ground methodologically, and has both theoretical and practical implications. In the rest of this chapter, we discuss in more detail the methodological, theoretical and applied contributions of this book, or in other words: what we did and developed, what we found and how this can all be used in practice. These subsequent sections are organised so that they are most relevant for our three main audiences—respectively corpus linguists, metaphor scholars and healthcare practitioners.

11.2 Methodological Contribution: Corpus-Based and Computational Approaches to the Study of Metaphor

A key area of progress in research on metaphor in the last decade has involved the use of authentic data and of rigorous, explicit methods of identification and analysis, including corpus-based methods. However, there is as yet no reliable and exhaustive automatic approach to metaphor identification. This poses a challenge for the kind of large-scale analysis that we embarked upon in this study. As shown in the course of the book, we addressed this challenge by developing and applying an innovative mixed-methods approach that combines qualitative and quantitative corpus-based analysis to identify patterns of metaphor in our corpus.

We manually identified and classified all relevant metaphors in a 92,000-word sample, carefully chosen to cover both genres and all three participant groups. We used the findings of the manual analysis to carry out both lexical (word-level) and semantic concordances in the complete corpus (cf. Cameron and Deignan 2003; Charteris-Black 2004). Corpus methods allowed us to take a rigorous approach to designing the complete dataset by scaling up the interviews and scaling down the forum data. They also enabled us to obtain large numbers of potential instances of metaphor (e.g. all uses of the word 'journey' and all instances of the semantic domain 'Sports'), which we could analyse manually for actual metaphoricity according to our standardised identification procedure (Pragglejaz Group 2007).

The use of semantic concordances, in particular, addresses the limitations of word-level corpus searches, and further develops an approach to the corpus-based study of metaphor previously piloted by a team including three of the present authors (Hardie et al. 2007; Koller et al. 2008; Semino et al. 2009). This approach is especially appropriate for specialised corpora, where it can be reasonably expected that certain semantic domains will contain a high proportion of metaphorical expressions or similes (e.g. 'Warfare, defence and the army' in our corpus), in contrast with others which are likely to include primarily literal expressions (e.g. 'Health and disease' in our corpus). As explained in Chapter 3, we made selective use of the 'broadsweep' function in Wmatrix, which makes it possible to identify all the lexical items that have been annotated for a particular semantic tag, whether or not it is the first-choice tag in the sequence allocated to each lexical item.

To achieve the specific goals of the case studies presented in Chapters 7–10, we additionally applied the following corpus techniques:

- Concordancing expressions corresponding to topics that may be discussed metaphorically: e.g. 'doctors' in the patient data (Chapter 7; see also Stefanowitsch 2006);
- Concordancing semantic domains corresponding to topics that may be discussed metaphorically: e.g. E4.1– (Sad) in the carer data (Chapter 9);
- Analysing key parts of speech in a particular dataset for patterns that may be related to metaphor use: e.g. NNB (Preceding noun of title) in the Warped thread (Chapter 10);
- Analysing key semantic domains in a particular dataset for patterns that may be related to metaphor use: e.g. G3 (Warfare, defence and the army; weapons) in the Warped thread (Chapter 10; see also L'Hôte 2014);
- Searching for particular combinations of parts of speech and semantic tags to identify topics that may be discussed metaphorically: e.g. JJ (general adjective) with L1– (Dead) (Chapter 8);
- Concordancing 'signals' of figurativeness: e.g. 'like' as a preposition to introduce a simile (see also Partington et al. 2013).

In each case, the outputs of the corpus tools were manually analysed for actual instances of metaphoricity in concordance lines, and selected instances were analysed qualitatively in their full co-text.

Overall, we have demonstrated the use of keyness analysis combined with part-of-speech and semantic tagging and how it can assist with the comparison of metaphor frequencies in our subcorpora. By doing so, we have made a contribution to computational linguistics research—which has so far failed to engage significantly with corpus-based studies of metaphor, instead focusing on narrow domains or construction types (e.g. verbs in Beigman Klebanov et al. 2016). Our results have been achieved through scaling a bottom-up classification of metaphor to a larger corpus, and through a data-driven computational analysis encompassing a wide range of word classes and semantic fields. This is the first time that such a method has been explicitly described, applied and tested on such a scale. With the exception of the custom-made database that we used to link our preliminary classification of metaphors in the sample corpus to the USAS (UCREL Semantic Analysis System) semantic tagset, we made use of only standard and widely available corpus software. Thus, this mixed-methods approach is one that other researchers could follow and apply within corpus-based research on metaphor more generally.

While we cannot claim to have found *all* relevant instances of metaphoricity in the corpus, we have been able to identify many thousands of linguistic metaphors in our data much more rapidly and systematically than would have been possible through manual analysis alone. In this way, we are able not only to compare the different sections of our corpus, but also to draw conclusions that are relevant to metaphor theory and analysis more generally.

11.3 Theoretical Contribution: Metaphor in Discourse

Our findings are relevant to metaphor analysis and theory more generally, particularly in relation to: variation in metaphor use across text types and discourse communities; the personal and interpersonal dimensions of metaphor; and methodological and theoretical approaches to the framing function of metaphor. We now consider each of these contributions in turn.

11.3.1 Metaphor, Text Types and Discourse Communities

Our approach and findings in this book contribute to an important strand in metaphor research that considers how, why and to what extent the use of metaphor varies depending on the type of text and the participants involved in communication (e.g. Steen et al. 2010; Deignan et al. 2013; Caballero 2017). At a very general level, our corpus is consistent in terms of the topics of communication, but there are important differences between the subcorpora that can be captured in terms of 'genre' and 'register'. As explained in Chapter 1, 'genre' captures differences between texts based on their structural characteristics, their communicative purposes and their association with members of different discourse communities (Swales 1990; Deignan et al. 2013; Semino et al. 2013). 'Register' captures differences between texts in terms of linguistic characteristics related to topic, the relationships between participants in communication, and the roles that language plays in the communication (Halliday 1985; Deignan et al. 2013; Semino et al. 2013). Within our corpus, the online forum data and the interviews differ in both genre and register. The three online forum subcorpora also differ in terms of the discourse communities involved (patients, carers or healthcare professionals), and the relationship between participants in interaction (similarity of life experiences for patients and carers versus similarities of profession for healthcare professionals). Within the patient online data, there is further variation between Warped, with its explicitly humorous, informal register, and patient contributions to the other threads on the forum, which are more mixed in tone. In addition, the interviews with healthcare professionals differ from the interviews with patients and carers in terms of the topics of discussion and the role of the interviewee (users of healthcare services versus providers of healthcare services).

The results presented in this book confirm that metaphor use is sensitive to variation in both genre and register, and add further insights to the findings of previous studies. We have identified differences across the subcorpora with regard to frequencies, forms and functions of metaphor use.

In Chapter 4, we showed how the overall frequencies of different types of metaphors are lower in the patient and carer interviews than in other sections of the corpus. We linked this to two aspects of these interviews. First, the topics elicited by the interview questions were to do with people's concrete experiences of healthcare services and therefore less conducive to metaphor use than the more sensitive and complex topics of the interviews with healthcare professionals (which included questions about quality of death and dying, among others) and the wider variety of topics discussed in the online fora. Second, the relationships among people contributing (semi-)anonymously to peer-to-peer online fora tend to be perceived and constructed as more informal and intimate than those in interviews, and particularly in interviews involving patients and carers as users of healthcare services. Overall, therefore, our analysis provides further evidence for a connection between metaphoricity and certain topics (such as death and the emotions; e.g. Lakoff and Turner 1989), and between metaphoricity and intimacy in relationships among participants in communication (e.g. Katz 2017).

The breakdown of frequencies of different types of metaphors in Chapter 4 shows broad similarities among the subcorpora. For example, Violence and Journey metaphors are the top two most frequent types of metaphors in all subcorpora. At a general level, this reflects the dominance and versatility of these metaphors in English generally, and can be linked to their basis in embodied experiences of physical struggle and movement. At a more specific level, we have shown that these metaphors are used more often than other types of metaphors for topics such as illness and death, which are central in our data. However, we have also shown that patients use both Violence and Journey metaphors considerably more frequently than healthcare professionals do, and that each group uses these and other metaphors in their own idiosyncratic ways. For example, patients sometimes describe their interactions with healthcare professionals as violent struggles, but this does not apply the other way round. Likewise, some healthcare professionals talk about themselves as fighting for the survival of patients and travelling alongside them, but patients seldom describe healthcare professionals that way. Even more specifically, particular metaphorical expressions within these broad types are only or predominantly used by one group in our data. For example, 'fighter' as a term of praise for oneself or others is typical usage only for patients and carers in our online data, while using 'pathway' for a structured care plan is part of the healthcare professionals' technical vocabulary and does not extend to patients and carers in our corpus.

Some types of metaphor are also associated with particular subcorpora and/or groups. For example, Openness metaphors used for the willingness to talk explicitly about death are characteristic of the interviews with healthcare professionals. This reflects both a particular hospice/palliative care-specific professional view about communication at the end of life and an interview question about quality of death. On the other hand, the high relative frequency of Animal metaphors in the carer online data results from the creative extension and exploitation of animal-related usernames by some carers on the online forum. In other words, this pattern emerges dynamically from interactions in the particular online environment that is included in our data—a phenomenon that has recently been recognised as important in metaphor use in a variety of discourse contexts (Cameron and Deignan 2006; Gibbs and Cameron 2008; Gibbs 2017).

Our findings therefore provide further insights into the relationship between metaphor use, text types and discourse communities. Metaphor use can both reflect and reinforce the views and attitudes that result from shared experiences (e.g. patients and carers) or shared professional perspectives (e.g. healthcare professionals). From a methodological point of view, it is important to combine observations about frequencies of metaphor use with analysis of specific expressions in context; similar frequencies of a particular type of metaphor among members of different discourse communities may potentially disguise considerable differences in terms of what expressions are used and how. From the point of view of practice, it is important to be aware of the potential implications of differences in metaphor use, especially for communication between healthcare professionals, on the one hand, and patients and their families, on the other. We return to these implications in the following.

11.3.2 *Personal and Interpersonal Aspects of Metaphor Use*

The metaphors that we identified in our analysis are used to perform a variety of functions. Our conclusions concerning the general function of framing are discussed in the next section. Here we reflect on the personal and interpersonal functions of some metaphors in our corpus.

A central and well-known function of metaphor which is prominent in our data is the expression of subjective experiences, and particularly emotions. Aside from emotional expression, some metaphors—such as humorous personifications of cancer—can also be used to reduce one's own anxiety, regain a sense of control and maintain identity in the face of rapidly changing circumstances.

Throughout the book, we have often pointed out the emotional implications of particular metaphor choices. In some cases, however, expressing a specific emotional state is the main function of metaphorical expressions. This applies particularly clearly to the metaphors for the experience of grief we discussed in Chapter 9, as in the case of similes such as 'you feel like your whole world is falling apart' and 'it still hits like a sledgehammer sometimes'. We have pointed out that, as well as expressing what the experience feels like, these uses of metaphor also suggest other aspects of the experience, such as lack of control over one's emotions. We also noted how the online forum provides a space in which both patients and carers can reveal their most negative emotions, because they feel that others will understand them but also not be as deeply affected as their own family and friends might be. This affordance of the online forum is explicitly mentioned by several contributors, among both patients and carers.

Another set of functions of metaphors in our corpus which is particularly prominent in the online data relates to the interpersonal dimension of language use. Online forum contributors use metaphors to:

- Explain things to one another, including through reconceptualisation (e.g. some Journey metaphors in Chapter 6);
- Provide advice (e.g. responses to the thread on emotional resilience initiated by the trainee doctor in Chapter 9);
- Comfort or explicitly support one another (e.g. some humorous metaphors in Chapter 10);
- Validate one another's feelings (e.g. some metaphors for grieving in Chapter 9);
- Encourage one another (e.g. some Violence metaphors in Chapter 5);
- Praise one another (e.g. the description of a forum contributor as a breast cancer 'gold medallist' in Chapter 4);
- Entertain one another (e.g. humorous metaphors in Chapter 10).

All of these different functions can contribute to mutual empowerment, building a sense of community and strengthening social bonds on the various threads of the online fora. However, metaphors can also be used to convey criticisms, as in the case of the Violence metaphors for the approach of some patients to life and death in the professional interviews (Chapter 8), or some metaphors for Western medicine or the UK healthcare system in Chapter 7. Overall, our study confirms the need to consider the functional and interpersonal dimensions of metaphor use alongside the representational and conceptual dimensions, which have traditionally received more attention.

11.3.3 Metaphor and Framing

Our study highlights the importance of the framing function of metaphor—the process whereby metaphor choices reflect and reinforce different ways of perceiving, understanding and evaluating our experiences, by highlighting some aspects of experiences while backgrounding others. Our findings also have implications for how best to account for such framing effects against the background of different theoretical approaches.

Our data contains many examples of how different people use different metaphors to express different views of the same topics or experiences. When discussing the healthcare professional data, for example, we contrasted different metaphorical framings of professional goals in relation to patients, such as 'fighting for patient survival' as opposed to 'accompanying' them on their 'uncertain journey' (Chapter 7). We pointed out that, among other things, these different framings lead to contrasting perceptions of patients' deaths (as professional failure versus a natural part of life) and may also suggest different approaches to care.

We have also shown, however, how the same individuals can use different metaphors to express different aspects of their experiences or of their own identities. For example, the extract from a bereaved carer's forum post that we used to introduce our study in Chapter 1 includes two contrasting metaphorical framings of the person's experience of his wife's cancer (as a journey and as a fight). Each framing conveys different aspects of the experience and casts the person in a different role, capturing different facets of his own self-perception (e.g. helplessness versus resilience). In Chapter 6, we showed in more detail how some people with cancer use both Violence and Journey metaphors, either separately or in combination, to highlight different dimensions of their experience of illness, such as intense effort and determination in the case of Violence metaphors, and long-term perseverance in the case of Journey metaphors. These observations suggest that it is too simplistic to treat Violence and Journey metaphors for cancer as straightforwardly alternative framings, as they can in fact complement each other.

A Multi-Level Approach to Metaphor and Framing

Overall, our analyses in this book suggest that no single existing theory can fully account for the framing function of metaphor in discourse. Rather, a multi-level approach is needed, drawing from and combining different approaches to metaphor use (see also Semino et al. 2016). At a general level, the notion of conceptual metaphors as initially proposed by Lakoff and Johnson (1980) can be applied to our data to capture broad contrasts in metaphorical framings. For example, the data discussed in Chapters 5 and 6 can be seen as evidence of two different conceptual metaphors, which can be expressed as BEING ILL WITH CANCER IS A VIOLENT

CONFRONTATION WITH THE DISEASE and BEING ILL WITH CANCER IS A JOURNEY. At this broad level, we can say that the illness is typically cast in different positions within the two broad metaphors (as an enemy versus a road), with potentially different implications for the position and feelings of patients. However, our study shows how different specific scenarios within these (and other) broad metaphors can involve very different framings, including in terms of (dis)empowerment and emotional and evaluative implications. In this sense, our findings support the focus on metaphor scenarios in some recent research on metaphor in discourse (e.g. Musolff 2006, 2016; Semino 2008). In addition, specific expressions (and particular co-texts) can sometimes be associated with specific framings in the interactions among members of particular discourse communities, as in the case of the positive use of 'fighter' on the patient online forum. This kind of emergent regularity in how a metaphorical expression is used by the members of particular groups can be described in terms of Cameron and Deignan's (2006) notion of 'metaphoreme'—a 'bundle of stabilizing linguistic, semantic, pragmatic, and affective patterns in the use of [a] word as metaphor, together with its possibilities for variation' (Cameron and Deignan 2006: 678).

Our study therefore argues for a multi-level approach to framing in relation to metaphor, including conceptual metaphors, metaphorical scenarios and linguistic expressions. Within this approach, an analysis can in principle be conducted in terms of each level separately, as long as analysts are aware of what conclusions can and cannot be safely drawn at each level. Ideally, however, all three levels need to be considered together, as they shed light on different aspects of and explanations for metaphor use. This is especially important where there is a concern for the practical implications of metaphors, as in the case of healthcare.

Aspects of Metaphor and Framing

Our analyses have also demonstrated a rich approach to metaphor and framing, which includes aspects such as identities, evaluation, agency and (dis)empowerment. We discussed the implications of different metaphors for how people construct their own identities throughout this book, and found this to be particularly important after a traumatic event, such as a death. Some of the metaphors used by bereaved carers (Chapter 9), for example, powerfully convey a dramatic change in people's perceptions of themselves, including in relation to other people (e.g. 'you realise you are only half a person' and 'I still feel like I am sitting on the edge'). Metaphors such as these also suggest emotional distress or discomfort even though they are not primarily or exclusively to do with emotions.

The evaluative implications of different metaphorical framings have been pointed out throughout the book (see also Deignan 2010), but are particularly evident in metaphorical descriptions of oneself and others. In

Chapter 4, for example, we noted how Animal metaphors can be used by patients to evaluate negatively their own approach to the illness, while in Chapters 4 and 5 we showed how Sports and Violence metaphors can be used to describe others positively, resulting in the praise and encouragement we discussed in the previous section. In Chapter 7, we showed how metaphors are used by some healthcare professionals to critique what they see as the depersonalisation of patients in some healthcare systems. In Chapter 8, we pointed out that some of our interviewees seem to use metaphors for the attitudes they see as unhelpful for patients at the end of life (e.g. 'they want to keep fighting fighting fighting'), without going on record with explicit criticism.

A further aspect of metaphorical framings that has proved particularly important in our data is to do with who is constructed as active and empowered in metaphorical scenarios and, conversely, who is presented as disempowered and how. For example, in Chapter 7 we showed how patients' metaphors often place them in a disempowered position in relation to healthcare professionals (e.g. 'I felt like my body was no longer mine and all the doctors were going to get access to it'). We also pointed out, however, that the (dis)empowering effects of metaphors need to be discussed at the level of specific scenarios and uses in context. As we showed in Chapters 5 and 6, both Violence and Journey metaphors can have (dis)empowering implications, depending on how they are used. More specifically, we argued that, while there are no straightforwardly 'good' or 'bad' metaphors for everyone, some metaphorical framings can tend towards negative implications for the people involved. This applies, for example, to the associations of failure with the framing of incurable illness as 'losing the battle' (Chapter 5), and with the framing of grieving as a linear journey in which re-experiencing negative emotions involves 'step[ping] backwards' (Chapter 9). These are instances of metaphors that could be explicitly challenged in the context of healthcare.

Overall, the findings of our analyses support and contribute to recent approaches to metaphor that focus on authentic uses in context, consider variation depending on text type and discourse community, and explain metaphor use in terms of the dynamic interaction of multiple factors, including not just general conceptual metaphors but also the roles and identities of speakers and writers, their mutual relationships, the topic, the previous co-text and so on (e.g. Gibbs and Cameron 2008; Cameron 2011; Deignan et al. 2013).

11.4 Applied Contribution: Understanding and Improving (Communication in) Cancer and End-of-Life Care

In this section, we draw out selected conclusions from our study that are particularly relevant to healthcare and social care professionals as well as, more generally, charitable organisations and patient groups. We begin by considering each participant group in turn. We then reflect on insights regarding the use of online fora by members of all three groups, and conclude with the practical implications and applications of our study.

11.4.1 Understanding Patients

One of the key findings of this study is a recognition of the diversity of metaphors used by people with cancer—a diversity that applies both across individuals and within an individual's own contributions to interviews and online fora. We were interested from the outset in whether and how patients use Violence and Journey metaphors, because of the controversy around the former and the recent promotion of the latter in the UK National Health Service and beyond. What we found, however, was a much more complex and varied picture. Patients draw on a wide variety of metaphors to describe and arguably construct their experiences of having cancer, including Sports metaphors, Restraint metaphors, Animal metaphors and others (see Chapter 4). Different metaphors capture different aspects and facets of the experience of illness and dying. The importance of this cannot be over-stated. Media reports, policy decisions and the like present a kind of duality, an either/or scenario of 'battle' versus 'journey'. This is simply not borne out by our study of how different people, and specifically patients, actually talk about their illness experiences.

In addition, we found that the degree of agency implied by metaphor choices in context has larger potential implications for patient self-efficacy, self-empowerment and mastery than does the choice of type of metaphor per se. The passive positioning of the self in relation to more powerful others such as medical professionals—or, indeed, the personification of cancer as an entity within the body—has a resonance with earlier categorical models of cancer coping styles such as helplessness or hopelessness (Greer and Watson 1987). Alternative ways to position the self as having agency and power are associated with both Violence and Journey metaphors, depending on how they are used in context. Importantly, we therefore argue that the actual choice of metaphor is less important than the degree of agency that patients ascribe to themselves, assuming that agency is desired by the patient.

There is substantial evidence that the diagnosis, treatment and survivorship phases of cancer are likely to be experienced in the context of heightened emotions (Osborn et al. 2006). For example, the description of cancer experiences as an emotional 'roller coaster' highlights the alternating periods of hopefulness following active treatment, and despondency when recurrence of the disease is identified. Patients may find it difficult to live with and express these mixed emotions. They may at times seek to protect family and friends from their anguish as it may add to their distress. Moreover, they may feel an obligation to appear grateful and compliant in interactions with healthcare professionals even though, as our analysis suggests, they often describe those interactions as antagonistic and/or entirely under the healthcare professionals' control (see Chapter 7).

The use of humour for emotional release and social bonding is a complex, dynamic phenomenon that we found in some online interactions among patients in our data. Our analysis suggests that spontaneous humour is appreciated by patients and is regarded as a helpful way to deal with distressing or embarrassing circumstances. This may in principle suggest that healthcare staff could initiate and reciprocate humour more often, but, as pointed out by McCreaddie and Payne (2014), there is a degree of risk for all parties in engaging in humorous exchanges. The potential for misjudging the situation and offending others means that it is appropriate for humour use by doctors and nurses to be confined to well-established patient relationships and to be based on initiation by patients (or carers) in newer relationships. What is crucial, however, is the avoidance of any kind of censorship.

11.4.2 Understanding Family Carers

Our study also revealed the importance and diversity of metaphors used by family carers. Family carers have been described both as providers of care for the person with cancer and as recipients of service provision, since caregiving impacts upon their health, emotional and social well-being (Grande et al. 2009). Vicarious suffering by family carers is known to be as severe as that of patients (cf. Grande et al. 2009), as shown by the metaphors we discussed in Chapters 4, 5 and 6 in particular. Within many cancer clinical contexts, family carers are often positioned as marginalised and silent witnesses of patients' suffering, with insufficient recognition of their needs for information and support. Surviving and coping with the experience of witnessing the illness and loss of their relative demands emotional resources. Some of our data provides retrospective accounts of experiences of caregiving and the death of the patient. The intensity of the emotions experienced during care provision and in bereavement are played out in the use of metaphor and in the advice that is shared with others on the online forum (see Chapter 9). In addition, some of the metaphors used for grieving (e.g. grieving as a linear journey) suggest unrealistic expectations that may lead to feelings of inadequacy and therefore negatively affect quality of life. This could be usefully drawn out and discussed in interactions between carers and healthcare professionals.

11.4.3 Understanding Healthcare Professionals

The variety of metaphors used by healthcare professionals in our data reveals a diversity of professional challenges and views, particularly concerning the goals of healthcare (Chapters 5, 6 and 7); communication with patients (Chapters 4, 7 and 8); emotional responses to, and involvement with, patients' circumstances and deaths (Chapter 7); and the demands and constraints of healthcare systems (Chapter 7). Our findings also show that healthcare professionals use Violence metaphors differently and less frequently than patients and carers, which may suggest awareness of their potentially problematic consequences and changes in normative language and metaphors in the UK healthcare system.

Given that end-of-life care is one of the concerns of this book, we devoted Chapter 8 to healthcare professionals' descriptions of 'good' and 'bad' deaths, particularly in response to our interview questions. We found evidence that very similar professional metaphors and narratives of both good and bad deaths within hospices were offered in the interviews conducted around England (see also Semino et al. 2014; Demjén et al. 2016). This suggests that these healthcare professionals drew upon wider cultural and professional discourses of dying. While this is understandable given that our interviewees will have gone through similar training and were interviewed in their own professional contexts, we tentatively drew attention to the potential pitfalls of such a unified view. It has the potential to limit the range of options deemed suitable for patients and their families, which can be particularly problematic in a multicultural context such as the UK. In addition, the applicability of such constructions to older people and those with non-cancer conditions is questionable (see, for example, Gott et al. 2008). On the one hand, palliative care professionals' constructions of a good death may challenge other biomedical models, where active life-sustaining—but often invasive, dehumanising and expensive, and ultimately futile—treatments are played out in intensive care environments. On the other hand, there is potentially little flexibility in the models suggested by the metaphors we identified, as well as the narratives told by our interviewees (see Semino et al. 2014).

11.4.4 Understanding Online Forum Communication About Illness and Healthcare

Our findings contribute further insights into how members of the three participant groups use peer-to-peer online fora, and into the role of those interactions in their lives.

Our data suggests that online fora such as the one we studied provide patients and carers who elect to use them with a mechanism to develop a sense of community and a place of emotional release in the context of anonymity, while not adding a further burden of disclosure within their families. These are therefore social spaces where active sharing of lived experience occurs, and mutual support is provided (see, e.g., Allen et al. 2016; Zhang et al. 2017). For example, we found evidence of how novice patients start to learn more about the likely trajectory of their disease and the implications for ongoing medical surveillance (follow-up clinics), investigations and treatment, and, ultimately, the outcome. In some cases, metaphors were offered as potentially helpful ways of reconceptualising or finding meaning in negative experiences (e.g. Example 6.2 in Chapter 6 for patients; and Example 9.5 in Chapter 9 for carers). The online forum also provides an environment where there are shared understandings of socially taboo or sensitive topics such as bowel function (see our examples in Chapter 10 from patients with colostomies), using potentially risky forms of humour. Patients appeared to use online exchanges to enhance their perceived control and coping, again including by means of humour.

Family members in particular appeared to use online interactions not only to find, variously, meaning in their experiences, recognition of their sometimes marginal role, and understanding of organisational and healthcare systems; but also to establish solidarity with others in a similar position. More specifically, bereaved family members appeared to appreciate the opportunity to share difficult emotions and experiences with one another without adding to the burden of relatives and friends. Currently, however, the potential advantages of online fora for carers do not seem to be exploited by most support services for cancer and other illnesses. These advantages include an opportunity to provide and receive reciprocal peer support, without leaving the cared-for person alone at home, and without divulging their personal identity. The 'anytime' nature of interaction online may be particularly appropriate for family caregivers, who may have limited opportunity to organise their daily lives around anything except the needs of the cared-for person. Loneliness and social isolation may to some extent be overcome through supportive virtual interactions. Similarly, disparate patterns of grieving may not fit well with structured programmes of face-to-face bereavement support services, unlike the flexibility offered by online fora, which are available day and night and are to a certain extent user generated/controlled.

However, the limitations of these online environments should also be acknowledged. For example, they may not be accessible to those with minimal information technology skills, limited Internet access or little or no access to appropriate hardware. Moreover, the dominance of particular perspectives in online fora may serve to construct cancer and/or end-of-life experiences in ways that are unhelpful, insensitive or potentially alarming to those who do not share those dominant perspectives. Online fora should therefore be regarded as additional sources of support for families; they cannot substitute for direct information provision by health professionals within a relationship where continuity of care is prioritised.

Not surprisingly, our analyses show that professionals' online communication appears to be constrained by professional codes of conduct, particularly in respect of patient confidentiality. However, the anonymity of online fora enabled some professionals to express their own views, evaluations, frustrations and negative emotions, including feelings of loss and powerlessness. These virtual environments may provide an important opportunity for healthcare professionals to support one another and to share concerns and understandings which go beyond job performance, organisational targets and clinical technicalities.

11.4.5 Implications for Practice

We have provided the most extensive evidence to date of patterns of metaphor use for cancer and the end of life, and have reflected on their functions and implications. We have attempted to spell out the potential applications of our findings throughout. Here we provide a summary of our recommendations, for the benefit of healthcare and social care professionals, and particularly for policy makers and those in health service management roles.

In the UK, there has been a major transition in cultural norms that makes talking about cancer much more acceptable than it was 30 years ago. However, there is controversy over the appropriateness of the dominant Violence metaphors, and policy documents have adopted instead the metaphor of cancer as a 'journey'. We confirmed that Violence metaphors can indeed be demoralising and disempowering, so that it is appropriate not just to avoid imposing them on patients (including through media and charity campaigns), but also potentially to challenge them if they seem unhelpful or detrimental to the person who is using them (e.g. when patients describe themselves as 'losing the battle').

However, our main finding is that no metaphor can be straightforwardly promoted as helpful for everyone or censored as harmful for everyone. Whether metaphors are helpful or harmful, empowering or disempowering, depends on who uses them and how. This emphasises the importance of paying attention to the specific metaphors that people actually use, and responding in ways that acknowledge or even exploit what seems to be helpful to each individual, while sensitively questioning what seems to be unhelpful. In this context, providing alternative metaphors as additional resources for communication and thinking may also be appropriate. On the basis of our findings, we have developed a 'Metaphor Menu for people with cancer'—a collection of quotes from our data and other sources which, at the time of writing, is being piloted as a patient resource in the North West of England (see Demjén and Semino 2017). We chose the metaphor of a 'menu' precisely to suggest that different metaphors will suit different people, and that there are no value judgements associated with preferring one metaphor over another.

Our findings pointed out other areas where attention or action may be needed. These include, for example, the potentially detrimental effects of some carers' metaphors for grieving (e.g. the Journey metaphors that suggest a straightforward linear process), of some healthcare professionals' metaphors for a patient's death (e.g. those that suggest that death is a professional defeat) and of the high degree of professional consensus on what is a 'good' or a 'bad' death, which may not sufficiently value and cater for alternative approaches. Some of the metaphors used for communication in clinical settings, especially by patients, also suggest that greater sensitivity to the needs of people who use healthcare services may be required.

Overall, one advantage of greater attention to the nuances of language use may be in providing 'value'-based targets for assessing outcomes of care, rather than institutional indicators, as has been argued within 'Realistic Medicine' (Catherwood 2016). For example, health services have recently been required to deliver services in line with measurable structural targets such as 'waiting' times. An alternative is to identify targets that relate more closely to what patients and their families value, such as the quality of interactions with health professionals. 'Realistic Medicine' has recently emerged as a new approach to measuring outcomes and goals in healthcare services in Scotland. It seeks to move away from structural and institutional targets such as measuring 'bed days' or waiting times in Accident and Emergency, to prioritise patient and family values such as quality of communication during clinical consultations. This initiative has important implications for personalising healthcare, and as such links with the findings presented in our book. Finally, providing opportunities for professional staff to tell their stories of vicarious and personal suffering may enable them to sustain compassionate care.

In conclusion, we have demonstrated how a corpus-based approach to metaphors for illness and dying can make important methodological, theoretical and applied contributions. We hope that further interdisciplinary research will build on the work we have presented here.

References

Allen, C., Vassilev, I., Kennedy, A., r Rogers, A. (2016). Long-term condition self-management support in online communities: A meta-synthesis of qualitative papers. *Journal of Medical Internet Research*, *18*(3), e61.

Beigman Klebanov, B., Leong, C. W., Dario Gutierrez, E., Shutova, E., and Flor, M. (2016). Semantic classifications for detection of verb metaphors. In *Proceedings of the 54th Annual Meeting of the Association for Computational Linguistics*, Berlin, Germany, pp. 101–106.

Caballero, R. (2017). Genre and metaphor: Use and variation across usage events. In E. Semino and Z. Demjén (Eds.), *The Routledge handbook of metaphor and language* (pp. 193–205). London and New York: Routledge.

Cameron, L. (2011). *Metaphor and reconciliation*. New York: Routledge.

Cameron, L., and Deignan, A. (2003). Combining large and small corpora to investigate tuning devices around metaphor in spoken discourse. *Metaphor and Symbol*, *18*(3), 149–160.

Cameron, L., and Deignan, A. (2006). The emergence of metaphor in discourse. *Applied Linguistics*, *27*(4), 671–690.

Cancer Research UK. (2017). *Cancer statistics for the UK*. Retrieved April 2017, from www.cancerresearchuk.org/health-professional/cancer-statistics

Catherwood, C. (2016). *Realistic medicine*. Report from the Chief Medical Officer for Scotland.

Charon, R. (2006). *Narrative medicine: Honoring the stories of illness*. Oxford: Oxford University Press.

Charteris-Black, J. (2004). *Corpus approaches to critical metaphor analysis*. Basingstoke: Palgrave Macmillan.

Deignan, A. (2010). The evaluative properties of metaphors. In Z. Todd, A. Deignan, and L. Cameron (Eds.), *Researching and applying metaphor in use* (pp. 357–373). Amsterdam and Philadelphia: John Benjamins.

Deignan, A., Littlemore, J., and Semino, E. (2013). *Figurative language, genre and register*. Cambridge: Cambridge University Press.

Demjén, Z., and Semino, E. (2017). Using metaphor in healthcare: Physical health. In E. Semino and Z. Demjén (Eds.), *The Routledge handbook of metaphor and language* (pp. 385–399). London and New York: Routledge.

Demjén, Z., Semino, E., and Koller, V. (2016). Metaphors for 'good' or 'bad' deaths: A health professional view. *Metaphor and the Social World*, *6*(1), 1–19.

Gibbs, R., and Cameron, L. (2008). The social-cognitive dynamics of metaphor performance. *Journal of Cognitive Systems Research*, *9*(1–2), 64–75.

Gibbs, R. W., Jr. (2017). Metaphor, language and dynamical systems. In E. Semino and Z. Demjén (Eds.), *The Routledge handbook of metaphor and language* (pp. 56–70). London and New York: Routledge.

Gott, M., Small, N., Barnes, S., Payne, S., and Seamark, D. (2008). Older people's views of a good death in heart failure: Implications for palliative care provision. *Social Science and Medicine*, *67*(7), 1113–1121.

Grande, G., Stajduhar, K., Aoun, S., Toye, C., Funk, L., Addington-Hall, J., Payne, S., and Todd, C. (2009). Supporting lay carers in end of life care: Current gaps and future priorities. *Palliative Medicine*, *23*(4), 339–344.

Greenhalgh, T. (2016). *Cultural contexts of health: The use of narrative research in the health sector* (Health Evidence Network (HEN) synthesis report 49). Copenhagen: WHO Regional Office for Europe.

Greer, S., and Watson, M. (1987). Mental adjustment to cancer: Its measurement and prognostic significance. *Cancer Surveys*, *6*, 439–453.

Halliday, M. A. K., and Hasan, R. (1985). *Language, context and text: A social semiotic perspective*. Geelong: Deakin University Press.

Hardie, A., Koller, V., Rayson, P., and Semino, E. (2007). Exploiting a semantic annotation tool for metaphor analysis. In *Proceedings of Corpus Linguistics 2007*, University of Birmingham.

Katz, A. N. (2017). Psycholinguistic approaches to metaphor acquisition and use. In E. Semino and Z. Demjén (Eds.), *The Routledge handbook of metaphor and language* (pp. 472–485). London and New York: Routledge.

Koller, V., Hardie, A., Rayson, P., and Semino, E. (2008). Using a semantic annotation tool for the analysis of metaphor in discourse. *Metaphorik.de*, *15*, 141–160.

Lakoff, G., and Johnson, M. (1980). *Metaphors we live by*. Chicago: University of Chicago Press.

Lakoff, G., and Turner, M. (1989). *More than cool reason: A field guide to poetic metaphor*. Chicago: University of Chicago Press.
L'Hôte, E. (2014). *Identity, narrative and metaphor: A corpus-based cognitive analysis of new labour discourse*. Basingstoke: Palgrave Macmillan.
McCreaddie, M., and Payne, S. (2014). Humour in health-care interactions: A risk worth taking. *Health Expectations*, *17*(3), 332–344.
Musolff, A. (2006). Metaphor scenarios in public discourse. *Metaphor and Symbol*, *21*(1), 23–38.
Musolff, A. (2016). *Political metaphor analysis: Discourse and scenarios*. London: Bloomsbury.
Osborn, R. L., Demoncade, A. C., and Feuerstein, M. (2006). Psychosocial interventions for depression, anxiety, and quality of life in cancer survivors: Meta-analyses. *International Journal of Psychiatry in Medicine*, *36*(1), 13–34.
Partington, A., Duguid, A., and Taylor, C. (2013). *Patterns and meanings in discourse: Theory and practice in corpus-assisted discourse studies*. Amsterdam: John Benjamins.
Pragglejaz Group. (2007). MIP: A method for identifying metaphorically used words in discourse. *Metaphor and Symbol*, *22*(1), 1–39.
Semino, E. (2008). *Metaphor in discourse*. Cambridge: Cambridge University Press.
Semino, E., Deignan, A., and Littlemore, J. (2013). Metaphor, genre and recontextualization. *Metaphor and Symbol*, *28*(1), 41–59.
Semino, E., Demjén, Z., and Demmen, J. (2016 advance access). An integrated approach to metaphor and framing in cognition, discourse and practice, with an application to metaphors for cancer. *Applied Linguistics*.
Semino, E., Demjén, Z., and Koller, V. (2014). 'Good' and 'bad' deaths: Narratives and professional identities in interviews with hospice managers. *Discourse Studies*, *16*(5), 667–685.
Semino, E., Hardie, A., Koller, V., and Rayson, P. (2009). A computer-assisted approach to the analysis of metaphor variation across genres. In *Proceedings of Corpus Linguistics 2009*, University of Birmingham.
Sontag, S. (1979). *Illness as metaphor*. London: Allen Lane.
Steen, G. J., Dorst, A. G., Herrmann, J. B., Kaal, A. A., Krennmayr, T., and Pasma, T. (2010). *A method for linguistic metaphor identification: From MIP to MIPVU*. Amsterdam: John Benjamins.
Stefanowitsch, A. (2006). Words and their metaphors: A corpus-based approach. In A. Stefanowitsch and S. T. Gries (Eds.), *Corpus-based approaches to metaphor and metonymy* (pp. 63–105). Berlin: Mouton de Gruyter.
Swales, J. (1990). *Genre analysis*. Cambridge: Cambridge University Press.
World Health Organization. (2017). *Cancer fact sheet*. Retrieved August 2017, from www.who.int/mediacentre/factsheets/fs297/en/
Zhang, S., O'Carroll, E. B., Owen, J., Bakken, S., and Elhadad, N. (2017). Online cancer communities as informatics intervention for social support: Conceptualization, characterization, and impact. *Journal of the American Informatics Association*, *24*(2), 451–459.

Glossary[1]

Annotation In work on corpus data, *annotation* refers to the practice of assigning analytic labels to elements of the language data in the corpus. This practice is also known as *tagging*. The most common form is word-level annotation, where each word is labelled according to its categorisation in some analytic scheme: for instance *part-of-speech tagging* is the process of assigning each word to a grammatical category, and *semantic tagging* is the process of assigning each word to a category of meaning. Annotation can also be applied above the level of the word; for example, semantic tags can be applied to phrases which form semantically meaningful chunks, e.g. idiomatic expressions. Annotation can be fully automated (i.e. carried out entirely by computer software), partially automated or fully manual.

Collocation A co-occurrence pattern observable in corpus data: that is, a trend for a certain pair of items to occur more often in the vicinity of one another than would be expected by chance alone. Typically, when investigating collocation, we look at co-occurrence patterns among words, though co-occurrence links among other kinds of entities (semantic or grammatical patterns) can be investigated too. When looking at collocations among words, we refer to the word under investigation as the *node*, and other words observed to co-occur with the node as its *collocates*. Collocational links between words are thought to be indicative of aspects of their meaning which may not be obvious to introspection by speakers of the language.

Conceptual domain Knowledge about a particular area of experience, normally including rich and complex networks of elements and relations, such as our knowledge about war, life, journeys, illness and so on.

Conceptual metaphor The cognitive phenomenon whereby one ***conceptual domain*** (the ***target domain***) is understood in terms of another (the ***source domain***). Conceptual metaphors involve mappings, or sets of correspondences, from source to target domain. They are usually expressed in terms of A IS B equivalences, such as LIFE IS A JOURNEY.

Concordance (lexical and semantic) A basic output of computer processing of a corpus. It is a visual representation of the results of some query that the computer has carried out across the corpus. This query can be for a single specific word, but it can also be for some aspect of the ***annotation***, for instance a ***semantic tag***. In the customary *keyword-in-context*, or KWIC, layout of a concordance, the matches are arranged vertically in the centre of the display: to the left and right of the query match is presented a limited amount of the text that is directly adjacent to the query match, so that the user is able to see how the item that they have queried relates to the language immediately before and after it. Concordances are typically used to allow an analyst to investigate aspects of an item's usage in terms of patterns of meaning, grammar or discourse behaviour.

Corpus A corpus (plural *corpora*) is a collection of textual data that is designed to represent some variety of language. The texts in a corpus are natural language data, that is, language produced in a real communicative context by users of the language. The variety of language that a corpus represents could be very broadly defined—e.g. English as a whole, or English as used in the UK—or very narrowly defined—e.g. the particular form of English usage produced by a particular group of people in a particular context of communication. The texts within a corpus are held in digital form to enable computer-assisted analyses, both quantitative and qualitative, that would be prohibitively time-consuming to carry out by manual processing. Corpora can be of any size in principle, although in practice the benefits of quantitative analysis are only realised with corpora of at least several tens of thousands of running words; the largest corpora are much vaster.

Discourse community A group of people who come together for a particular purpose and share texts and communicative practices.

(Dis)empowerment (in language) The process through which linguistic choices reflect, facilitate and/or undermine different kinds and degrees of agency, validation, evaluation and control, with implications for identities, emotions and relationships.

Extended metaphor The occurrence of several words in close proximity that express the same metaphorical comparison.

Framing (in relation to metaphor) The ability of different metaphors to reflect and facilitate different ways of making sense of and evaluating a particular topic or experience, by foregrounding some aspects, while backgrounding others.

Genre Any conventionalised use of language that has distinctive structural characteristics and communicative purposes, and involves particular discourse communities (e.g. a lecture or a news report).

Mappings (or conceptual mappings) Correspondences between elements of ***source*** and ***target domains*** in ***conceptual metaphors***. For example, in the conceptual metaphor LIFE IS A JOURNEY, the person living their life corresponds to a traveller.

Metaphor The phenomenon whereby we talk and think about one thing in terms of another, as when trying to recover from an illness is described as a 'battle'.

Metaphorical expression A linguistic expression that, in context, is used to mean something that contrasts with (one of) its more basic meaning(s). This applies, for example, to the use of the expression 'battle' in the phrase 'her battle against cancer'. Here the contextual meaning of 'battle' (someone's attempt to recover from or cope with cancer) contrasts with the basic meaning (a physical fight involving weapons). The contextual and basic meanings of a metaphorical expression belong to different ***conceptual domains***, and the contextual meaning can be understood in terms of the basic meaning. In the case of the expression just given, a difficult enterprise is understood in terms of a physical fight.

Metonymy The phenomenon whereby we refer to one thing in terms of something else that is closely associated (or contiguous) with it, as when the expression 'The White House' is used to refer to the US President and administration.

Scenario Knowledge about a particular type of situation, including a setting, entities, participants, goals and actions, such as our knowledge of travelling on a train or being at a party.

Semantic tag A label applied to a word or phrase in a ***corpus*** indicating its coarse-grained meaning or sense. The labels used in the UCREL Semantic Analysis System (USAS) are drawn from a taxonomy of 232 tags arranged in a hierarchy within 21 major semantic domains such as 'emotion' or 'government and public'. The taxonomy uses the linguistic theory of semantic fields as an organising principle which cuts across part-of-speech boundaries to group words together into sets of related concepts.

Simile The explicit linguistic formulation of a comparison between two unlike entities, usually signalled by expressions such as 'like' or 'as if', as in 'Cancer is like a journey'.

Source domain A ***conceptual domain*** that is used to think and talk metaphorically about another conceptual domain. In the ***conceptual metaphor*** LIFE IS A JOURNEY, JOURNEY is the source domain.

Target domain A conceptual domain that is metaphorically thought and talked about in terms of another conceptual domain. In the conceptual metaphor LIFE IS A JOURNEY, LIFE is the target domain.

Note

1. The descriptions of the following entries draw from the glossary in Semino (2008): conceptual domain, conceptual metaphor, mapping, metaphorical expression, metonymy, scenario, simile, source domain, target domain.

Reference

Semino, E. (2008). *Metaphor in discourse.* Cambridge: Cambridge University Press.

Appendix 1
Interview Questions

1. Patient Interviews

Introductory Statement

Well, first of all I would like to thank you for agreeing to take part in this interview and share your cancer experiences with me. My name is (Researcher's name), and I am from Lancaster University. We have been funded by Dimbleby Cancer Care to look at the concerns, perspectives and resilience of older people as they face the diagnosis of cancer. The aim is to develop some guidelines for people providing services so that they will be relevant and helpful to other people in the same situation. It is important that we get the views from people who have used cancer care service and find out if their needs have been met. We will be talking to a number of people like you in Sheffield, Manchester, London and Plymouth. There are no right or wrong answers because we just want to understand your views.

We are using a tape recorder so that we do not miss anything that is said. I would like to say that anything that is said is confidential to me and the Research Team and will not be repeated outside this interview. So, I would like you to feel at ease with the interview. When the results of the research are published I want to assure you that you will not be identified, just the general themes that emerge from the interviews.

Are there any questions you would like to ask before I continue?

Okay, I would just give you a brief account of what we will talk about. I would like to begin by asking you to tell me about your cancer experiences.

Then, I would like you to tell me a little bit about yourself and your background, a bit about your life experiences.

I am also interested to find out how you have coped with the situation; what services were/are available to you; how you were/are helped; what were your concerns and perspectives; what could have been done to help you coping with the situation.

Is there anything you would like to clarify before we start the interview? If not, I will now turn the recorder on.

First Interview—Questions Guide

Information About the Experiences With the Cancer Diagnosis

1. We would like you to tell us your story. Can you start by saying how you knew there was something wrong?

   (Probe: When was that? How did you feel about that?)

2. Could you tell me what happened starting from the time you were diagnosed?

   (Probe: How did you find out? Who told you? What were your reactions? Did you understand what they told you? Were you given explanations? Were you asked if you wanted to know everything? How did you find the person(s) who gave you the diagnosis?)

2. Carer Interviews

Interview Structure—Carers Who Have Accepted the Offer of Services

The interview is in two sections. In the first section I would like you to answer a few general questions about yourself, and in the second part of the interview I would like you to answer a few general questions about the carers' service. This information will remain anonymous and confidential to the research team.

Section One

QUESTIONS ABOUT YOU

What is your name?
What age are you?
What is your marital status? (*Married, divorced/separated, widowed, living with a partner, single, other*)

QUESTIONS ABOUT YOUR EMPLOYMENT STATUS

EMPLOYMENT STATUS

Are you employed, unemployed, retired, self-employed, other?
What best describes your current (or last) employment occupation?

ETHNICITY

Which ethnic group would you say you belong too? (*White, Indian, Pakistani/Bangladeshi, Black Caribbean, Chinese, Other*)[1]

CARER'S HEALTH

In general, how do you describe your health? *(Excellent, very good, good, fair, poor)*

RELIGIOUS BELIEFS

Do you have religious beliefs? (*Yes, no*) If yes, please tell me your religion? If yes, do you draw support from your beliefs?

SERVICE/PROJECT

Where did you hear about (Name of Service)? *(Local Hospice, local community, local carers' organisation, local church, local library, other)*

Section Two

QUESTIONS ABOUT YOUR CARING SITUATION

Who are you caring for? *(Spouse, son, daughter, mother, father, child, grandchild, friend/ neighbour, other)*
How long have you been caring for the person?
Are you the main carer?
Does anyone help you? *(Other family members, social services, palliative care team, other)*
How old are they?
How long have they been ill? Tell me the story about their illness.

Section Three

QUESTIONS ABOUT THE SUPPORT RECEIVED FROM (NAME OF ORGANISATION)

Please tell me which of the carers' support services you have received, or are currently receiving from *(Name of Organisation)*, e.g. Social Day Centre, Bereavement Support, Information Advisory Service, Complementary Therapies, Drop-In Centres, Respite Services/Sitters etc.

Please answer the following questions on the main service you received.

EXPECTATIONS FROM THE SERVICE

What did you hope to gain from using the service?
Was the service relevant to your needs?
Were your expectations of the service met?

FREQUENCY AND CONVENIENCE OF THE SERVICE

How often did you receive the service? *(Weekly, monthly, other)*
How long have you had this service? *(A week. several weeks, several months, other)*
What do/did you think of the frequency of the service? *(Too often, not often enough, about right)*
How often do/did you attend the service? *(Every time it was available, frequently, rarely, other)*
Is/was the service held at a time that is convenient for you?
Is/was the service held at a convenient location for you?
What did you think of the length of each of the sessions? *(Too long, too short, about right, other)*

RELEVANCE OF THE SERVICE TO YOU

Would you recommend the service to other carers?
Is there another service that you feel would more appropriately meet your needs, (*for example, someone to do your garden, or shopping for you*)?
Did you benefit from the service(s)? *(A lot, a little, not at all)*
Do you think the service could be improved?
Are/were the numbers of people attending the service: about right, too many, or too few?
If the service involves attending a social group, do/did you feel that you were listened to:
By the other **carers** attending the group?
By the **professionals/volunteers** facilitating the group?
Do/did you feel able to express yourself within the group, and to what degree *(a lot, a little, not at all)*?
If the service was 'respite care', were you satisfied that your relative/ friend was cared for well during your respite?

CLOSING QUESTIONS

Do/did you receive similar services from any other people or organisation?
Do you have any help to care for the person you are caring for?

Is there anything else you would like to add, or say, that you feel has not been discussed so far in this interview?
Are there any questions you want to ask me?

ADDITIONAL QUESTIONS GUIDE FOR THE INTERVIEW WITH FAMILY CARERS WHO HAVE REFUSED THE OFFER OF SERVICES

(*To be asked following the questions in section one*)

What services were offered to you?
Why did you refuse the offer of the services?
Are there any services that you would have accepted if they had been offered? If so, tell me about that.
Have you received any similar services in the past?
If yes, tell me about them.
What (if any) support do you have to help you in your caring responsibilities?
Thank you for taking part in this interview. Is there anything else you would like to say?

3. Professional Interviews

Preliminaries

Info sheet and consent form
Record date, name and position

Questions

- What is your professional background?
- Tell me a bit about end-of-life care in the UK, how does it work?
- What services do you provide at the hospice you work for?
- What is your experience with end-of-life care?
- Can you highlight the three main issues for family carers and for patients? [probe for emotions]
- Working in this area, what are the main challenges for you as a person? [listen to the interviewee's use of terms, e.g. 'palliative care', 'support care', 'end-of-life care', and ask how they define them]
- Tell me about a good and/or [depends on how much time is left] about a difficult death that a patient at your hospice has had.
- What issues would you highlight when it comes to communicating with patients and family carers?
- Is there anything you would wish to add?

Closing

Thank you.

Note

1. All interviewees in our data described themselves as white.

Appendix 2

Key Semantic Domains in Three Main Subcorpora

1. Key Semantic Tags in the Patient Subcorpus

SEM Tag Code	*SEM Tag Description*	*Raw Frequency in Patient Data*	*Normalised Frequency per 100 Words in Patient Data*	*Raw Frequency in Carer and Professional Data Combined*	*Normalised Frequency per 100 Words in Carer and Professional Data Combined*	*Log Likelihood*	*Log Ratio*
Z8	Pronouns	96,722	16.68	135,798	15.41	355.08	0.11
B1	Anatomy and physiology	5,964	1.03	6,517	0.74	336.22	0.48
A5.1	Evaluation: Good	5,846	1.01	6,670	0.76	254.03	0.41
F1	Food	1,764	0.30	1,543	0.18	251.29	0.80
B5	Clothes and personal belongings	976	0.17	699	0.08	234.94	1.09
Z4	Discourse bin	12,455	2.15	16,083	1.82	185.36	0.24
A9	Getting and possession	11,324	1.95	14,666	1.66	162.68	0.23
M1	Moving, coming and going	7,003	1.21	8,836	1.00	134.44	0.27
E4.1	Happy	1,745	0.30	1,838	0.21	119.44	0.53
W4	Weather	372	0.06	239	0.03	111.48	1.24
T1.1.3	Time: Future	5,717	0.99	7,273	0.83	100.65	0.26
A1.4	Chance, luck	712	0.12	637	0.07	94.30	0.76
Z6	Negative	10,657	1.84	14,448	1.64	79.84	0.17
A13.7	Degree: Minimisers	656	0.11	612	0.07	75.15	0.70
O2	Objects generally	3,239	0.56	4,025	0.46	72.25	0.29
S1.2.6–	Foolish	315	0.05	236	0.03	68.44	1.02
X3.4	Sensory: Sight	2,418	0.42	2,930	0.33	67.47	0.33
O4.3	Colour and colour patterns	503	0.09	449	0.05	67.12	0.77
E5–	Fear/shock	928	0.16	981	0.11	62.38	0.52
K5.1	Sports	491	0.08	449	0.05	60.39	0.73
O1	Substances and materials	322	0.06	260	0.03	57.92	0.91

Y2	Information technology and computing	474	0.08	440	0.05	55.29	0.71
S3.1	Personal relationship: General	1,392	0.24	1,649	0.19	46.49	0.36
F2	Drinks and alcohol	608	0.10	631	0.07	44.73	0.55
O4.4	Shape	593	0.10	616	0.07	43.43	0.55
A5.1	Evaluation: Good	894	0.15	1,010	0.11	41.37	0.43
N5.1	Entire; maximum	4,406	0.76	5,914	0.67	38.84	0.18
S2.1	People: Female	553	0.10	592	0.07	34.84	0.51
X3.4	Seen	107	0.02	75	0.01	26.98	1.12
M4	Sailing, swimming, etc.	211	0.04	191	0.02	26.87	0.75
A13.6	Degree: Diminishers	995	0.17	1,223	0.14	24.54	0.31
N4	Linear order	3,784	0.65	5,184	0.59	23.52	0.15
A1.4	Lucky	207	0.04	197	0.02	22.02	0.68
B4	Cleaning and personal care	488	0.08	554	0.06	21.90	0.42
O4.6–	Temperature: Cold	150	0.03	131	0.01	21.47	0.80
B2	Healthy	397	0.07	439	0.05	20.91	0.46
Z3	Other proper names	1,200	0.21	1,532	0.17	20.33	0.25
X2.2	Knowledgeable	4,485	0.77	6,245	0.71	20.00	0.13
T1.3	Time: Period	6,234	1.08	8,801	1.00	19.87	0.11
O4.2–	Judgement of appearance: Negative	535	0.09	629	0.07	18.90	0.37
O4.6	Temperature: Hot/ On fire	9	0.00	0	0.00	16.64	4.77
N3.2–	Size: Small	533	0.09	642	0.07	15.63	0.34
M7	Places	1,161	0.20	1,513	0.17	15.46	0.22

2. Key Semantic Tags in the Carer Subcorpus

SEM Tag Code	*SEM Tag Description*	*Raw Frequency in Carer Data*	*Normalised Frequency per 100 Words in Carer Data*	*Raw Frequency in Patient and Professional Data Combined*	*Normalised Frequency per 100 Words in Patient and Professional Data Combined*	*Log Likelihood*	*Log Ratio*
S4	Kin	6,533	1.18	5,059	0.56	1,621.98	1.08
Z8	Pronouns	96,625	17.46	135,887	14.97	1,332.57	0.22
Z1	Personal names	6,295	1.14	6,512	0.72	673.88	0.67
S3.2	Relationship: Intimacy and sex	1,636	0.30	1,096	0.12	540.82	1.29
T1.1.2	Time: Present; simultaneous	4,429	0.80	4,522	0.50	498.44	0.68
T1.3	Time: Period	7,040	1.27	8,003	0.88	498.14	0.53
X2.6	Expected	2,701	0.49	2,622	0.29	363.54	0.76
E2	Like	2,808	0.51	2,794	0.31	347.14	0.72
A14	Exclusivisers/particularisers	4,148	0.75	5,009	0.55	210.63	0.44
A13.3	Degree: Boosters	7,024	1.27	9,219	1.02	196.59	0.32
E4.1–	Sad	1,741	0.31	1,808	0.20	183.59	0.66
T1.1.3	Time: Future	5,562	1.01	7,427	0.82	133.64	0.30
S1.2.5	Tough/strong	608	0.11	500	0.06	131.32	1.00
A9	Getting and possession	10,681	1.93	15,310	1.69	114.17	0.20
M8	Stationary	709	0.13	693	0.08	93.24	0.75
E4.2	Content	686	0.12	682	0.08	85.06	0.72
X9.2–	Failure	648	0.12	651	0.07	77.40	0.71
M1	Moving, coming and going	6,491	1.17	9,347	1.03	64.88	0.19
O4.2	Judgement of appearance: Positive	1,246	0.23	1,503	0.17	63.69	0.44
T1.1.1	Time: Past	1,895	0.34	2,445	0.27	60.99	0.35
T1	Time	1,861	0.34	2,405	0.26	59.14	0.34

T1.2	Time: Momentary	838	0.15	962	0.11	56.43	0.52
O4.5	Texture	491	0.09	531	0.06	43.81	0.60
X3.2	Sensory: Sound	1,012	0.18	1,257	0.14	42.93	0.40
Q1.3	Telecommunications	526	0.10	583	0.06	42.04	0.57
H5	Furniture and household fittings	602	0.11	695	0.08	39.37	0.51
N6	Frequent	1,657	0.30	2,221	0.24	38.43	0.29
T2	Time: Beginning	1,709	0.31	2,300	0.25	38.14	0.29
S1.2.4	Polite	530	0.10	607	0.07	36.12	0.52
N5.1	Entire; maximum	4,181	0.76	6,139	0.68	30.54	0.16
I1.2	Money: Debts	566	0.10	687	0.08	27.85	0.44
X2.1	Thought, belief	6,023	1.09	9,108	1.00	24.10	0.12
A5.1	Evaluation: Good	761	0.14	990	0.11	22.93	0.34
X2.2–	No knowledge	279	0.05	310	0.03	22.04	0.56
E4.1	Happy	1,493	0.27	2,094	0.23	21.29	0.23
T1.1	Time: General	442	0.08	541	0.06	20.64	0.42
B4	Cleaning and personal care	466	0.08	576	0.06	20.42	0.41
A5.1	Evaluation: Good	4,983	0.90	7,533	0.83	20.09	0.12
N5.2	Exceed; waste	710	0.13	938	0.10	18.78	0.31
A5.3–	Evaluation: Inaccurate	467	0.08	586	0.06	18.47	0.39
G2.1–	Crime	226	0.04	250	0.03	18.23	0.57
S1.2	Personality traits	229	0.04	256	0.03	17.58	0.55
S3.1	Personal relationship: General	1,263	0.23	1,778	0.20	17.20	0.22
W2	Light	225	0.04	252	0.03	17.12	0.55
X8	Trying hard	1,171	0.21	1,654	0.18	15.28	0.22

3. Key Semantic Tags in the Professional Subcorpus

SEM Tag Code	*SEM Tag Description*	*Raw Frequency in Professional Data*	*Normalised Frequency per 100 Words in Professional Data*	*Raw Frequency in Carer and Patient Data Combined*	*Normalised Frequency per 100 Words in Carer and Patient Data Combined*	*Log Likelihood*	*Log Ratio*
L1–	Dead	3,907	1.19	1,850	0.16	5,383.26	2.87
Z5	Grammatical bin	96,516	29.42	284,462	25.10	1,763.01	0.23
L1	Alive	1,473	0.45	1,431	0.13	1,103.05	1.83
B3	Medicines and medical treatment	6,245	1.90	12,732	1.12	1,086.91	0.76
B2–	Disease	4,468	1.36	9,152	0.81	765.29	0.75
S8	Helping	3,728	1.14	7,231	0.64	761.92	0.83
A11.1	Important	960	0.29	892	0.08	756.66	1.89
S2	People	2,303	0.70	3,855	0.34	699.23	1.04
S5	Belonging to a group	1,227	0.37	1,516	0.13	664.48	1.48
P1	Education in general	1,028	0.31	1,219	0.11	592.28	1.54
G2.1	Law and order	742	0.23	700	0.06	574.86	1.87
A4.1	Generally kinds, groups, examples	1,398	0.43	2,219	0.20	478.73	1.12
X4.1	Mental object: Conceptual object	1,144	0.35	1,728	0.15	434.59	1.19
S9	Religion and the supernatural	1,147	0.35	1,736	0.15	433.97	1.19
A2.2	Cause and effect/connection	1,852	0.56	3,460	0.31	422.90	0.89
A1.8	Inclusion	423	0.13	331	0.03	398.00	2.14
G1.1	Government	443	0.14	365	0.03	396.47	2.07
I3.2	Professional	180	0.05	50	0.00	322.31	3.64
G1.2	Politics	183	0.06	77	0.01	269.92	3.04
X6	Decided	502	0.15	664	0.06	243.55	1.38
Q2.2	Speech acts	3,339	1.02	8,388	0.74	230.50	0.46
Q4.2	The media: Newspapers etc.	232	0.07	173	0.02	228.24	2.21

Q4	The media	146	0.04	58	0.01	222.09	3.12
G2.2	General	91	0.03	8	0.00	220.34	5.30
S7.1	In power	928	0.28	1,738	0.15	210.42	0.88
G2.2	Ethical	234	0.07	208	0.02	193.63	1.96
X5.2	Interested/excited/energetic	516	0.16	789	0.07	191.20	1.18
A9–	Giving	1,353	0.41	2,939	0.26	186.94	0.67
I3.1	Work and employment: Generally	1,210	0.37	2,554	0.23	186.36	0.71
A12–	Difficult	745	0.23	1,365	0.12	179.67	0.91
X4.2	Mental object: Means, method	719	0.22	1,322	0.12	171.72	0.91
S7.2	Respected	235	0.07	237	0.02	168.25	1.78
Z2	Geographical names	1,407	0.43	3,232	0.29	153.78	0.59
A2.1	Change	1,406	0.43	3,237	0.29	152.11	0.59
A15–	Danger	168	0.05	141	0.01	147.59	2.04
X2.4	Investigate, examine, test, search	579	0.18	1,050	0.09	143.61	0.93
A5.1	Evaluation: Good/bad	181	0.06	172	0.02	139.07	1.86
Y1	Science and technology in general	250	0.08	308	0.03	135.99	1.49
S7.4	Allowed	664	0.20	1,293	0.11	134.07	0.83
A1.5.1	Using	404	0.12	662	0.06	128.88	1.08
W5	Green issues	88	0.03	39	0.00	126.07	2.96
S7.1	In power	54	0.02	7	0.00	121.41	4.74
X2.2	Knowledge	69	0.02	21	0.00	119.02	3.50
A7	Likely	5,901	1.80	17,297	1.53	115.12	0.24
X9.1	Able/intelligent	487	0.15	901	0.08	114.32	0.90
Q4.1	The media: Books	223	0.07	288	0.03	112.56	1.42
A4.2	Detailed	482	0.15	900	0.08	110.24	0.89
S7.1–	No power	54	0.02	13	0.00	102.00	3.84
N5.1–	Part	334	0.10	558	0.05	101.87	1.05
E1	Emotional actions, states and processes general	415	0.13	791	0.07	89.41	0.86
I3.2	Work and employment: Professionalism	121	0.04	119	0.01	89.30	1.81

(*Continued*)

3. Key Semantic Tags in the Professional Subcorpus (Continued)

SEM Tag Code	*SEM Tag Description*	*Raw Frequency in Professional Data*	*Normalised Frequency per 100 Words in Professional Data*	*Raw Frequency in Carer and Patient Data Combined*	*Normalised Frequency per 100 Words in Carer and Patient Data Combined*	*Log Likelihood*	*Log Ratio*
A6.3	Comparing: Varied	158	0.05	191	0.02	88.46	1.51
A5.2	Evaluation: True	480	0.15	967	0.09	86.95	0.78
I1.1	Money and pay	285	0.09	480	0.04	85.28	1.04
A4.2–	General	77	0.02	51	0.00	83.84	2.38
E2	Like	106	0.03	99	0.01	83.06	1.89
B2	Health and disease	160	0.05	204	0.02	82.46	1.44
A6.1–	Comparing: Different	1,680	0.51	4,455	0.39	81.66	0.38
X9.1	Ability and intelligence	25	0.01	0	0.00	74.69	7.43
X5.1	Attentive	176	0.05	261	0.02	69.36	1.22
A6.1	Comparing: Similar	507	0.15	1,113	0.10	67.18	0.65
G2.1	Lawful	46	0.01	20	0.00	66.62	2.99
K4	Drama, the theatre and show business	123	0.04	154	0.01	65.25	1.46
A7–	Unlikely	172	0.05	276	0.02	57.51	1.11
A6.2	Comparing: Usual	618	0.19	1,474	0.13	56.51	0.53
A1.6	Concrete/abstract	75	0.02	75	0.01	54.26	1.79
A1.2	Suitable	169	0.05	277	0.02	53.88	1.08
N3.1	Measurement: General	82	0.02	89	0.01	53.46	1.67
A3	Being	22	0.01	2	0.00	52.97	5.25
X7	Wanted	2,094	0.64	6,005	0.53	52.02	0.27
X1	Psychological actions, states and processes	140	0.04	217	0.02	50.43	1.16
S1.1.1	Social actions, states and processes	559	0.17	1,339	0.12	50.03	0.53

O4.1	General appearance and physical properties	532	0.16	1,262	0.11	49.98	0.54
L1	Life and living things	45	0.01	31	0.00	47.43	2.33
A7	Likely	164	0.05	281	0.02	47.08	1.01
A1.7	Constraint	200	0.06	371	0.03	46.60	0.90
A5.4	Evaluation: Authentic	442	0.13	1,031	0.09	45.02	0.57
N3.7	Measurement: Length and height	118	0.04	178	0.02	44.95	1.19
S7.4–	Not allowed	51	0.02	43	0.00	44.60	2.03
X9.2	Success	304	0.09	654	0.06	43.60	0.68
S7.2–	No respect	35	0.01	20	0.00	42.63	2.60
G3	Warfare, defence and the army: Weapons	166	0.05	299	0.03	41.93	0.94
C1	Arts and crafts	316	0.10	694	0.06	41.80	0.65
N3.7	Long, tall and wide	48	0.01	41	0.00	41.42	2.02
A10	Open; finding; showing	959	0.29	2,592	0.23	40.44	0.35
N5	Quantities: Many/much	211	0.06	421	0.04	39.45	0.79
T3	Time: Old; grown-up	82	0.02	113	0.01	37.06	1.33
S6	Strong obligation or necessity	2,363	0.72	7,057	0.62	36.47	0.21
S1.1.3–	Non-participating	43	0.01	38	0.00	35.80	1.97
T1.3	Time period: Long	108	0.03	174	0.02	35.79	1.10
W1	The universe	188	0.06	375	0.03	35.18	0.79
S7.1	Power, organising	32	0.01	22	0.00	33.79	2.33
I1	Money generally	396	0.12	962	0.08	32.95	0.51
S9–	Non-religious	16	0.00	3	0.00	32.75	4.20
A1.2–	Unsuitable	30	0.01	20	0.00	32.49	2.37
A1.9	Avoiding	124	0.04	221	0.02	32.21	0.95
S1.2.1	Informal/friendly	84	0.03	127	0.01	31.85	1.19
A12	Easy	211	0.06	448	0.04	31.80	0.70
S1.2.5–	Weak	106	0.03	181	0.02	30.68	1.02
N5–	Quantities: Little	70	0.02	101	0.01	29.08	1.26
S5–	Not part of a group	325	0.10	781	0.07	28.61	0.52

(Continued)

3. Key Semantic Tags in the Professional Subcorpus (Continued)

SEM Tag Code	*SEM Tag Description*	*Raw Frequency in Professional Data*	*Normalised Frequency per 100 Words in Professional Data*	*Raw Frequency in Carer and Patient Data Combined*	*Normalised Frequency per 100 Words in Carer and Patient Data Combined*	*Log Likelihood*	*Log Ratio*
S1.2.1–	Formal/unfriendly	45	0.01	51	0.00	27.66	1.61
S6–	No obligation or necessity	89	0.03	148	0.01	27.44	1.05
A13.5	Degree: Compromisers	444	0.14	1,136	0.10	27.43	0.43
O1.3	Substances and materials: Gas	88	0.03	147	0.01	26.85	1.05
X3.2–	Sound: Quiet	90	0.03	153	0.01	26.33	1.02
E6–	Worry	821	0.25	2,294	0.20	26.22	0.31
W3	Geographical terms	252	0.08	587	0.05	25.83	0.57
X6	Deciding	20	0.01	11	0.00	25.02	2.65
S8–	Hindering	271	0.08	651	0.06	23.90	0.52
A6.1	Comparing: Similar/different	51	0.02	69	0.01	23.81	1.35
S1.2.6	Sensible	84	0.03	148	0.01	22.48	0.97
N3.8	Measurement: Speed	66	0.02	108	0.01	21.12	1.08
I3.2–	Unprofessional	18	0.01	11	0.00	20.87	2.50
T3–	Time: New and young	516	0.16	1,405	0.12	20.53	0.34
Z3	Other proper names	732	0.22	2,084	0.18	19.57	0.28
T3	Time: Old; grown-up	53	0.02	82	0.01	19.17	1.16
X7–	Unwanted	67	0.02	116	0.01	18.74	1.00
E6	Confident	198	0.06	469	0.04	18.74	0.54
X9.1–	Inability/unintelligence	77	0.02	142	0.01	18.24	0.91
A1.5.2	Useful	91	0.03	178	0.02	18.12	0.82
S1.1.3	Participating	226	0.07	554	0.05	17.92	0.49
A1.7–	No constraint	153	0.05	348	0.03	17.47	0.60

Appendix 3

Metaphor Groups and SEM Tags

Metaphor Groups	*Semantic Tags*
Violence	G3 (Warfare)
	S8+ (Helping)
	S8– (Hindering)
	E3– (Violent/aggressive)
	X8+ (Trying hard)
	A1.1.1 (General actions, making)
	A1.1.2 (Damaging and destroying)
Journey	M1 (Moving)
	M2 (Coming and going)
	M3 (Movement/transportation: land)
	M6 (Location and direction)
	M7 (Places)
Restraint	A1.7+ (Constraint)
	A1.7– (No constraint)
	S7.1+ (In power)
	S6– (No obligation or necessity)
Animal	L2 (Living creatures)
Openness	A10+ (Open)
	A10– (Closed; hidden)
	Q2.1– (Speech: not communicating)
Sports and Games	K5.1 (Sports)
	K5.2 (Games)
	X9.2+ (Success)
Religion and the Supernatural	S9 (Religion and the supernatural)
Obstacles	O2 (Objects generally)
	S8– (Hindering)
	W3 (Geographical terms)
Wholeness	N5.1+ (Entirety, maximum)
	A13.2 (Degree: maximisers)
	S5+ (Groups and affiliation)
	S5– (Groups and affiliation)
Machines	A2.1+ (Change)
	I3.1 (Work and employment: generally)
	O3 (Electricity and electrical equipment)
	X9.2– (Failure)

Index

Note: **Boldface** page references indicate tables. *Italic* references indicate figures.

Contributors

Zsófia Demjén is Senior Lecturer in Applied Linguistics at the UCL Centre for Applied Linguistics, specialising in language and communication around illness. She is author of *Sylvia Plath and the Language of Affective States: Written Discourse and the Experience of Depression* (2015, Bloomsbury) and co-editor of *The Routledge Handbook of Metaphor and Language* (2017).

Andrew Hardie is Reader in Linguistics at Lancaster University. His main research interests are the theory and methodology of corpus linguistics; the descriptive and theoretical study of grammar using corpus data; the languages of Asia; and applications of corpus methods in the humanities and social sciences. He is one of the lead developers of the *Corpus Workbench* software for indexing and analysing corpus data, and the creator of its online interface, CQPweb. He is co-author, with Tony McEnery, of the book *Corpus Linguistics: Method, Theory and Practice* (2012).

Sheila Payne is Emeritus Chair in Palliative Care at the International Observatory on End of Life Care at Lancaster University, and Visiting Professor at Ulster University and Zurich University of Applied Sciences. She is a health psychologist with a background in nursing, and research interests in palliative care and ageing.

Paul Rayson is Director of the UCREL Research Centre and Reader in Natural Language Processing (NLP) at Lancaster University. His long-term research focus is semantic-based NLP with noisy language, e.g. historical and computer-mediated communication varieties. His applied research is in dementia detection, learner dictionaries, text mining of historical corpora and annual financial reports.

Elena Semino is Professor of Linguistics and Verbal Art in the Department of Linguistics and English Language and Director of the ESRC Centre for Corpus Approaches to Social Science at Lancaster University, and Visiting Professor at the University of Fuzhou (China). Her interests are in: stylistics, medical humanities, health communication, corpus linguistics, narratology and metaphor theory and analysis. She is author of, among others, *Metaphor in Discourse* (CUP, 2008) and co-editor of *The Routledge Handbook of Metaphor and Language* (2017).

FSC
www.fsc.org
MIX
Papier | Fördert gute Waldnutzung
FSC® C083411

Kolibri 360 GmbH
Ferdinand-Jühlke-Straße 7
99095 Erfurt, Deutschland
produktsicherheit@kolibri360.de